Advance Praise for *Healing Pai*

———○———

"If you've ever been sick, hurt or simply frustrated with your doctor's limited explanation of what's wrong with you . . . this is the book for you. You will learn, in a humorous and interesting way, how to help yourself out of a place of pain and into a place of peace."

LUCINDA WATSON
Author: *How They Achieved: Stories of Personal Achievement and Business Success*

"Dr. Nerman transforms the reader from victim to advocate, from patient to master. This book is a must-read."

PAMELA MARTIN, MD
Associate Clinical Professor of Psychiatry, UC San Francisco

"Dr. Nerman has written a beautiful treatise describing the significance of trauma as a cause of human suffering. This is the hallmark of osteopathy, a uniquely American medical system that has proven to be profoundly relevant in the care of the whole person."

MARK E. ROSEN, DO, FCA
Past President and Senior Faculty, The Osteopathic Cranial Academy

"Dr. Nerman changed my life and ended decades of trauma pain. Reading *Healing Pain and Injury* helped me understand why she succeeded when dozens of other health care professionals had failed. All this time I thought it was magic!"

DEBRA DELANEY
Software Company CEO

———○———

more **Advance Praise:**

———o———

"Maud Nerman is a famously skilled clinician—both as an osteopath and a homeopath. Weaving personal anecdotes with solid clinical information, the book is both fascinating and useful. I highly recommend it for both clinicians and the lay public."

ROGER MORRISON, MD
Cofounder: Hahnemann Medical Clinic, Hahnemann College of Homeopathy
Author: *The Desktop Guide, Desktop Companion to Physical Pathology*

"Dr. Nerman provides phenomenal insight into the causes and treatment of trauma as well as useful guides for prevention. As an integrative physician, this book will be one of my recommendations for my patients and colleagues."

MICHELLE PERRO, MD, DHOM
Integrative Physician, Sutter Pacific Medical Foundation,
Institute for Health and Healing

"If you continue to experience pain despite treatment, this book may unlock the doors to relief."

ALAN CARUBA, *Bookviews*
Founding Member, National Book Critics Circle

"Dr. Nerman has compiled a truly eye-opening treatise on the devastating effects of trauma and injury shock on our health. The interconnectedness of every organ and energy system of the body, and the pivotal role that osteopathy can play in healing are deftly described in practical and readily understandable language."

MICHAEL E. ROSENBAUM, MD
Author: *Super Supplements*
Past President, The Healthy Foundation

———o———

HEALING PAIN
and INJURY

Maud Nerman, DO, CSPOMM, CA

BAY TREE PUBLISHING
Pt. Richmond, CA

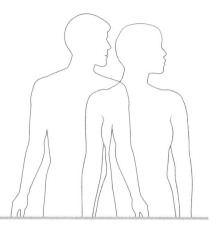

The information provided in this book is designed to provide helpful information on the subjects discussed. This book is not meant to be used, nor should it be used, to diagnose or treat any medical condition. Neither the author nor the publisher is engaged in rendering medical, psychological, general health, or any other kind of professional services in this publication. For diagnosis or treatment of any medical problem, consult your physician. The author and the publisher specifically disclaim responsibility for any liability, loss, or risk, personal or otherwise, that is incurred directly or indirectly as a consequence of the use and application of the contents of this book.

BAY TREE PUBLISHING
1400 Pinnacle Court, #406
Pt. Richmond, CA 94801
www.baytreepublish.com

Printed in the United States

EDITOR: Adrienne Larkin
BOOK DESIGN: Laura Lovett | By Design
ILLUSTRATION: Sarah Chen
PHOTOGRAPHY: William Gordh

Library of Congress Cataloging-in-Publication Data
Nerman, Maud.
  Healing pain and injury / by Maud Nerman, DO, CSPOMM, CA.
    pages   cm
  ISBN 978-0-9859399-0-8 (pbk.)
  1. Osteopathic medicine. 2. Chronic pain—Treatment.
    3. Wounds and injuries—Treatment. I. Title.
  RZ301.N47 2013
  615.8'528--dc23   2013032105

"To find health should be the object of the doctor. Anyone can find disease."

—ANDREW TAYLOR STILL, MD
Founder of osteopathic medicine

———○———

Dedicated to three brilliant lights of osteopathy—

although there are many others:

MURIEL CHAPMAN, DO

REBECCA LIPPINCOTT, DO

STANLEY SCHIOWITZ, DO, FAAO

I thank them for their generosity, wisdom, and kindness.

And to my patients, who are my constant teachers.

———○———

CONTENTS

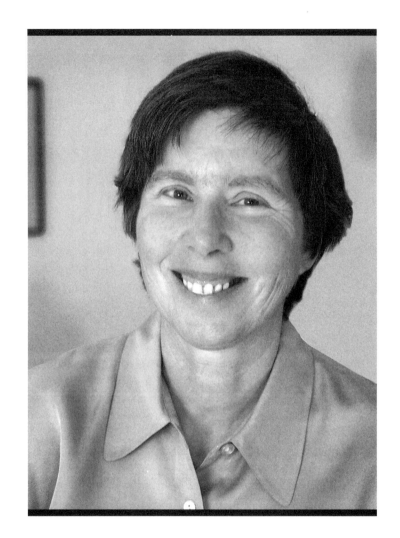

Maud Nerman, DO, CSPOMM, CA

Preface

I have been practicing as an osteopathic physician for over three decades. During that time, I have successfully treated thousands of patients who have come to my door suffering from the hidden symptoms of traumatic injury. Many of these courageous people have suffered for years from mysterious ailments for which no one could give them an answer, bouncing from practitioner to practitioner in an endless quest to get well.

They suffer from crippling headaches, debilitating fatigue, mysterious weight gain, insomnia, neck and back pain, sexual dysfunction, depression, anxiety, vertigo, memory problems, digestive problems, vision problems, immune disorders, heart arrhythmias, chronic pain, and a host of other maladies that seem to have appeared out of nowhere. Most of the time no one realized there was any connection between the patient's spiral of suffering and the injury that started it. Desperately trying to get well, the patient is often dismissed as a "head case" whose suffering is all imagined or emotionally based.

To me these gallant souls are not head cases. The effects of traumatic injury on the human body and spirit can be insidious, causing problems far away from the site of the original insult, affecting almost any organ system, and throwing its victims into a spiral of loneliness, isolation, and despair.

None of it is necessary.

It takes listening carefully to the patient, as the patient almost always holds the clues that lead to the real problem. Over the years I have learned that my patients are my greatest teachers—they, plus a thorough knowledge of anatomy and an awareness of how the body works to heal itself. I've learned that most people in pain are suffering from the sequelae of traumatic injury. In many cases the trauma was seemingly minor, and had occurred months or even years earlier.

When these patients at last received the correct diagnosis and the right kind of help, their recovery seemed almost miraculous. But not to me. For I know the body has a remarkable ability to heal from trauma with the right kind of help.

After helping many people who have suffered so needlessly, and knowing that there are countless others who could so easily be helped, I became determined to share what I've learned. And it is to you that I primarily address this book. However, it will also assist practitioners. I wish I'd had something like this to read during my first twenty years of practice.

HOW THIS BOOK CAN HELP YOU HEAL

As you read this book, you will discover the surprising and little-recognized ways that trauma damages health. You will see how the body's unique heroes of health are often the keys to well-being, and you will learn the three steps to healing the damage done by trauma. This book will help you take control of your journey back to health.

There are many things that you can do on your own. You may already be doing some of them. If you are, this book will help you to see them in a new light so you can utilize them in the most beneficial way. For some problems, you will need assistance from a trained practitioner. And if you are doing everything right but still cannot completely regain your health, you may find the answer in the chapters on hidden obstacles to cure.

Though my main focus arises from my work as an osteopathic physician specializing in manual medicine, I've also practiced homeopathy for thirty years and find it invaluable in treating trauma. I mention some of its uses throughout this book.

Here, you'll find chapters on everything from sleep to sexual healing to taking charge of your recovery, because I want you to have the right tools for your journey back to health. I have always believed that you, the patient, are the key participant in this healing process. Of course, I cannot address in this book all the possible health problems that might contribute to your suffering. But I can help you make some critical decisions so you can find the tools to help yourself.

WHY I'M AN EXCELLENT GUIDE ON YOUR JOURNEY

I'm an excellent guide on this journey, not only because I'm a physician who has specialized in helping people recover from traumatic injury but also because I have suffered from serious illness. Though my problem did not result from traumatic injury, the skills I learned helped me become not only a better physician but also a better guide for you.

As a child, my asthmatic lungs often burned with each breath. My mother's fierce determination to keep me alive, coupled with the wisdom of several doctors, taught me much about the necessary tools for healing. Over time I incorporated exercise, fresh air, and nutrition to help keep my lungs healthy. My childhood experience with illness taught me that significant illness and injury demand patience, persistence, and determination. I recommend mixing those attributes with a large dose of curiosity. Grateful for my recovery, I wanted to help other people regain their health. I considered many branches of medicine, from traditional medicine to physical therapy to chiropractic training, before deciding to become an osteopathic physician.

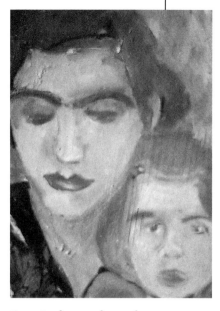

Portrait of my mother and me. Painted by my mother, Joann Haimson.

OSTEOPATHIC MEDICINE:
A Complete Philosophy of Healing

Osteopathic medicine is a uniquely American form of medicine. It is practical, sensible, and grounded in a profound knowledge of human anatomy. Osteopathic physicians are trained with a traditional four-year medical school curriculum. Like our MD colleagues, we complete our training in clinics and hospital residencies.

But here is a critical difference: though osteopathic physicians pay attention to disease and trauma, we focus on assisting the body's amazing self-healing ability. As the physician who created osteopathic medicine, Andrew Taylor Still, MD, told his students, "To find health should be the object of the doctor. Anyone can find disease." Osteopathic physicians are also steeped in a complete philosophy of healing that sees the patient as a whole human organism, not as a collection of diseases or symptoms to be dissected and drugged piece by piece. Osteopathic medicine understands that the body's structure and function are intimately related and that to heal, a person must heal structure in order for function to improve.

To underscore the importance of the musculoskeletal and neurological systems in health, osteopathic medical students spend approximately five hundred additional hours studying anatomy, kinesiology (mechanics of bodily motion), and manual medicine so that they can repair structure and function with their hands and design a more complete healing protocol. After medical school we osteopathic physicians go on to specialize in our chosen fields as cardiac surgeons, internists, neurologists, and manual medicine specialists or in any of the other branches of medicine.

Before I knew anything about osteopathic medicine, I had figured out that to keep my lungs happily able to absorb air, my ribs had to move freely. By swimming regularly, I kept my chest flexible. When I discovered the power of osteopathic manual medicine, I found that a good treatment from an osteopathic physician also freed up my ribs and improved my breathing. Since I love working with my hands and have directly experienced osteopathic manual medicine's remarkable healing power, I chose to specialize in that aspect of osteopathic medicine.

Many people know that osteopathic manual medicine can help back pain and other structural problems. Few realize that manual medicine is a complex healing modality that can work directly with the pulsations of the nervous system and the brain to treat brain injury and many neurological problems. Manual medicine can lower blood pressure, enhance the complex fluid dynamics of the body, reduce inflammation, and improve immune function. It can cure conditions like esophageal reflux, bronchitis, colic in infants, constipation, and migraine headaches, accelerate healing from surgery and from such problems as brain injury, heart arrhythmias, ulcers, and asthma. Osteopathic care is especially effective after injury compromises health, because osteopathic physicians understand the dynamics of trauma and pay attention to five critical parts of the body that are often overlooked. Time after time I've found that by addressing hidden injuries I can help restore people to health, even if they come in for a seemingly unrelated medical problem.

I love that osteopathic medicine has such a complete and comprehensive view of health and healing that it often makes seemingly untreatable problems dissolve. But the greatest power of osteopathic medicine is its recognition of the body's great natural healing power.

HOMEOPATHY: The Perfect Complement

Long before I decided to become a physician, a friend of mine who had suffered from a severe epileptic disorder was cured of her condition by homeopathy. I recall being skeptical but also intrigued. Her recovery certainly put homeopathy on my radar.

Years later, when I finished my internship and began my medical practice, the last thing I wanted to do was learn another complex system of medicine with a voluminous knowledge base. But then one of my patients changed my mind. Alexandra was a young woman who kept having infections that responded to neither antibiotics nor osteopathic manual medicine. She finally called her homeopathic physician. Twelve hours after taking the dose of homeopathic *Sepia* (cuttlefish ink) he prescribed, her infection resolved completely. I knew then I had to add homeopathy to my medical tool chest. I am so glad I did. Now, I would feel severely limited in my medical practice if I did not know homeopathic medicine. I have included a chapter in the book on homeopathy, and throughout the book I briefly refer to the homeopathic remedies I used in a particular case.

Like osteopathic medicine, homeopathic medicine is based on recognition of the body's remarkable healing power, which homeopathy calls the "vital force." Homeopathic medicine was created by Samuel Hahnemann, a physician and scholar who refined the 2,000-year-old tradition of medicine described by Hippocrates as "like cures like." Hahnemann found that when a common substance like salt or a poison like arsenic is extraordinarily diluted and shaken, it could cure the very symptoms that a larger dose would cause. Homeopathy is now practiced all over the world and used by hundreds of millions of people.

Remember that the body always moves toward health. No matter how long ago it happened, and no matter how serious the injury that damaged your health, *you can get better.*

Welcome to your healing journey.

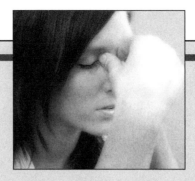

Symptoms of Trauma

Do you suffer from any of the following?

- Anxiety
- Inflammation
- Sexual dysfunction
- Fatigue
- Menstrual problems
- Uncontrolled anger
- Mood swings
- Back pain
- Memory problems
- Headaches
- Sinusitis
- Bloating
- TMJ
- Heart arrhythmias
- Shortness of breath
- Inability to focus
- Pelvic pain

- Chronic pain
- Migraines
- Depression
- Insomnia
- Vision problems
- Dizziness
- Neck pain
- Sciatica
- Immune dysfunction
- Weight gain
- Slow healing
- Tinnitus
- Chronic lung infections
- Constipation
- Acid reflux
- Hormonal imbalance
- Asthma

If so, keep reading.
Your symptoms may be the result
of an accident or injury.

1

You Can Get Better!

Trauma—injury to living tissue caused by an external force—is something we all face at some point in our lives. Millions of years of evolution have designed our bodies to heal in the face of trauma. We have an ingenious autonomic nervous system that instantaneously switches on our "fight-or-flight" response in the face of danger, a complex immune system that is primed to seal off injured tissues from healthy ones and heal them, and a brilliantly engineered musculoskeletal system that can absorb and redistribute the tremendous forces to which our bodies are constantly subjected.

But sometimes the process of healing from injury goes powerfully awry. The life-saving fight-or-flight response of the autonomic nervous system fails to turn off. The inflammatory response essential for healing overwhelms the body's ability to manage it. And the distortions forced upon the musculoskeletal system by trauma are too great for the body to accommodate. All too often a patient shows up at my office after months or years of suffering, and I find that trauma has shocked their nervous system, fired up their inflammatory response, and disrupted their structural integrity. The result can be a host of seemingly unrelated and surprising symptoms, including the list that begins this chapter.

Once the patient unravels the journey that catapulted their body into suffering, their health dramatically improves. I know this because I have helped thousands of suffering patients, and because I have taken this journey myself.

It helps to know that the body is your biggest ally, always working to restore your health. Every moment, every cell in your body fights to make you healthy. Every cell constantly throws out the waste products of life and injury. Blood continually bathes every cell, bringing it the nutrients of healing. With these perfectly designed resources rushing in, the body continuously rebuilds itself.

Though this book focuses on the effects of physical trauma, know that illness is often a trauma to the body. Much of what I say about treating trauma can also apply to disease. Full recovery often includes calming the nervous system, controlling inflammation, and restoring motion to areas restricted by illness.

THE THREE PRINCIPLES OF HEALING FROM TRAUMA

Trauma does three things to your body that over time can devastate your health. Yet these three things are invisible to most people—including most medical practitioners. Treat these three things, and seemingly miraculous recovery occurs.

1 Trauma Shocks the Nervous System

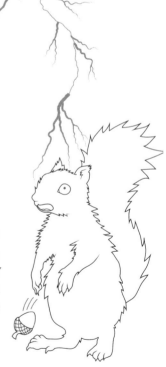

The body is wise. Immediately after trauma or injury, adrenaline and other stress chemicals pour into your bloodstream so that you can fight off a lion or flee a burning car. You become hypervigilant and alert. This response helps you survive.

All too often the body cannot turn off this fight-or-flight reaction. Days, weeks, even months go by and the body still pours fight-or-flight chemicals into your system. You feel wired and tired at the same time. Sleep is disrupted, digestion is poor. Your breathing continues to be rapid and shallow. You are inflamed, anxious, irritable, and depressed. Your nervous system is wearing itself out responding to a threat that no longer exists. Nothing seems to help. I call this being stuck in "injury shock." If this situation persists for weeks, months, or years people feel exhausted, healing grinds to a halt, they are constantly inflamed, and other health problems—such as arthritis, digestive problems, insomnia, or autoimmune disease—can rear up.

Treat the injury shock and return the nervous system back to balance: then you can begin to heal.

If your body cannot turn off the fight-or-flight reaction after trauma, your nervous system can get stuck in injury shock.

16

2 Trauma Provokes a Firestorm of Inflammation

Inflammation is a necessary and normal response to trauma. After an injury, powerful cells from the immune system rush in to contain the problem. The body increases blood flow to the damaged region, sends in garbage collectors to remove debris, and then sets contractors to work to rebuild the damaged muscles, blood vessels, nerves, and connective tissue. We experience this repair process as swelling and inflammation.

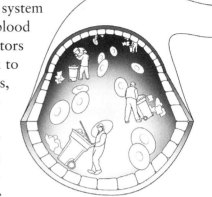

Sometimes trauma overwhelms the body's ability to manage its own healing. Then inflammation takes off like a runaway train. This firestorm of inflammation can cause constant burning pain, chronic muscle spasm, loss of joint mobility, and more inflammation. Ultimately, chronic inflammation may contribute to diseases such as diabetes, Alzheimer's disease, and heart disease. In order to get well, you must turn off this runaway inflammation.

All too often, trauma overwhelms the body's ability to manage its own healing. Then inflammation takes off like a runaway train.

3 Trauma Jams Up the Body's System of Motion

Life is motion. Optimum health depends upon the free movement of the joints, bones, organs, muscles, and connective tissues. The heart must beat fully and the lungs must expand freely for vibrant health. But other organs also must move in their natural rhythms. The gut must pulsate enthusiastically as it pulls in nutrients. The liver must rock as it processes toxins to make them harmless. And the most essential organ—the brain—must expand and contract six to fourteen times a minute to enliven the whole body. Trauma can restrict any of these critical motions and damage health.

Because the body is so deeply interconnected, restriction of motion in one area can have profound effects elsewhere. An ankle sprain doesn't just restrict the normal range of motion of the foot. It can have a ripple effect elsewhere, as other joints are strained, stretched, and pushed out of alignment as they try to pick up the ankle's workload. I often trace low-back pain to ankle problems. As the pelvis tilts up or down to compensate for the foot's instability, the sacrum rotates out of alignment, twisting the vertebrae above, trapping nerves and causing sciatica, low-back pain, headaches, and even pain in the opposite shoulder.

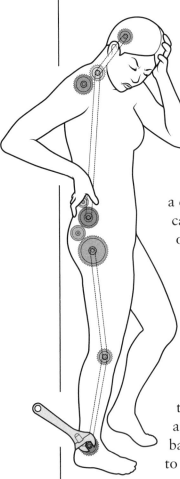

The body is so interrelated that problems in one system can reverberate in a distant system or structure.

Injury to one kind of structure can also cause a problem in a completely different system of the body. A blow to the chest can squeeze blood vessels and drive up blood pressure. A fall off a chair can deliver a bony karate chop to the spinal nerves that feed the uterus and genitals and can cause painful menstrual cramps or even impotence.

Just as essential as the motion of the tissues is the free flow of the fluids that permeate the body. Trauma can twist the blood vessels that bring nutrients to damaged tissue and the lymphatic channels that float away inflammation-causing debris. The injured site then becomes like a New York garbage collector's strike, with all that putrid junk left to fester in the sun. Trauma also can squeeze the nerves that are valiantly trying to orchestrate the complex task of healing, basically handcuffing the conductor's hands. Restoring motion to all these systems, not just to the joints, is essential to healing.

To stop this cascade of injury, the primary injury must be identified. Then it must be properly aligned, and balanced with the rest of the body, and its fluid pathways restored. Otherwise, pain and dysfunction can spring up in seemingly unrelated parts and even unrelated systems of the body.

Remove injury shock, control inflammation, and restore motion: these are the three keys to getting back your health.

2

The Story of a Mysterious Illness

"Every day for four years, I woke up determined to find out what was wrong with me. I was in terrible pain, exhausted, dizzy, unable to focus, with terrible spasms in my hand. Every doctor had an opinion. None of them helped me. Eventually, they sent me to a psychiatrist."

In 1985, a thirty-eight-year-old woman sat on the edge of a chair in my office determined to find out why her health had collapsed. She had a pile of X-rays on her lap and a notebook full of reports. She looked vibrant enough, but I knew better than to assume. I listened.

"I feel like my body has rusted together," Samantha (or Sam, as she liked to be called) said. She held the base of her skull. "I get dizzy when I eat, and my arm becomes so weak I drop things. But what's really odd is that just before I drop things, my sinuses start to drain. I've been everywhere. One doctor said I had food allergies. I gave up all kinds of food, including sugar. My husband said, 'You may not live longer, but it will certainly seem longer.' Funny. The changes didn't make any difference. No one knows what's going on, so the last doctor sent me to a psychiatrist."

"That's because they gave up," I said. "We'll try to figure out what's wrong."

I put Sam's cervical (neck) X-rays up on my viewbox. They showed a bit of arthritis but basically looked normal. Even though her X-rays did not reveal the source of her problems, that was okay with me. I trusted her history as well as what my hands would soon tell me, because touch senses not just the position of structures but also joint motion and the quality of the body's tissues.

Sam's medical history was fairly unremarkable except for her history of trauma. A type A personality and ferocious athlete, Sam had discounted the significance to her health of the various concussions she had sustained and the multiple car accidents she had been in. "Everyone gets their bell rung in sports," she said with a smile.

Sam lay down on the table, and I examined critical areas of her body. The base of her skull felt like it was welded to her spine. I did not feel the healthy, normal motion that this important joint should have, making me suspect she had suffered a blow to the base of her head. The fact that the weld felt so solid meant that the injury was years old.

Then I put my hands around her skull. The healthy brain beats six to fourteen times a minute, reflected in the subtle but easily discernable expansion and contraction of the skull. Her skull had only slightly better motion than a rock. By now I suspected significant trauma to both her head and neck. And since trauma to either the head or neck can cause dizziness as well as sinus problems, the reasons for her suffering were becoming clearer. I also knew that problems in the neck can cause problems with nerves going to the hand. Anatomy and physiology always explain a lot.

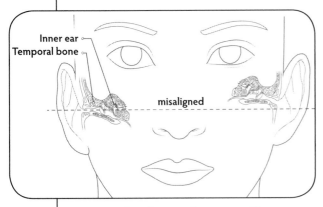

Inner ear
Temporal bone

misaligned

Sam was dizzy because her temporal bones were out of alignment. When she ate, her moving jaw rocked the temporal bones and aggravated the misalignment, making her dizziness worse.

When I put my hands to the sides of her head, the mystery of her dizziness further unraveled. Her temporal bones—the fan-shaped bones containing the inner ear and all the components necessary for balance—were way out of alignment. This misalignment gave Sam's brain conflicting information about her position in space. I told Sam, "Your dizziness is probably not caused by food allergies. The balance centers in your inner ear are being affected by your crooked temporal bones. When you chew, your jaw rocks the temporal bones and makes the imbalance worse. That's why you feel dizzy. Once the bones are positioned properly, the dizziness should go away."

As I moved down her body I found that her very straight neck had lost its natural curve. I suspected that the problem came from her car accidents, when the back of her head had slammed against the headrest and her neck was violently snapped backward and forward. Her too-straight neck explained why her sinuses drained just before her hand cramped. Without the natural cervical curve, she had less room for nerves to exit from their bony homes. Every spasm in her neck muscles compressed the nerves in her upper neck going up to the sinuses and in her lower neck going down to the arms.

"That's why your sinuses drain before you drop things," I told her. "Both sets of nerves are getting compressed. It's simple anatomy."

After I treated her, she said her neck didn't hurt quite so much. Given how long she had been suffering, I knew she would need more treatments to recover her health.

As time went on, we unraveled the whole story of this mysterious illness. It's a fascinating story about the importance of persistence. You must insist on an explanation even when everyone is telling you there's nothing wrong. So let's go back in time and find out how this all started.

A LONG SEARCH FOR ANSWERS

Samantha Robertson, Esq., known to the gym rats at the downtown YMCA as Razor because of her exceedingly sharp passing skills, was a fixture at lunchtime basketball games, weekend softball games, and tournament tennis. Sam lived for her sports.

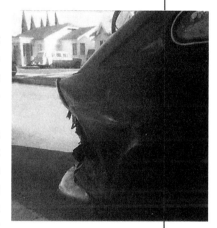

One day, six years before she walked through my office door, she had been cruising to work down La Cienega Boulevard in Los Angeles. As she approached a busy intersection, Sam stopped to let an ambulance through. Unfortunately, the driver in the car behind her had the radio up too loud to hear the sirens. She slammed into the lawyer's Volkswagen fastback. Sam felt shaken and sore, but the next day she was back at her sixty-hour-a-week job. She never saw a doctor.

Sam never connected her deteriorating health to the collision that had crushed her small car.

In the months that followed, Sam's first step on the basketball court was slower. Her neck would bother her after a particularly grueling week at the office. Her husband became very concerned.

She gradually got worse. Eventually, she was in constant pain. All her joints started to ache, and her jaw hurt all the time. The base of her skull was painful and tender. She kept dropping things. She couldn't focus. She was exhausted. Her balance was so poor that she stopped playing sports. She considered going on disability because she could not work.

She never connected any of it to the accident.

Coming from a family of physicians, she had great faith in medicine to make her well. In those days before the Internet, she went to the medical library and researched every symptom and condition she could. She made appointments with every kind of specialist. A neurologist told her that it was a neurological problem and suspected MS. The MRI he ordered was negative, and the powerful drugs he put her on did not help.

An endocrinologist ordered thousands of dollars' worth of blood tests, including tests for diabetes, and couldn't find anything wrong but prescribed more powerful drugs anyway. She fired him and tried another doctor. As the medical professionals were hunting for a solution, she was spending her money like water and getting sicker and sicker.

Finally, when her family physician gently suggested that she see a psychotherapist, she realized he was telling her, "I can't figure out what's wrong with you. Therefore, nothing is wrong with you. It's all in your head."

She knew it wasn't in her head. She continued to ask everyone she knew for recommendations to any health care practitioner who might help. Eventually, after both her midwife and her dentist told her to see me, she called for an appointment.

HOW SAM HEALED

From the fibrotic and immobile quality of the tissues in her neck and head, I concluded that Sam's neck problems were long-standing. Her fatigue, along with her chronically shallow breathing, made me suspect that the car accident had sent her nervous system into a fight-or-flight response that had never quite turned off. Its effects were now chronically embedded in her nervous system and made her feel like her body had rusted, keeping her exhausted and in pain.

To treat her, I had to release the spasm in her neck so the nerves to her sinuses and her arms did not have so much pressure on them. I coaxed her overtaxed nervous system to calm down, and I realigned her crooked temporal bones. Then I restored motion to the tiny sinus bones so that the chronic inflammation in her sinuses could heal. I also had to restore motion to the stuck base of her skull. As always, I worked on all of that together, so that after four treatments, plus a good homeopathic remedy (*Sepia*), Sam did feel somewhat better. Later in the book, I explain how I treat. Right now, I want to focus on Sam's healing journey.

Three months after her first osteopathic treatment, Sam tentatively resumed light physical activity. After five months, she stepped gingerly onto a tennis court to test her newfound health. She wondered, "Will I pass out again like I did the last time? Will everything spin? Will I drop the racquet?"

She hit the ball. Felt good. Then another. Fifteen minutes later, she still felt fine. She told me later that she started to cry. She had gotten her life back.

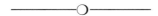

I start with Sam's story because it highlights many critical points:

- Traumatic injury causes much needless—and treatable—suffering.
- Most health problems make sense if the practitioner listens carefully to the patient and understands the relevant anatomy, and how the body functions as a whole.
- Healing takes time. Patience matters.
- Persistence matters, too, both for patients and the practitioners who treat them.

My primary tools are osteopathic medicine and homeopathy, but you have access to many other tools which I will introduce in the coming chapters. Throughout this book, I provide simple and practical ways for you to participate in your healing journey. Let's get started.

I.

Why Injury Shock
Prevents Healing

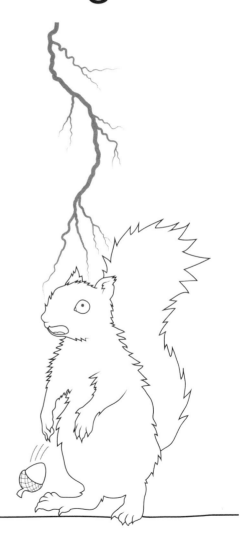

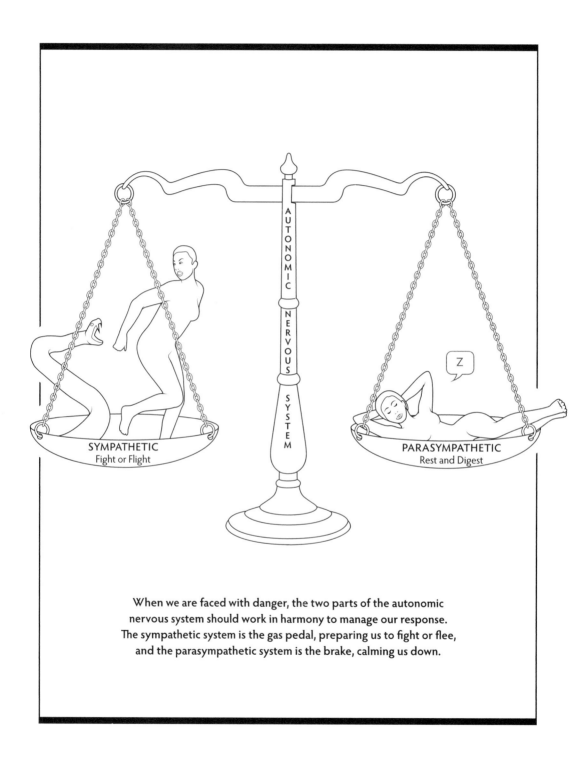

When we are faced with danger, the two parts of the autonomic
nervous system should work in harmony to manage our response.
The sympathetic system is the gas pedal, preparing us to fight or flee,
and the parasympathetic system is the brake, calming us down.

3

The Devastating Consequences
of Injury Shock

CHARLIE was running hard toward the soccer ball when he collided with his opponent. They both crashed to the ground. Momentarily stunned and with the wind knocked out of him, twenty-eight-year-old Charlie took a few minutes to climb to his feet.

Charlie thought little of the soreness in his neck and chest over the next few days. But then a month passed. He came to see me because his sore neck was not getting better. He was feeling extremely anxious and was having terrible trouble sleeping. His asthma, which had been under control for years, was bothering him again. Charlie's other practitioners were mystified. Charlie was stuck in injury shock. As I describe later, once I treated his injury shock, his symptoms resolved fairly quickly.

I see countless patients like Charlie who cannot get well after trauma or injury, and no one can tell them why. While some treatments and drugs give them temporary relief, nothing sticks. Like Charlie, these patients come in exhausted, irritable, anxious, and depressed. Some are in terrible pain. Some, like Charlie, cannot sleep. Others sleep too much and still wake up tired. Despite exemplary diets, rigorous exercise programs, and dozens of visits to medical specialists, their health deteriorates. Their lives have become a blur of exhaustion and pain.

I became most successful at helping patients like Charlie when I recognized that injury had catapulted their nervous systems into a state of injury shock. To help them heal, I had to work to remove any remnants of this injury shock.

I am not talking about the kind of shock that paramedics and emergency room physicians deal with. That kind of shock involves a life-threatening collapse of the cardiovascular system and is a true medical emergency. What I call injury shock is different. It is the inability of the nervous system to restore itself to balance in the aftermath of a trauma. For someone to heal from trauma, the first order of business must be to calm the nervous system and restore it to balance. Once I do that, my patients recover much more quickly, whether from an old trauma or new.

THE BODY'S RESPONSE TO DANGER

To understand injury shock, we need to look at how the nervous system responds when we are faced with danger or trauma.

Inside us, a powerful internal system called the *autonomic nervous system* (ANS) regulates heart rate, breathing, blood pressure, immune response, digestion, reproduction, and millions of other critical processes that go on without our conscious control. The ANS is the key player in the body's response to trauma and danger and in the orchestration of healing afterward.

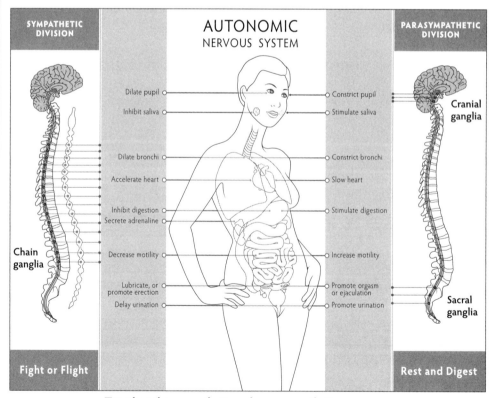

Together, the sympathetic and parasympathetic nervous systems control much of what goes on inside our bodies.

The autonomic system has two parts. The *sympathetic* pathway is like the gas pedal, instantaneously readying the body's fight-or-flight response in the presence of danger or threat. Working together with and balancing the sympathetic pathway is the *parasympathetic,* or rest-and-digest, pathway. This pathway acts like the brake on our hypervigilant reaction to danger. It calms down the sympathetic pathway and restores the nervous system to balance. When these two pathways work in harmony, the body is able to deal with the emergency presented by the trauma and then mobilize the body's healing processes afterward. But when they do not work in harmony, a cascade of pain, inflammation, and chronic ill health will result.

Symptoms of Injury Shock

- Fatigue
- Depression
- Anxiety and panic
- Insomnia
- Shortness of breath
- Digestive disorders
- Chronic pain
- Reproductive impairment
- Frequent infections
- Inflammation
- Mental confusion
- Slow healing

THE SYMPATHETIC NERVOUS SYSTEM: Fight-or-Flight

When a person is faced with danger or trauma, the brain instantly activates the sympathetic nervous system (SNS). Within seconds, the body biochemically shifts into hyperdrive. The SNS signals the adrenal glands to release the stress hormones epinephrine (adrenaline) and norepinephrine (noradrenaline) into the bloodstream. Steroid hormones called glucocorticoids, which include cortisol, flow into the blood. The stress hormones create dramatic changes in the body so it can deal with the threat to survival:

- The heart beats faster and harder.

- Blood flow to the brain, the gut, and the skin is constricted as blood is diverted to the powerful skeletal muscles to ready them for action. Blood pressure rises.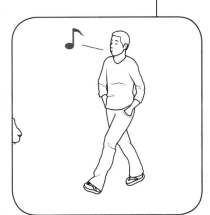

- The alveoli in the lungs dilate and breathing becomes rapid and shallow in preparation for increased oxygen demand from the major skeletal muscles. This breathing pattern pours adrenaline into the body and diminishes pain to enable escape from danger despite grievous injuries.

- The pupils of the eyes dilate to take in as much

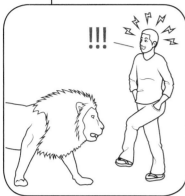

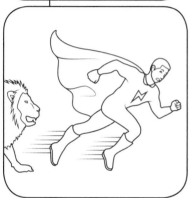

light as possible so that potential threats can be rapidly identified.

• The liver and muscles release fatty acids and glucose (sugar) into the bloodstream to provide quick sources of energy.

• Insulin production is inhibited to prevent glucose and fat from being stored, and muscles and fat cells become temporarily resistant to insulin's effects. The spike in glucose levels and stress hormones provides a surge of superhuman energy so that a person can run from a lion or climb from a burning car.

• Clotting factors in the blood increase to prevent excessive blood loss in case of injury.

• The brain loses some ability to focus on details, and higher cognitive functions are suppressed as the brain directs its focus to the big picture so that the person can survive the threat.

• Body systems that are nonessential for immediate survival—such as the digestive, growth, and reproductive systems—are shut down. Instead, the body redirects its energy to functions deemed necessary for survival. Even parts of the immune system are shut down.

• The sleep system is disrupted so the person can remain alert.

• Memory of the traumatic event is stored in long-term memory so it can be retrieved quickly if a similar danger is faced again.

This powerful, ancient, and instantaneous response orchestrated by the SNS is vital to our ability to survive an immediate threat. It enables us to act quickly and decisively in an emergency situation. However, this is designed to be a short-term response. When the response persists even after the threat is over, it creates havoc with our health.

THE PARASYMPATHETIC NERVOUS SYSTEM: Rest-and-Digest

After the immediate danger has passed, the brain should reverse the course of action by activating the parasympathetic branch of the autonomic nervous system (ANS). The slower-acting parasympathic nervous system, or PNS, restores the body's ability to heal. The PNS is in charge of the nutritive, life-giving functions of the body and brings the nervous system back into balance:

- The PNS slows down the furiously beating heart, restoring it to a normal rhythm.

- The PNS dilates (expands) critical blood vessels, particularly those in the brain, gut, and injured areas, so that oxygen, immune factors, and critical nutrients can be transported where they are needed.

- The PNS slows down and deepens rapid, shallow breathing and restores normal breathing patterns.

- The PNS revives the digestive system, including food absorption and gut motility, so the body can provide nutrients to damaged tissues.

- The PNS reawakens other life-giving functions such as reproduction, sleep, and growth.

- The PNS restores the part of immune function that was suppressed by the stress hormones. Restoration of full immune function allows the immune system to efficiently and effectively destroy and remove pathogens, toxins, and damaged tissues.

How Injury Shock Happens

Like a political party in power, the powerful fight-or-flight SNS hates to relinquish control after the danger has passed. It often fails to turn off the flood of raging chemicals that keep us hyperalert and agitated. I call this situation injury shock, and it can damage health long after the trauma has passed:

- The heart continues to beat too fast, contributing to high blood pressure and feelings of anxiety and panic. Insomnia, depression, and fatigue soon follow.

- Oxygen flow to the brain is compromised, which can result in mental confusion and memory problems.

- Digestion remains poor, unable to provide the body with the necessary nutrients to heal injured tissues.

- Breathing remains too fast and too shallow, signaling the brain to continue producing more stress hormones. Rapid, shallow breathing also drastically alters blood chemistry so that the body's tissues become oxygen-starved.

- Chronically high levels of the stress hormone cortisol impair both long-term and short-term memory functions. They also contribute to insulin resistance, which can lead to diabetes and heart disease.

- Infertility, decreased sperm production, premature ejaculation, and impotence can also result from chronically high cortisol levels, partially through cortisol's inhibition of reproductive hormones.

- Chronically high levels of cortisol can cause inflammation to spin out of control. In a short-term crisis, cortisol is essential to control excessive inflammation that could cause serious tissue damage. However, if cortisol levels remain too high, the body's immune cells become resistant to its anti-inflammatory effects, and inflammation explodes. As I discuss later, out-of-control inflammation is a health calamity and has been implicated in a host of chronic health problems, including heart disease, Alzheimer's disease, diabetes, and obesity.

- Resistant to the suppressive effects of cortisol, an out-of-control immune system can attack the body itself, causing serious autoimmune diseases.

- Ultimately, the immune system becomes weakened under the constant assault of stress hormones and inflammation. For anyone with an underlying health problem—such as an autoimmune disease, asthma, depression, and/or migraines—injury shock can spin these illnesses out of control and make the person sicker.

Without a well-balanced nervous system to orchestrate the complex job of controlling inflammation and mobilizing nutrients, immune factors, and lymphatic and blood flow to the injured area, the body cannot heal. As inflammation grows, it can slowly become systemic and starts attacking unrelated areas of the body, such as the heart. The region of injury itself loses mobility, and the surrounding connective tissue tightens and immobilizes it further. The body recruits other structures to take over the functions of the injured area. Eventually, these structures become overstressed and damaged, creating further inflammation and pain. A cascade of more injury, pain, and inflammation follows as the injured nervous system keeps the suffering patient exhausted.

THE FREEZE RESPONSE

There is another way our primitive response to trauma can interfere with healing: the freeze response.

Faced with a mountain lion, the opossum freezes and plays dead. Since many predators refuse to eat carrion, the lion, seeing the immobile body, assumes the creature is dead. The mountain lion walks away, giving the opossum a new lease on life. Human beings are also imbued with this freeze response. The freeze response may explain why so many people sit paralyzed

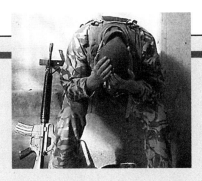

The Long Reach of Injury Shock

The chemical cascade that can spin the sympathetic nervous system out of control can also be provoked by the mere anticipation of danger or death. A near-miss car crash can send the nervous system into the same cascade of harmful physiological changes as an actual one. Soldiers who missed the bullet often experience a severe stress reaction called posttraumatic stress disorder (PTSD), which I consider to be a severe aspect of injury shock.

An unexpected accident, no matter how small, can provoke a powerful sense of danger, triggering a too-powerful fight-or-flight response from the SNS and just as fiercely catapulting the body into injury shock. This is perhaps the reason that if someone does not see a car collision coming before impact, they are fifteen times more likely to be injured. The injury shock can be profound. I believe that this powerful injury shock and its frequent companion, the frozen state, are critical factors that cause many people to be slow or unable to recover fully from injury.

And, necessary as surgery may be, the body often reacts to surgery as though it were a sudden dangerous accident, sending the body into a shocked state that needs to be resolved before full healing can take place.

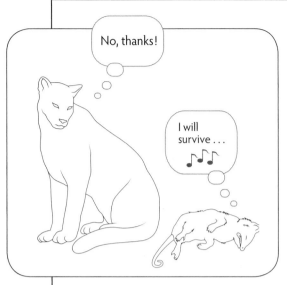

in a crisis. But even if a person sits frozen in a car after a collision, their heart still races, and though paralyzed, they are filled with panic as the SNS tries to kick them into action and make them escape the car before it burns. It's like pushing the brake and the gas pedal at the same time, grinding the gears of the psyche. The result is a terrifying feeling of frenzied paralysis in the face of danger.

This frozen state further compresses areas of the body already jammed together by trauma, locking up the diaphragm and compromising the breath. Joints, bones, muscles, and organs can remain frozen deep inside the body, slowing down their ability to regain their normal motion. In the worst-case scenario, the war between the racing sympathetic nervous system and the braking parasympathetic nervous system can lead to posttraumatic stress disorder.

Once safe, people need to reawaken the parts of their body that remain frozen. These areas are often deep and hidden, locking up connective tissue, blood vessels, and lymphatics as well as the organs and muscles, especially the diaphragm.

If the trauma is fairly recent, the nervous system reacts to injury shock like a meth addict full of speed. It becomes weak, jittery, and erratic, like Charlie's did. If the trauma is old, over time, chemical changes exhaust the poor body. If there is a frozen component to the shock, this further complicates the picture, as the body becomes rigid and the person often complains of fatigue. This is what I felt in Sam's body when she complained that she felt like she had rusted.

Whether the injury is new or old, the treatment is similar: the sympathetic nervous system must be calmed, the parasympathetic nervous system must be activated, the entire autonomic nervous system must be returned to balance, and frozen tissues must be awakened. Once that happens, extraordinary healing can take place. I turn to that in the next chapter.

4

Restore the Breath, Restore Health

Fix the breath and the patient will heal. It took me many years to grasp this wisdom repeated by my osteopathic teachers. In the Old Testament, when God gave Adam life, God didn't jump-start Adam's heart or brain. No! God breathed life into Adam.

Restoring the breath is only part of what I do to calm and balance the nervous system, but because it is so important, I address it first.

Breathing is not just the great life-giving force. Physiologically, it is a key modulator of the dance between the sympathetic and the parasympathetic nervous systems. Rapid, shallow breathing keeps the fight-or-flight SNS overactive. Deep, slower breathing activates the restorative PNS and rebalances the two systems, allowing the body to heal. Slower breathing quiets the heart rate, drops blood pressure, oxygenates the tissues, and helps restore sleep, digestion, and immune function. Working with the breath gives us a direct way to break the cycle of hyperagitation and stress pounded into the nervous system by trauma.

There is much you can do yourself to restore a slower, more regular breathing pattern and reawaken the healing PNS. The simple act of focusing attention on breathing can sometimes help restore the breath to calm. You will find many simple and powerful approaches to restoring the breath at the end of this section.

Sometimes, the force of trauma also restricts the free movement of two critical structures required for full breathing—the diaphragm and the rib cage. Then, hands-on work is usually required to restore the breath. That's some of what I do. Through osteopathic manipulative treatment, I free up restricted areas—particularly the diaphragm and the rib cage—to restore the breath and bring the nervous system to balance.

RAPID, SHALLOW BREATHING: A Health Catastrophe

When a person is faced with danger, the nervous system switches the body to rapid, shallow breathing. Breathing rates increase from eight to sixteen breaths per minute to twenty-four breaths per minute and higher. The person breathes high in the chest rather than deep in the lungs, relying more on the intercostal muscles in the upper chest rather than the diaphragm to expand lung capacity.

Rapid, shallow breathing has survival value in the short term. It prepares the body to send large amounts of oxygen to the major skeletal muscles that are being readied for vigorous physical action so you can escape from a predator. It signals to the body that there is danger. It keeps the SNS pouring stress chemicals into the blood.

In the longer term, however, rapid, shallow breathing is a health catastrophe. It causes a cascade of devastating biochemical changes that can cripple health.

Chronic rapid, shallow breathing starves the tissues of oxygen. When you breathe too rapidly, you reduce the amount of carbon dioxide in the blood below its optimum levels. Red blood cells release their payload of oxygen to the tissues only in the presence of carbon dioxide, a phenomenon known as the Bohr effect. The more hard work muscles do, the more carbon dioxide they produce. The more carbon dioxide they produce, the more oxygen is released to them. This wise mechanism ensures that the body releases the right amount of oxygen to the tissues that need it most.

But if breathing stays rapid and shallow, you end up exhaling too much carbon dioxide. Then red blood cells greedily hold on to their oxygen molecules. Despite your taking many breaths, your tissues become oxygen starved. Muscle spasm, poor healing, asthma, dizziness, numbness, sleep disruption, immune dysfunction, and anxiety are some of the problems that result from low oxygen levels.

The lack of available oxygen caused by rapid, shallow breathing signals the brain that the danger has not passed. The SNS continues to pour stress hormones into the body. The stress hormones keep blood pressure high, the heart beating too fast, insulin production chaotic, the digestive and reproductive systems functioning poorly, the brain unable to think clearly, and the immune system unbalanced. Anxiety, fatigue, depression, and fear pervade your mood.

Lack of oxygen also signals the brain to increase the rate of breathing, making the problem worse. To reawaken healing, your breathing must slow down and deepen.

To assist the breath, I restore motion to compromised areas—in particular, the diaphragm and the rib cage. Then slower, deeper breathing can restore proper oxygen and carbon dioxide balance in the tissues, help shut off the flood of stress hormones, and revitalize the nutritive parasympathetic nervous system. With the PNS active, the body can marshal blood flow, nutrients, and immune cells to the sites of injury so that healing can take place.

THE FIRST KEY: Free Up the Diaphragm

When the diaphragm moves freely, the rib cage can expand, the lungs can fill more fully, and the PNS powerfully wakes up. The diaphragm lies at the heart of breathing. It is an awe-inspiring, amazing muscle, one of the five critical heroes of health. I focus later on the diaphragm's essential role in the fluid dynamics of immune function, hormonal balance, digestion, heart health, and blood flow. Right now I'll talk about the diaphragm's role in breathing.

Full breath requires a freely moving diaphragm. The diaphragm sits like a large muscular umbrella on top of the abdominal organs and underneath the lungs and heart, to which it is attached. As with a giant bellows, its downward movement as we inhale creates a vacuum that pulls air into the lungs. Its upward movement allows us to exhale.

There is an intimate connection between the diaphragm and the rib cage. The diaphragm attaches in front to the lower ribs and to the bottom of the breastbone. In back it attaches to the lower six ribs and the upper lumbar vertebrae. The diaphragm's powerful pumping widens and lifts the lower ribs, creating more room for the lungs to expand and fill with air.

Trauma can restrict the free movement of the diaphragm in many ways, drastically affecting the vigor and the rate of the diaphragm's pumping:

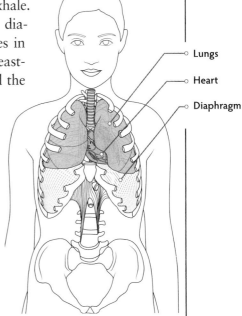

Lungs

Heart

Diaphragm

As the diaphragm descends, it expands the rib cage and creates more room for breath to fill the lungs.

37

• Like any muscle, the diaphragm can go into spasm. Direct trauma to the chest can cause spasm. The forceful gasp we involuntarily take when faced with danger can lock the diaphragm in spasm. When spasm occurs, exhaling becomes more difficult.

• Since the diaphragm is attached to the ribs, the lungs, the spine, and the breastbone, as well as to the liver, the heart, and the stomach, any injury to the diaphragm can affect these organs. A restricted diaphragm can cause heart problems, reflux and indigestion, chest pain, asthma, bronchitis, and back and rib pain. Conversely, heart and digestive problems, chest pain, lung problems, and distorted ribs or vertebrae can cause the diaphragm to become restricted.

People who flip over their bicycle handlebars often slam part of the diaphragm against its rib attachments. A rear-end collision can slam the seat into the spine's attachments to the diaphragm as well as compress the breastbone against the seatbelt. These and similar forces can twist the diaphragm and can cause the diaphragm to spasm, restricting its free movement. A cascade of health problems result when the diaphragm does not move well.

• A restricted diaphragm cannot move air in the lungs efficiently, and other muscles are recruited to help us breathe. We breathe higher in the chest, expelling too much carbon dioxide, triggering the vicious cycle of stress hormones pouring into the bloodstream.

• The movement of the diaphragm is critical to lifting and enlarging the rib cage; a poorly moving diaphragm generally means a poorly moving rib cage. The lungs cannot inflate as fully and we cannot get a full breath.

• The pumping of the diaphragm moves critical lymphatic fluid throughout the body; a poorly moving diaphragm means that the lymphatic system stagnates, resulting in increased inflammation, lung infections, immune problems, and poor healing.

• The diaphragm's intimate connection with the heart, the liver, and the digestive system means that all these systems suffer when the diaphragm does not move properly.

Osteopathic medicine has always focused intently on the health of the diaphragm, and osteopathic physicians have developed many techniques for restoring the diaphragm to its full function. When I attend to the diaphragm, I put gentle and firm pressure directly on the lowest part of this muscle. I am always careful not to disrupt the placement of the lower ribs, which link rather delicately to the rib cage. I use this technique as long as there has been no recent trauma to the internal organs like the liver or spleen. Trauma that injures those or other organs can be deadly, and pressure near these organs after trauma can therefore be potentially dangerous.

If there has been recent trauma, I am more cautious, and I release the diaphragm indirectly by using a technique my mentor, Robert Fulford, DO, taught. This technique releases the abdominal fascia to which the diaphragm attaches. This is not a technique for inexperienced practitioners. A practitioner must be very careful to avoid pressure on the lower ribs or the aorta, especially after trauma may have injured one or both of them.

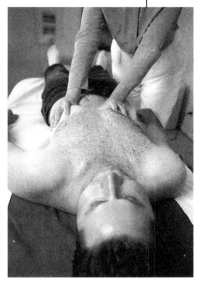

After I release the diaphragm my patients often tell me, "I didn't know breathing could feel so good."

Once spasm in the diaphragm is released and mobility restored to the structures to which it attaches, breathing automatically deepens and slows. As the breath returns to its normal pattern, the PNS is powerfully reawakened. The SNS calms down and the flood of stress hormones slows. Digestion and immune function are restored and the body can once again successfully orchestrate the process of healing from injury.

THE SECOND KEY: Free Up the Ribs

Free breath requires a flexible rib cage. With each breath, the ribs should move up and expand outward, turning in their joints with the spine. This movement allows the lungs to expand and fill with air. When the ribs can't pivot or articulate easily in their joints, this restriction dampens the ribs' ability to expand and lift and prevents the lungs from fully inflating. So the second thing I do to restore the breath is make sure that the ribs are moving freely.

The ribs fit in the back between the spinal vertebrae, where each rib has multiple connections to the vertebra above and below it. In the front, the upper ribs connect to the sternum (breastbone), and most of the lower ribs connect via cartilage to each other. The rib cage, though it looks solid, actually has over 150 articulations (joints). There are literally more than a hundred places where the ribs can get stuck or their motion restricted.

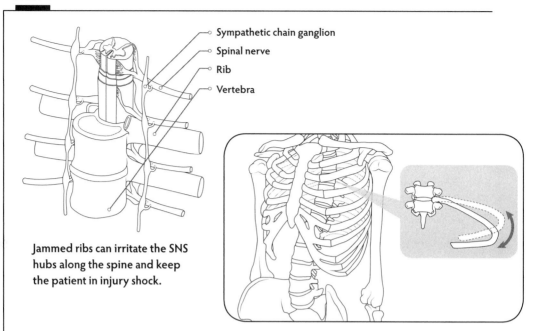

Sympathetic chain ganglion
Spinal nerve
Rib
Vertebra

Jammed ribs can irritate the SNS hubs along the spine and keep the patient in injury shock.

When the ribs can't pivot easily in their joints between the vertabrae, they trap the lungs and prevent their full inflation.

Blows to the chest can also push the ribs backward toward their joints with the spine, where the ribs get caught more easily than in the front. When the ribs get jammed into their spinal joints, they can irritate the ganglia, or hubs, of the sympathetic nervous system (SNS) that run nearby. The ganglia are a series of way stations along the spine where the SNS hangs out before it goes to work. Since the SNS is the orchestrator of the fight-or-flight stress response, jammed (restricted) ribs that irritate the ganglia can fire up the stress response, with all the problems that this causes:

- Car accidents are a main source of problems with the ribs. Although seat belts and shoulder harnesses save lives, the occupants often twist around the restraining shoulder harness, which torques and compresses the rib cage.

- Falls are another source of problems because they compress the ribs and tend to twist and distort the torso. We rarely fall without twisting, too, and the combination of twisting and jamming significantly locks up the motion of the rib cage.

- Direct blows to the chest—from a steering wheel, a punch, or a sports collision like Charlie's—also jam the ribs into their joints with the spinal vertebrae, markedly decreasing chest flexibility and ultimately breathing power. The stagnant lungs can become a Petri dish for harmful bacteria and viruses, resulting in bronchitis and other lung infections.

When I treat the ribs (once I know nothing is broken), I gently and gradually pull the jammed ribs away from the vertebrae. This helps the lungs inflate and releases pressure on the nearby sympathetic chain ganglia, calming down the stress response. I also remove twists and torques in the ribs by gently side-bending the torso to enlarge the space between the vertebrae so the ribs can get free. Once the ribs expand more freely, precious oxygen can flow more easily into the lungs, pressure is taken off the ganglia, and the breath and the nervous system can return to balance.

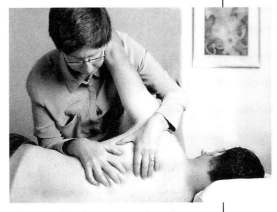

Releasing the ribs improves breathing and helps shut down the flood of stress hormones following trauma.

WHAT YOU CAN DO

Use the resources at the end of this section to help restore your breath. My wonderful yoga teacher, Patricia Sullivan, has put together a program for this book that will help you relax, overcome anxiety, restore the breath, and awaken the nutritive PNS. I have added my favorite breathing exercise, which is taught by Andrew Weil, MD.

I will simply add one thing: there is nothing better than swimming to expand the rib cage, relax the diaphragm, restore full breathing, and help calm the nervous system. Because it requires regular, deep inhalations and longer exhalations, swimming can help the ANS return to normal. The gentle twisting motion of the typical Australian crawl stroke (freestyle) helps expand the rib cage and release the diaphragm. Swim only if you can do so without pain. If you have neck problems or problems turning your head, use a mask and snorkel. The crawl and the sidestroke are usually okay. The breaststroke can be hard on the neck and low back, and please, no butterfly. That's too vigorous and causes too much arching of the low back and the neck. Don't swim if it causes numbness in your hands or your feet, or hurts your shoulder.

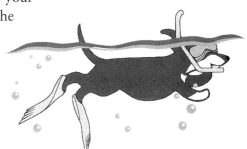

By now you are no doubt beginning to understand why Charlie, whom we met in the last chapter, had recurring asthma and was still anxious, sleep deprived, and in pain weeks after colliding with his opponent on the soccer field.

As you may have guessed, I found during my examination that Charlie's breathing was rapid and shallow. When I put my hands on him, I found his ribs distorted, either by the collision with the other player or by his subsequent fall to the ground. Neither his ribs nor his diaphragm moved very much with his breath. His diaphragm was locked up, either because of the trauma to his chest or because, like many people faced with sudden trauma, Charlie had gasped. With his diaphragm in spasm, full breath was not possible.

Charlie's shallow breathing had left his tissues oxygen starved and his SNS in overdrive. With the calming PNS overwhelmed by its powerful twin, Charlie remained in injury shock, causing his sleep problems, anxiety, breathing problems, poor healing, and continuing pain.

Over three visits, I gently released the spasm in his diaphragm and coaxed his ribs back into their proper place. As his diaphragm began to work better, his ribs widened and began to move more fully. He began to breathe much better, and soon his asthma resolved.

As Charlie's breathing returned to a normal rhythm, the SNS calmed down and the nurturing PNS asserted itself. His anxiety started to go away and his sleep and digestion improved. Soon the trajectory of his healing took off, and shortly thereafter he became completely well.

— 5 —

Treating the Nervous System

Sometimes hands-on work is required to bring balance to the nervous system. That's some of what I do. Through osteopathic manipulative treatment, I work directly to restore the nervous system to balance.

To explain this further, I'll tell you about Stephanie and Mike. They suffered trauma that ranged from the truly horrific to the relatively minor, yet, working with each of them, I was able to calm their exhausted nervous systems and put them on the path to health.

STEPHANIE was almost killed in a terrible head-on collision. When I first saw her, the forty-two-year-old mother of two was unable to sleep, in tremendous pain, and exhausted no matter how much she rested.

A truck crossed over the median and slammed into the family's car. Stephanie was thrown against the steering column, breaking her ribs, smashing her skull, and fracturing her spine. The firefighters and medics extracted her from the twisted wreckage and rushed her by medevac helicopter to a trauma center, where her life was saved.

She came to see me four months later. She had done a wonderful job of recovering from her trauma, but her health had stopped improving. She was still suffering from tremendous pain, had lost her sense of smell and taste, and was profoundly exhausted. Her symptoms, particularly her inability to fully heal, told me that that her nervous system was still in injury shock.

Stephanie's breathing was shallow and her color was poor. This was not surprising, given the serious injuries to her chest and ribs, which would have made full breathing difficult. The trauma had also twisted her heavy diaphragm and sent it into spasm, further limiting the excursion of her lungs. And, like many people faced with sudden danger, Stephanie had gasped, forcefully pulling her diaphragm down and partially locking it there. With her ribs, chest, and diaphragm compromised, full breath was not possible.

My physical exam corroborated my diagnosis. Her broken ribs had healed in a distorted pattern. Her spasmed diaphragm helped maintain the

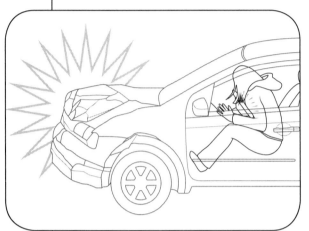

contorted pattern. The trauma had also pushed the back of her ribs up against the vertebrae they attached to, squeezing the sympathetic nervous system's hubs (the ganglia). The mechanical pressure against the ganglia, combined with her rapid, shallow breathing pattern, had helped keep her fight-or-flight sympathetic nervous system (SNS) in overdrive. With her nervous system out of balance, her healing had stalled.

The injuries to her ribs and diaphragm were not the only reason Stephanie's nervous system was functioning poorly. The accident had profoundly battered her brain, as evidenced by the damage to the olfactory nerves, which had resulted in her loss of the sense of smell. Her tissues, including her brain, had been flooded for months with stress hormones that had kept the SNS working at a fever pitch. When I put my hands on her skull to palpate the pulsations of the brain, I felt like I had plugged my hands into an electric socket. Her tissues literally vibrated under my hands. Her nervous system was continuing to react as if the accident was still happening.

I gave Stephanie high doses of homeopathic *Arnica montana* and *Aconitum napellus*, the two homeopathic wonder remedies for treating injury and injury shock. Immediately her body started to relax. Then I put my hands to work.

I first gently released the spasm in her diaphragm and coaxed her ribs and other structures back into their proper places. That process not only helped her lungs inflate but also released the mechanical pressure that kept her SNS firing as if she were still in danger. The diaphragm began working more easily, and her ribs widened and moved more fully, giving her a better ability to breathe. She began to take deeper breaths and became much more relaxed.

With fuller, slower breath, her nervous system calmed down significantly.

Even so, the impulses of her nervous system were still weak, jagged, and rapid, not smooth and regular, as they are in a healthy person. Restoring her breath was a necessary first step to restoring the balance to her nervous system, but it was not enough.

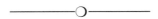

MIKE was riding his bicycle down the city street when a woman opened her car door in front of him. He crashed into the door and flipped over it onto the pavement, landing hard on his side. The blow twisted and compressed his ribs.

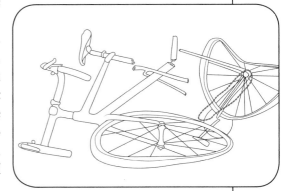

Mike came to see me a month later. "I didn't break anything, but I feel terrible. Eating makes me nauseous, and my neck still hurts all the time. But the worst part is, I can't sleep. I fall asleep for forty-five minutes and wake up in a panic. I'm taking sleeping pills to get through the night. It's crazy—even though I'm exhausted, I feel wired all day."

Like Stephanie, Mike was still in injury shock. His stomach problems, lingering neck injury, anxiety, and insomnia strongly suggested that the nutritive parasympathetic nervous system (PNS) was still in hibernation. Mike's SNS was in overdrive, where it was now stuck. The fall had compressed Mike's ribs and jammed them tightly into the thoracic vertebrae, where they irritated the nearby SNS ganglia. Bike accidents are notorious for squeezing this area.

I untwisted Mike's ribs and gently pulled the rib heads away from his spine. But this wasn't enough to fully restore Mike's nervous system. As with Stephanie, it was going to take more than simply restoring motion to his ribs and diaphragm to bring his nervous system back into balance and calm.

TREATING THE NERVOUS SYSTEM'S PULSATIONS

In a healthy person, the brain and the spinal cord—known together as the central nervous system—beat at between six and fourteen times a minute. Because we can feel this pulsation best at the skull, we call it the cranial rhythmic impulse (CRI). The pulsation of the CRI exists independent of the beating of the heart and the movement of the breath, though both influence it. After an injury, this smooth, full amplitude of motion often becomes chaotic and weak.

If the trauma is fairly recent, such as Stephanie's car crash or Mike's fall,

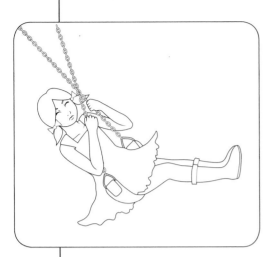

Sometimes the pulsations of the nervous system are chaotic and disjointed like the erratic movements of a child twisting on a swing.

the nervous system becomes erratic and weak and its pulsations get stuck in an ineffective pattern. To treat it, I steadily pull the nervous system toward calm and strength. I generally do this from either the sacrum, where much of the central nervous system ends, or by treating the brain through the skull.

Imagine the irritable central nervous system as though it were a young child at the playground swinging way too high. Her swings have become chaotic and disjointed and she is about to fly off the seat. If I try to abruptly stop the swing, she'll tumble off. To help her, I have to slowly dampen her swing and gently coax her down.

I do something similar with an over-firing, erratic nervous system. I first listen with my hands and acknowledge without judgment the existing pattern. This acknowledgment alone begins the healing process. Then I work with the chaotic pattern. By moving my fingers and my intention ever so gently along with the pattern, I slowly and gradually dampen the rapid, ineffective pulsations and pull the pattern toward a regular rhythm. I then stay with this healthier rhythm until the body claims this rhythm for its own. Once the body accepts this change, the strength and amplitude of the nervous system's pulsations become fuller and more powerful.

Each time I treat someone, my goal is partial improvement. I will do more on the next visit. If the neurological injury is significant, I might have to do this for a half dozen or more visits. After a neurological injury, the nervous system seems to easily forget part of what it learns from a treatment and needs repeated help.

In old encrusted problems like those of Sam, whom we met in the second chapter, the neurological components of injury have stopped being erratic and chaotic. It's as though the nervous system has exhausted itself and its amplitude has become slow and sluggish, beating one or two times a minute rather than eight. When the nervous system has weak, inactive pulsations, I slowly encourage it to pick up its frequency. I gently push the child on the swing into more powerful and frequent motions. As the CRI's amplitude and frequency move toward normal, so does the entire central nervous system. Then pain decreases and function improves.

Treating Stephanie's Nervous System

After working to restore Stephanie's breathing pattern, I addressed her chaotic, erratic, and suffering central nervous system. Because Stephanie had suffered a significant insult to the brain, the brain tissue was initially too vulnerable to treat directly. I started at her sacrum, where the central nervous system ends and the dural membrane that surrounds the brain has its ultimate anchor. The central nervous system's erratic, weak pulsations are palpable in the sacrum as well as in the skull. As I would with the child on the swing, I moved to slowly and gently steady these pulsations. My finger movements are so minuscule that some patients do not even feel them.

As the chaotic pattern under my hands evened out into a slightly more orderly one, the neurological pulsations through the spinal cord became firmer and fuller. This process took about seven minutes. Once I sensed a modest improvement, I moved up to treat the head.

Responding to the treatment, Stephanie's central nervous system no longer felt like it had been plugged into an electric socket; it felt more like a three-year-old struggling to learn how to swing. Because the dural membrane that embraces the brain feeds through the sutures of the skull and attaches to the scalp, I could feel how the brain was sitting inside the skull. The brain was slightly twisted and off-center. Using these dural membranes as if I were using guy wires to right a model ship in a glass bottle, I slowly and gently pulled the brain back toward center. Once the brain fit better in the skull, its erratic pattern calmed significantly. It's as though the brain was struggling the only way it knew how—through increased electrical discharge—to find its way home.

After I had adjusted the position of the brain in the skull and calmed its erratic pulsations, the brain's beat became much more even, and the amplitude

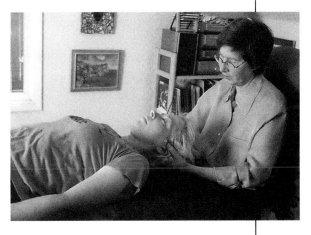

When I treat the central nervous system directly, I steadily pull it toward calm and strength. I generally do this from the sacrum, where much of the central nervous system ends, or by treating the brain through the skull.

of its pulsations increased. I talk much more about these details in the chapters on brain injury. Here, I want to emphasize that treating the neurological insult helps address a critical component of injury shock.

Though she had seen me only once, the treatment was so effective that a few weeks later Stephanie dropped me a note thanking me for the dramatic change in her health. She told me her pain had markedly diminished, her sleep had improved, her breathing was better, and her energy had started to return. When I saw her a month after our initial session, she said she was thinking much more clearly, and was able to work three to four hours a day, adding, "I feel like I've turned a corner." After several more treatments at two-week intervals, she was breathing more fully and her nervous system was restored to balance. She was well on her way back to health. Eventually, she also recovered most of her sense of taste and smell.

Mike did not suffer the head trauma that Stephanie had sustained. He was also younger, and his injuries were much less serious, so his nervous system dysfunction was milder. The nervous system's chaotic pattern wasn't nearly as palpable as Stephanie's. His was more like a child sitting on a swing that has a few kinks in the chain suspending it, so that its swing is slightly off-kilter. Because the overall trauma was far less severe and did not involve the brain, I started to work directly at the skull, slowly feeling and directing the nervous system's rhythm and rate back to normal.

Once Mike's injury shock resolved, his injured neck had fuller neurological input and was much more receptive to treatment; in three weeks it was significantly better. As his nutritive PNS woke up, his digestion and sleep slowly returned to normal.

Balancing the autonomic nervous system by restoring the breath and working with the nervous system directly are the first critical steps after trauma to restoring the patient to health.

Other Aids to Healing

There is much you can do on your own to help balance the autonomic nervous system.

Yoga postures can be profoundly helpful in restoring neurological balance. Chapter 7 includes specific poses I've found very helpful to my patients.

Movement can be a critical factor in helping resolve injury shock. Movement can resolve mechanical strains that promote neurological irritation. Regular aerobic exercise reduces levels of the stress hormones adrenaline and cortisol and promotes restful sleep. Exercise also increases the levels of endorphins, the body's natural mood elevators. Swimming probably is the best exercise for restoring normal breathing patterns, as it frees up the rib cage and diaphragm and promotes the long, slow exhalations that rebalance the oxygen–carbon dioxide chemistry of the blood.

Tai chi and qigong have a well-documented ability to lower blood pressure significantly and help maintain or lower cortisol levels. Research has also found that these practices can reduce the activity of the SNS and alter brain function in a way that stimulates the restorative PNS.

Besides their many other health benefits, all of these practices can profoundly help remove injury shock and allow the body to heal.

For millennia, *sound and music* have been used successfully as a powerful healing modality. Gregorian and other forms of chant, as well as many religious incantations and mantras, have a strong calming effect on the nervous system. They regulate the breath, increase blood oxygen levels, slow the heart rate, and decrease blood pressure as well as help rebalance the ANS and dissipate injury shock.

The Holosync Program (www.centerpointe.com) contains a sound pattern that includes rain and other water sounds that many of my patients have found very calming and healing. For more information on sound and healing, Joshua Leeds has written a book, *The Power of Sound*, which discusses this topic in more detail.

Injury shock, inflammation, and restricted motion all affect each other like an out-of-control mob, and each must be addressed for a patient to fully heal from injury. However, I have found that treatment is most effective when the nervous system is balanced first. Once injury shock is attended to, you are well on your way toward health.

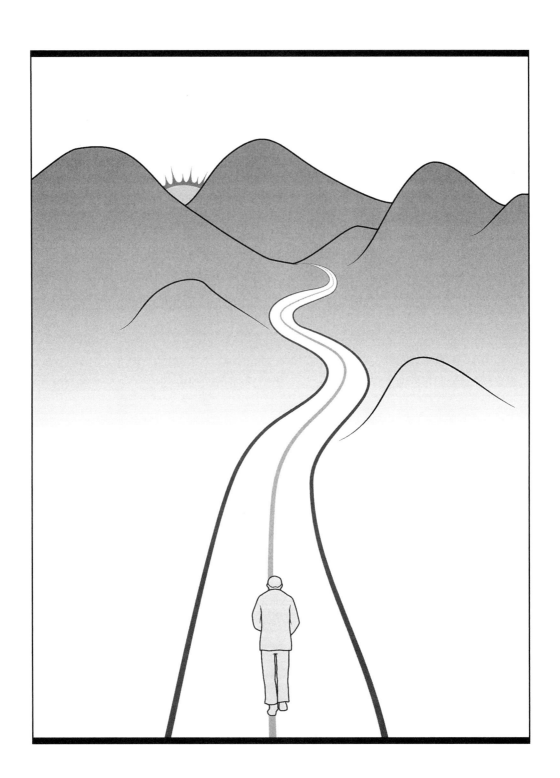

6

Healing the Psychological Wounds of Trauma

Our bodies are miraculously designed to protect us from harm. During times of threat, the body instantaneously pours enormous physical and psychological resources into survival. The sympathetic nervous system surges stress chemicals through us so we are prepared to fight or run. But sometimes we cannot act. We may see the truck coming toward us, but before we can react, it slams into us.

For some people, trauma profoundly shatters their sense of safety and predictability in the world. They become trapped in anxiety, fear, anger, or depression, no matter how conscientiously they attend to their healing. These powerful emotions can turn into posttraumatic stress disorder (PTSD), an anxiety disorder that can overwhelm their ability to cope with daily life.

People who find themselves both terrified and frozen in the face of trauma seem to be especially vulnerable to PTSD. Paralysis in the face of danger pounds a tremendous amount of undischarged fear, anger, or despair into the nervous system. Unless this energy is discharged in some way after the danger has passed, these damaging emotions can penetrate the body's tissues and permeate the person's emotional and physical well-being. A circuit of fear and agitation becomes hardwired into the nervous system. Eventually, seemingly minor stress can trigger outbursts of rage or spasms of fear, anxiety, and helplessness. The person may overreact to the ordinary difficulties of life for no apparent reason.

PTSD haunts soldiers and civilians in war, occurs in over a third of victims of motor vehicle accidents, and is a frequent complication of traumatic brain injury. Victims of childhood physical and sexual abuse pay an especially steep price. That trauma appears to etch changes into the nervous system that make them much more vulnerable to PTSD and chronic pain cycles later on. Acute symptoms of PTSD or a lingering hyperarousal state include hypervigilance, exaggerated startle, nightmares, sleep disturbance, and panic attacks. Later manifestations of PTSD can include pain, depression, mood swings, problems with thinking and concentrating, and sleep problems as well as other severe psychological pathology. Chronic pain syndromes have been linked to PTSD.

Though I deal with the psychological dimension of trauma every day in my practice, this is not my area of expertise. Over the years, I have seen my patients aided by good therapists who help them develop strategies for recovery. Patients suffering from PTSD have been helped by the sophisticated psychological treatments developed for this complex condition. This chapter will offer guidance as to why PTSD happens and some of the innovative approaches that can help victims of this debilitating condition.

THE CONFLICTING FORCES OF INJURY SHOCK

I talked earlier about how in even a minor accident or fear-provoking event, a basic and primitive part of ourselves often perceives that we could die. Sometimes, instead of running or fighting, we become paralyzed and unable to act. We are caught in a state of absolute helplessness while fight-or-flight chemicals surge through us. The autonomic nervous system goes to war with itself, pushing us to run at the same time that we are unable to move.

Peter Levine, PhD, in his book *Waking the Tiger: Healing Trauma,* talks about this response. He learned about one aspect of discharging trauma after talking to gamekeepers in Africa. These gamekeepers tranquilized wild animals to tag or examine them. If, after being captured and handled by game keepers, the released animals did not discharge their hyperarousal by trembling, running motions, diaphoresis (sweating), and/or deep breathing, they soon died. Levine speculates that their deaths result from their inability to properly discharge their hyperaroused state. The simultaneous hyperstimulation of the sympathetic nervous system and the parasympathetic nervous system is like pushing the gas pedal and the brake at the same time. It creates a cyclone of undischarged internal energy.

Unlike wild animals, people don't die from lack of release of this hyper-charged energy. But Levine and many other practitioners, including me, believe that if we cannot discharge the explosive energy caused by the frozen state, ongoing psychological and/or physical damage results.

As Levine points out, one of the effects of this hyperaroused state is to hard wire the recall of the dangerous situation into long-term memory. At one time in our evolutionary past, this had great value: future survival depended on quickly retrieving important lessons from life-threatening events. However, if the energy and fear generated during the crisis is not released quickly, the brain stores the experience in long-term memory with an emotional overlay of terror. Once a fear circuit has been embedded into the nervous system, it can react for decades and be triggered by any encounter with stress or helplessness.

Levine uses therapeutic guidance he has called Somatic Experiencing therapy to help the patient access their felt sense of the traumatic event. This is done in a secure and safe environment. At the same time the painful sensations arise, the therapist helps the patient access their own inner strength as it manifests in their body. From that place of inherent health within, the patient returns to the edge of the fearful or traumatic sensation or memory. By moving like a pendulum between the healthy side and the fearful side, the patient gradually dissipates the destructive energy trapped in their tissues. This process develops resilience in the nervous system so the person is not easily triggered by future stressful events.

Robert Scaer, MD, another expert on the psychological effects of trauma, also believes that humans frequently do not discharge their autonomic arousal state after trauma and that the combination of terror and freezing is the most devastating of the hyperarousal states. There are many reasons that discharge may have been suppressed. Unlike indigenous cultures that use dance, vocalization, ritual, and collective tribal attunement to discharge hyperarousal states after trauma, we have no communal rituals to help us downregulate the brain's fear response. Circumstances may not allow rapid discharge, as in the horrendous case of repeated childhood sexual abuse, where the victim has no escape. Failure to discharge this destructive arousal etches into the brain a neurologic circuit of fear, rage, or helplessness. Over time this highly destructive state can become PTSD.

Why would the incredibly wise body create this frozen state, which places almost impossible demands on the autonomic nervous system—like a car stuck in quicksand, spinning its wheels to escape while it slowly sinks into oblivion? There are some scenarios in which freezing might be a powerful survival mechanism. If there is insufficient oxygen in the atmosphere, from smoke or a cave-in, an animal has a much higher chance of survival by lying still, reducing its energy demands and not using up the limited supply of oxygen. Freezing may trick a predator into believing the animal is dead, causing it to leave the prey alone. In situations in which there is no escape, as in chronic childhood trauma, stillness and dissociation can be the keys to psychological survival. Whatever the cause, however, the discharge of the hyperaroused state is as vital to long-term survival as the frozen state itself.

PTSD represents an overreaction of the brain's emotional circuitry. These responses are centered in the amygdala, the part of the brain that orchestrates how we feel and how we interpret our responses to those feelings. The amygdala, which sits near the tip of each temporal lobe, assigns meaning and importance to experiences that it interprets as life-threatening. It then works with other brain regions to consolidate those experiences in our long-term memory. Controlling the amydala's response to trauma is a key to healing from PTSD.

Like Peter Levine, Robert Scaer offers solutions. He emphasizes the importance of regaining the body-brain balance and restoring balance between the two parts of the autonomic nervous system. He believes that fear circuits can be extinguished if exposure to the cues that trigger them occurs while the person is in a state of safety. Scaer also finds value in treatment systems that alternately stimulate one side of the brain in order to inhibit destructive patterns in the other side, such as Eye Movement Desensitization and Reprocessing (EMDR).

EMDR uses powerful neurological pathways to treat PTSD as well as lesser psychological and physical trauma. Francine Shapiro, PhD, worked in the Veterans Administration in the 1970s. She found that by using directed bilateral eye movements, she could help soldiers discharge some of the psychological trauma of war. In a sighted person, approximately fifty percent of the brain's nerves are involved in vision, so it makes sense that the brain can be profoundly affected by the use of visual cues.

Part of EMDR's power also comes from the intimate relationship between the eyes and the hormonal systems. After each optic nerve exits the back of the eye, it sends out neurological strands that run next to the pituitary gland, the body's master gland. I believe this anatomy is one of the many reasons the eyes can powerfully affect our hormones and our moods.

Of course, there is much more than bilateral eye movement involved in good EMDR therapy. Most EMDR practitioners also integrate other aspects of psychotherapy, such as cognitive, interpersonal, experiential, physiological, and somatic therapies into their practice.

I'm thrilled that Levine's Somatic Experiencing therapy and Scaer's work have recognized the profound damage that trauma can do to the nervous system and have designed effective methods to assist recovery from this debilitating condition.

OSTEOPATHY AND PTSD

I have treated many patients suffering from PTSD as a result of physical or psychological trauma. Like Levine and Scaer, I have found that the simultaneous triggering of the parasympathetically mediated freeze response and the sympathetically mediated fight-or-flight response creates the most damage to the nervous system if not released promptly afterward. I can feel this in people's bodies as a form of injury shock.

When I treat a patient after trauma, my first job has always been to calm and balance the autonomic nervous system. If fear lives in the amygdala, calm resides in the optimal functioning of the vagus nerve, the primary mover of the restorative parasympathetic nervous system. My work restores the vagus nerve to fuller function while quieting the chemicals of arousal and fear.

Just as deep breathing helps animals discharge their hyperaroused state, unfreezing the diaphragm and restoring deeper, slower breathing helps the vagus nerve regain its prominence in creating calm. Treatment at the base of the skull opens up the bony channels through which the vagus nerves pass as they exit the brain. These channels can be narrowed by the swelling of surrounding muscles and tightened by fear, pinching the nerves and hampering their work. By gently and bilaterally rocking the temporal bones using a technique developed by the founder of cranial osteopathy, William Sutherland, DO, and named the "pussyfoot," I can alternately massage each vagus nerve as it passes through the skull. This extremely calming technique, with its alternating motion, resembles the bilateral brain stimulation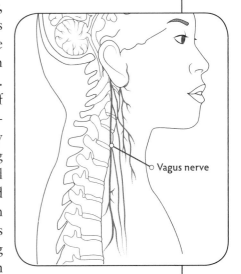

Vagus nerve

of modalities such as EMDR. Perhaps the central role of a happy vagus nerve in controlling PTSD explains why vagal nerve stimulation (VNS) is now being explored medically as a way to eradicate the fear circuits in the amygdala.

My attitude toward the patient shares a resemblance to the way Peter Levine encourages his patients to seek their grounding or inherent strength.

When I put my hands on a patient, I not only search for the areas of pathology, but even more importantly, I also focus on the health in their tissues. I then work to amplify that vibrant life force, in essence using the patient's own vitality to melt away the pathology.

If I can treat a person within the first forty-eight hours after a trauma, I find I can often release the hyperaroused state before it can etch a fear circuit into the nervous system. The sooner injury shock is removed and balance restored to the nervous system, the better chance a patient has of discharging this harmful energy, and the less likely that such a damaging circuit will take hold. But even if the first treatment is months or years after the trauma, I believe that osteopathic treatments can help remake the damaged circuitry in the brain. Bringing balance to the autonomic nervous system and amplifying the power of the vagus nerve can quiet down the troubled psyche's state of perpetual distress, regardless of when the trauma occurred. This work can support the work of psychotherapy and aid its success.

Besides relying on the guidance of a trained practitioner, there are ways that people suffering from PTSD can promote their own healing. I mention two of them here. The next chapter focuses on the power of yoga and the breath to restore balance to the nervous system.

Meditation. It has been known for years that meditation can dramatically reduce stress, anxiety, substance abuse, addiction, and depression. Recent studies have also shown that meditation can help overcome depression and anxiety both in combat veterans and in child survivors of natural disasters, and it is now being used to treat PTSD. A soldier who had been taught mindfulness meditation as part of a pilot study continued to meditate after he was deployed to Iraq. His fifteen minutes of daily practice was so helpful in controlling stress that others in his unit took up meditation as well.

Meditation is a powerful, simple method of recentering the mind and turning off the fear response. Meditation, especially Jon Kabat-Zinn's mindfulness meditation—which is both simple and powerful—has been shown to diminish pain, lower anxiety and stress, and significantly improve the sense of well-being. Even fifteen minutes a day of meditation can have powerful healing effects in the brain.

Tapping (EFT). Tapping (EFT, or Emotional Freedom Technique) is a resource for healing trauma by addressing pain and illness. EFT is a self-help technique that bears some similarity to EMDR. The teachers of this technique claim that EFT can help neutralize the impact or charge of trauma. Several of my patients have reported that it has helped them gain control over their lives after trauma and illness. While I lack personal experience with this technique, I always cheer on any effective technique that people can do for themselves. To learn more about tapping, see www.emofree.com.

Trauma can wound our emotional and spiritual well-being as surely as it harms our physical health. Never be afraid to seek help to reclaim your psychological health after trauma has damaged it, and remember that there are many compassionate professionals who can help you on that journey.

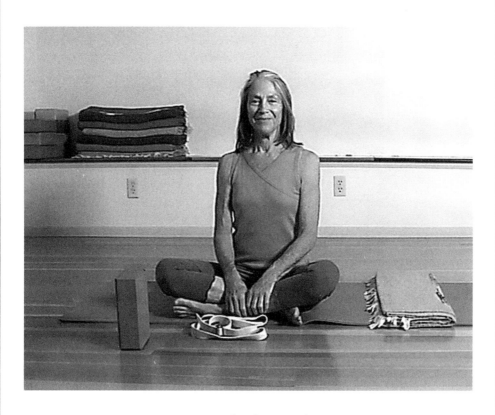

PATRICIA SULLIVAN *has been teaching yoga
and other movement therapies throughout the United
States for over thirty-five years. I have asked her
to share some simple poses and breathing practices
that can help heal injury shock, traumatic injury,
and chronic pain.*

7

A Program for Healing Injury Shock

It's amazing how a few minutes of movement a day reaps tremendous rewards. We are designed to move, and more than any other single thing, movement creates health. Once you start developing a movement activity, be it for five minutes or an hour a day, the body craves it. Like a puppy waiting to go outside, it will start to jump for joy at the opportunity to move. That joy heals as well.

Patricia Sullivan, a renowned teacher and practitioner of yoga and other movement modalities, including qigong and Egoscue, is my personal teacher. I have asked her to share her knowledge with the readers of this book. In this chapter, she will show you some simple poses that assist the diaphragm, calm the sympathetic nervous system, reawaken the nutritive parasympathetic nervous system, and restore the entire nervous system to balance.

Before you undertake this practice, or any other exercise after injury, a few gentle words of advice and caution:

- As with any injury, you must be cleared by your physician before you do the physical exercises.
- If an exercise hurts, don't do it.
- The more acute or recent your injuries, the slower you should progress with these exercises.
- Enjoy your wondrous breath and let it be your guide. Try not to force or pull your breath. That can irritate the tissue-paper-thin alveoli (the small grape-like air collectors in your lungs) and tightens the small muscles in the alveoli so they will absorb less oxygen.

• Do the easy ones first and then move on to the others. Start with one or two things that are comfortable and easy to do, and try to do them every day. These exercises are good for many problems and areas of the body, but because they so clearly help breathing, I put them here. I will be referring to them throughout the book.

I would like to add one of my favorite practices. I call it 4-7-8 breathing. It is an exercise Andrew Weil, MD, teaches to countless audiences. It is easy to do, and like an Olympic athlete taking calming breaths before a big event, you will find that it helps calm your nervous system. You can do it sitting in a comfortable position such as on a chair, or cross-legged with some height under your bottom. If you can't sit comfortably, lie down.

To start, tuck your tongue softly in back of your upper front teeth. Breathe in through your nose as deeply as you can for a count of four. Hold that breath for a count of seven. Then exhale for a count of eight, relaxing your tongue and slowly letting the breath out through the space between your tongue and your front teeth. Do this patterned breathing for two minutes a few times a day. It improves diaphragm motion, restores the natural rhythm of the breath, and helps calm the nervous system.

The key is to pause your breath for longer than you inhale, and exhale for twice as long as you inhale. However, feel free to modify this practice. At first, I had trouble holding my breath for a count of seven. Once I started to relax and breathe in more slowly and fully, I found it much easier to hold it for that long. You may not notice anything when you first start, but persevere. Breathing exercises pay off over time—days and weeks. The results can be dramatic.

And now I turn you over to Patricia!

BREATHING PRACTICES

I'd like to introduce some of the poses we do in my classes and some breath work that is fundamental to the way I teach. I have tailored these practices to help us balance our nervous system after injury or trauma. After a trauma or any kind of accident that shocks the nervous system, our breathing can get clenched up and not come back to normal. The nervous system can get clenched up, too. We want to work toward restoring normal breathing and the diaphragm's ability to move freely without us having to think about it—that's when it does its best work.

Yoga has been working with breathing exercises for thousands of years. One part of this work is simply to become more conscious of our breathing. When we are, we can tell when we're breathing more shallowly, when we're breathing quickly and so on. That awareness helps lead to fuller, more relaxed breathing. Specific practices to change breathing patterns, when used regularly, are also very helpful.

Hissing Breath

The first breathing exercise involves making a hissing sound, like a snake. The breath fills the lungs much more deeply and in a much more relaxed way. By doing this practice even a few times, you calm the heart and mind, and the body feels like it has plenty of energy. If the system is starved for oxygen, with this practice it gets a big drink.

▶ Take a deep breath, and for as long as you're exhaling, make a hissing sound. The belly flattens backward towards the spine and then relaxes. The breath floods back in and goes much deeper into the lungs, which means the diaphragm has really opened. This breaks the holding pattern of the diaphragm. Three to five times is usually enough. Take a resting breath between hissing breaths if you feel you need to.

Vowel Sounds

Making vowel sounds can be very helpful to restore the breath. When you breathe out normally, two or three or four seconds later, your breath is done. When you close your breathing apparatus around your larynx to make these sounds, it takes longer for the sound to come out—eight, ten, even fifteen seconds. This may seem surprising, but people do it all the time when they sing. When you breathe out for a long period of time, you stimulate the response in the body that says "Breathe deeply" in such a 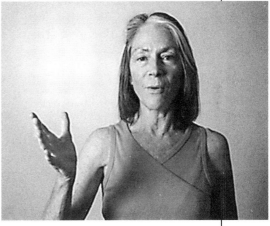 way that your habitual breathing patterns don't override it.

The sounds themselves are very soothing and calming to the brain. Some people work with high sounds; some people work with low sounds. You can carry on for quite a little while with these sounds in a joyful way.

▶ Start with the *oooooooh* sound. Breathe in normally, and as you exhale, make a long *oooooooh* sound. After three or four *oooooooh*s, move to *uuuuuuu,* and then *ahhhhhhh* and *aaaaaaaa* and *eeeeeee.*

I tend to start with the *oooh* and *uuuu* sounds as these help you to stay present in the belly area. You can do *oooh*s and *uuuu*s for a long time. *Aaah*s, *aaaa*s, and *eeee*s tend to bring the energy up. These, I feel, are from the solar plexus and the heart.

Inhale and Hold

When we're feeling anxious or a bit panicky, it's good to do this simple breathing practice. The Hissing Breath and the Vowel Sounds help us breathe out more slowly, which helps calm the nervous system. You can also find relief from anxiety or shortness of breath simply by holding the breath in. This practice helps improve the motion of the diaphragm and restore the natural rhythm of the breath. You can do this practice any time you find yourself feeling anxious.

▶ Take a deep, slow in-breath, gently directing the breath deep into the abdomen. Hold that breath for a number of seconds—four, five, six, up to ten seconds, whatever is easily doable for you—then let the breath out without allowing it to rush out. Don't hold the breath for so long that you can't let it out smoothly. You may want to take a normal, resting breath or two before you do it again. Repeat five or six times.

Alternate Nostril Breathing

This simple practice is a powerful way to balance the sympathetic and the parasympathetic nervous systems. You can do it sitting at your desk or lying in bed. Some people find that it helps lull them to sleep. There is no need to physically close off each nostril. It works very well just by focusing your attention.

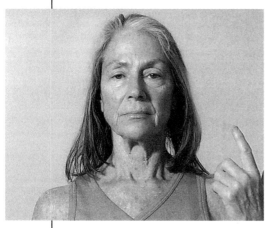

▶ Focus your awareness on your left nostril for three to four breaths. After a few cycles of inhaling and exhaling predominantly through the left nostril, pause at the end of an in-breath, then shift your focus and breathing emphasis to your right nostril. Exhale and inhale with the emphasis on the right nostril, then shift your focus and emphasis back to the left. Shift your focus gently back and forth, each time at the end of an in-breath. Repeat for at least six and up to twelve breaths.

RESTORATIVE POSES

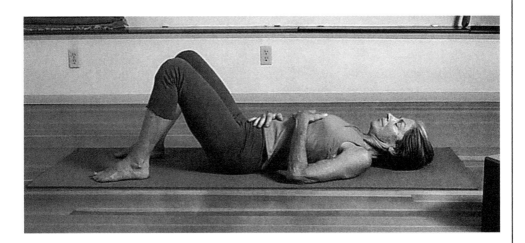

Reclining Pose

This pose helps loosen the ribs and diaphragm and draw air into the lobes of the lungs. It is very soothing to the nervous system.

▶ Lie down or sit on a comfortable surface. Place one hand gently on your belly and the other hand on your chest. Inhale slowly for a count of three and direct your breath into the hand on your belly. Feel your hand ride on your expanding belly. Hold for a count of three, then slowly exhale to a count of six, feeling your hand move down toward your spine as you exhale.

Then breathe slowly for a count of three into the hand resting on your chest. Hold for a count of three, and then slowly exhale for a count of six. Repeat this sequence five or six times, alternating your focus between your hands. You can also do this practice with your hands draped across the sides of your rib cage.

To relax the diaphragm even more, tighten your abdominal muscles for two seconds at the end of your exhale, then release. You will notice how your breath jumps into your lungs as your diaphragm starts to loosen up.

The next two poses quiet a very important bundle of nerves above the navel and just below the chest area that tend to get clenched up after a shock to the nervous system. Hugging a pillow or lying down on bolsters, pillows, or blankets feels like being held and comforted to our nervous system, even if it doesn't to our thinking mind. Sometimes the simplest things can help so much!

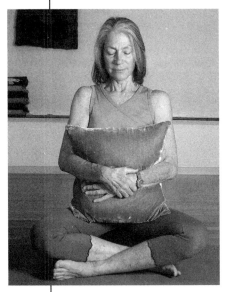

Hug a Pillow

◉ Take a nice couch or bed pillow, sit in a comfortable place, and hug it in—put your arms around it and breathe. Close your eyes and shut out the world. Stay with this for a few minutes.

Hug Some Blankets

It's wonderful to lie down and have the nerves in the belly soothed by lying on a supportive surface. I use blankets, but you can also use pillows or bolsters.

◉ Sit next to your pile of blankets or pillows, and as you exhale, turn your body and lie down on the pile. Your hip should be close to the pile, and your knees tucked up comfortably. One side of your torso should be completely supported on the blankets or pillows. As you breathe, the pressure of your upper body pushes the breath in toward the network of nerves in the belly, soothing them.

As you settle in, gently scan your body. Is there tension in your arms, and, if so, can you let it go? Are you holding something invisible in your hands? Can you let that go? Notice, too, the tongue and jaw and any other tense location.

You can set a timer for three to five minutes, but you might find you want to stay longer. Breathe in and feel the end of the in-breath. Feel the transition to the out-breath, then let it go. Just keep letting go. After a few minutes, turn and lie on your other side. If this position is hard on your neck, make a little rumple or wedge in the corner of your blanket so your head is on a slant. Your neck should never feel strained. Then close your eyes and continue to breathe and relax. It can be quite surprising how wonderful this is.

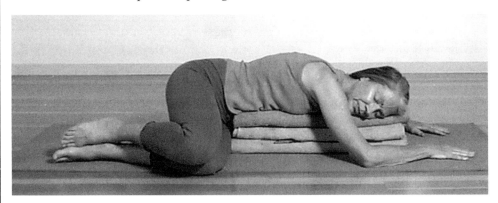

Legs on a Chair

This is one of my favorites. You can use a chair, a bed, a bench—anything that enables the lower leg from the knee to the heel to be resting. Your feet and knees shouldn't be too high. Try to have a straight line from knees to hips. Place your arms out from your sides. You may need to place a small blanket or towel on the chair so that your legs rest comfortably in a horizontal position. A small towel under your head also may help.

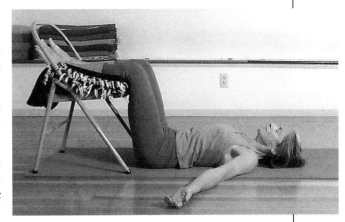

► You'll notice as you breathe out that your belly drops back toward the floor and then fills as you breathe in. After a few breaths, at the end of the exhalation, tighten all the muscles of the abdomen and pause for a second or two, and then release everything. Notice the way the breath comes back in. It can be delightfully surprising. Do eight to ten of these.

Legs Up the Wall

This pose is so relaxing! When you place your legs up the wall and your back flat on the floor, gravity helps you release leg tension and stretches and opens the diaphragm. This calming pose can be done to give you more energy during the day, or at the end of the workday. It can also be done to help you sleep. Yogis know this as a pose that reverses the constant daily downward pressure on our heart, legs, lungs, and diaphragm.

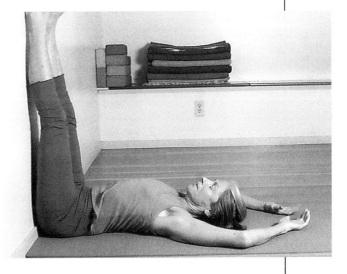

► Get as close to the wall as you comfortably can, keeping your bottom on the floor. Bring your legs up to rest on the wall. Breathe slowly and relax.

Cover your eyes if you like. A beanbag over the eyes is very nice! Try taking your arms up a little bit, either all the way overhead or just to the side. This can release the rib cage even more and help to smooth out and deepen the breath.

The companion DVD includes these and other exercises to help restore the breath and balance the nervous system.

I hope you find these poses helpful on your healing journey. For more information about my philosophy and practice, please visit my website at www.patriciasullivanyoga.com.

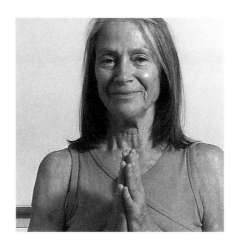

II.

Taming Inflammation

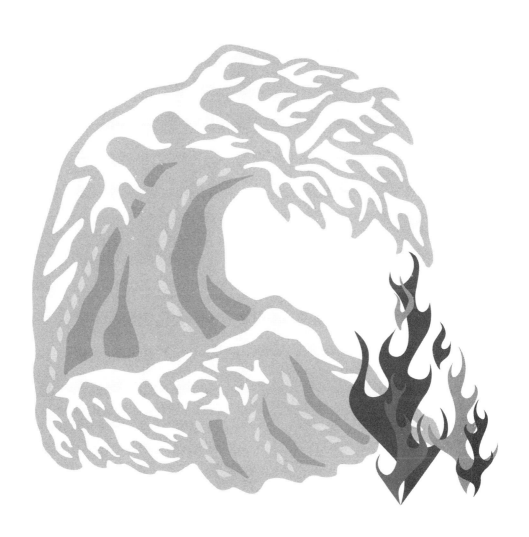

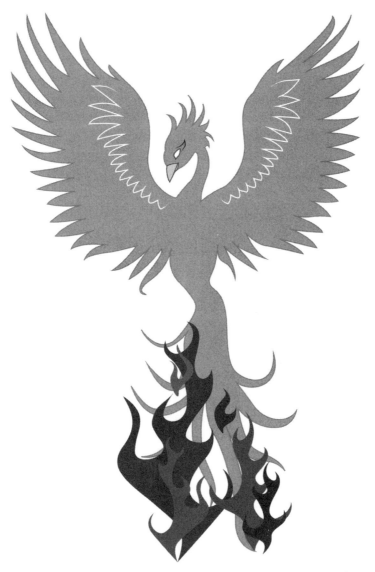

"*Let the lymphatics always receive and discharge naturally; if so, we have no substance detained long enough to produce fermentation, fever, sickness, and death. We strike at the source of life and death when we go to the lymphatics. Thus it behooves us to handle them with wisdom and tenderness . . .*"

—Andrew Taylor Still, 1899, Founder of osteopathic medicine

8

Phoenix Rising:
Inflammation and Healing

Inflammation is a valiant hero, constantly saving us. When injury attacks the body, the damaged cells cry out for help. The immune system, hearing the call, sends inflammatory warriors to the rescue. Thus begins the intricately choreographed cascade of activity that causes the characteristic heat, redness, swelling, and pain we experience as inflammation. Like the mythical phoenix that was consumed by fire and then reborn from the ashes, healing is born out of the fires of inflammation.

Healing from trauma is a complex dance orchestrated by a dizzying array of chemical messengers that shepherd the body through inflammation to health. Chemical messengers called cytokines and prostaglandins that fuel and quench the inflammatory fire communicate, interact, and switch each other on and off to achieve healing. Each stage of inflammation, from its powerful, destructive beginning to its eventual termination, is programmed to produce repair and healing as the end result. However, particularly at the beginning, the inflammatory assault is so powerful that it can inflict additional damage on injured tissues and cause collateral damage to nearby healthy ones. But if inflammation is allowed to complete its work, healing and repair arise inexorably from its pain, and both pain and inflammation gradually fade away.

Inflammation is the beginning of healing, yet diseases that are linked to it are killing us at an alarming rate. Heart disease, obesity, diabetes, atherosclerosis, Alzheimer's disease, stroke—it seems that every day, a new and deadly pestilence is linked to inflammation's fiery power. And even when inflammation is not killing us, out-of-control inflammation can cause searing and unrelenting pain. How did it come to pass that this primordial process, without which we cannot heal, has become the very thing that destroys our health?

The answer to that question has intrigued researchers who are beginning to delve into inflammation's secrets. There are some secrets, however, that are hiding in plain sight. Inflammation is a tightly regulated process in which each stage creates the conditions for the next to take hold. The body carefully balances inflammation's destructive power with its qualities of restoration and healing. Interrupt or prolong any step, starve the body of the nutrients necessary to turn inflammation off, dam up essential fluid flow necessary to sweep toxins away, or stop the motion of this elegant process, and instead of healing, inflammation and pain can consume the body.

In this section, I will explore ways to promote inflammation's healthy aspects while keeping it from taking off in a destructive direction. I will also offer solutions to quench damaging fires once inflammation goes haywire. In the process, I highlight the magical world of the ultimate Cinderella—the underappreciated and hardworking soul of recovery, the lymphatic system. To put this in a human context, I introduce Libby.

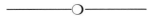

LIBBY had just gotten to sleep, that luxurious state where everything relaxes and we feel like a babe in arms. Then Libby's six-month-old baby screamed from the nursery down the hall. Half asleep, Libby rushed into the hallway, where four-year-old Timmy had left his toy truck. Libby slipped on the toy, twisting her upper body backward and hitting her shoulder against the wall as she fell.

Dazed and stunned, Libby finally stood up, holding her aching neck and arm. She did not sleep well that night. The next morning, ever the trooper, she went to her job as a cashier at the neighborhood supermarket. Since her neck burned and she had stabbing pain in her shoulders, she popped several non-steroidal anti-inflammatory drugs (NSAIDs), which cut down her pain and enabled her to do the twisting, turning, and lifting required at her job.

Two days later, still in a lot of pain, vaguely nauseated, and suffering a headache, Libby wondered if she had the flu. She went to see her doctor. He examined her and told her she had a bit of whiplash. He recommended continuing her regimen of NSAIDs and cleared her for work, saying, "You'll be fine in a couple weeks. Just go on with your life."

But Libby could not get on with her life. Soon the pain spread to her arms, back, hips, and feet and disturbed her sleep. She was in so much discomfort that she stopped taking her evening stroll with her children. Too tired to cook, she found herself surviving on fast food and diet soda. Finally, two months after her fall, one of her coworkers, seeing her pasty and swollen face, told her to see me.

I listened to Libby's history and examined her. Her neck muscles, especially in the front, were boggy and tender. The force of the trauma and the ensuing muscle spasm had restricted the normal movement of her upper ribs and neck. Libby's face looked swollen like a person after a long night of drinking, but she hadn't had a drink. I found other problems as well: her diaphragm was in spasm and her sympathetic nervous system was overstimulated.

Because Libby's injuries were extensive, the initial assault of inflammation was powerful. Even so, by now she should have been well on her way to recovery. Instead, her pain and inflammation were getting worse and spreading to other areas.

To understand why this was happening, I'll describe how the inflammatory process works and what it did to Libby. Though I discuss this process in a chronological order, inflammation is more like a ten-ring circus, with lots of these activities occurring together.

HOW INFLAMMATION WORKS

After Libby fell, her injured cells immediately sent out distress signals. Mast cells that live in the nearby connective tissue (fascia) picked up the call and released histamine, a chemical signal that the body is under attack. Chemicals produced by the injured cells, called cytokines and prostaglandins, caused the surrounding blood capillaries to become porous. Fluids and fibrous proteins flooded in through the leaky capillaries to wall off the injured areas. (This sealing-off process is critical to protect nearby tissues from any infection or toxins brewing at the injury site.) Platelets rushed in to stop bleeding. Nutrients and warrior cells of the immune system also entered the injury site. The flood of fluid, cells, and proteins caused the swelling in Libby's face and neck.

The prostaglandins and other chemicals released by the injured cells stimulated the already-activated pain receptors in the surrounding nerves, causing even more pain. The pain was warning Libby to rest so her body could heal. I would have expected Libby to have significant pain and inflammation in the first few days or even week after her fall. After that, inflammation should have started to resolve. But for reasons you will see in a moment, Libby continued to be swollen and inflamed.

ATTACK OF THE NEUTROPHILS:
Controlling Their Destructive Power

The body's first reaction to injury is ancient, fierce, and protective. Whether it is a sprained ankle or a deep wound, the body does not negotiate with injury: it goes to war. Along with a tsunami of proteins and fluids, highly destructive immune cells called neutrophils arrive quickly through the enlarged blood vessels. Billions of neutrophils are created every day in the bone marrow and float harmlessly in the blood until they are called into action. Then they undergo a Frankenstein-like transformation and become the body's shock troops. They flood into sites of injury or infection and destroy things. Do not be deceived by their innocuous name. Once activated, neutrophils are some of the most powerful healing and destructive cells in the body.

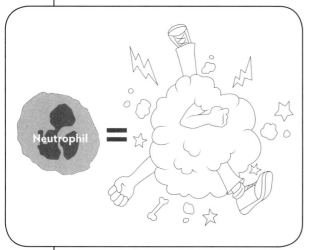

The body needs neutrophils to clean up debris at an injury site, but neutrophils are not particular about what they destroy in the process.

Neutrophils are like stupid bombs. Their job is to keep the situation from getting out of control until more sophisticated immune cells arrive. Neutrophils don't distinguish between injured tissues and healthy ones. They don't try to figure out if bacteria or viruses are contaminating an injury. Neutrophils do their job by releasing an explosion of highly reactive chemicals called free radicals, highly unstable molecules that are very good at killing pathogens but also cause damage and stress to healthy tissues. Neutrophils release powerful enzymes to dissolve dead and damaged tissue, and injure healthy tissue in the process. Then the neutrophils engulf and eat up what's left.

Neutrophils create so much destruction that inflammation will not turn off until they go away. Wisely, the body has built-in mechanisms to keep them under control and get rid of them. Neutrophils don't live very long at the injury site. They usually self-destruct after about forty-eight hours. By the third day, the chemical signals that called them to the injury site should be countermanded by different compounds with soothing names like protectins and resolvins. These healing compounds, which are made from omega-3 fatty acids in the diet, tell the neutrophils to stop coming to the injury site. They signal for other, less destructive cells to come into the tissues and gobble the neutrophils up. Amazingly, the neutrophils send out the same signals, heroically calling for their own demise. If all goes as it should, the neutrophils expire, the next cells eat them up, and the lymphatic system carts all of them away.

Anything that delays the removal of neutrophils sets the stage for continuing tissue damage, ongoing inflammation, and pain. There is growing evidence that neutrophils overstaying their welcome play a central role in joint destruction in such chronic, painful inflammatory conditions as rheumatoid arthritis. The less time the neutrophils spend in the inflamed tissue, the faster and more completely inflammation resolves.

THE HUNGRY MACROPHAGES:
Inflammation Ends When They Leave

The rescuing cells that gobble up neutrophils and coordinate the serious business of healing are called macrophages (*macrophage* means "big eater"), which live in the blood as cells called monocytes. Countless numbers of these tiny, seemingly weak cells travel around aimlessly in the blood. Like ninety-five-year-old vacationers in Florida floating on inner tubes in their swimming pools, daiquiris in hand, monocytes are having a good time in the ninety-eight-degree weather of the blood. Then they are called into action and transform into the hunks of the immune system—the big-eating macrophages.

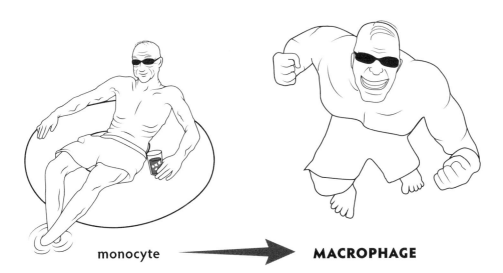

monocyte → **MACROPHAGE**

When summoned to the site of injury, monocytes transform from seemingly innocuous cells into ferocious warriors—the macrophages.

73

The hungry macrophages are much larger, more sophisticated, and longer lived than the neutrophils. While they also cause tissue destruction, they perform many other tasks. They scrub the injury site so that debris doesn't fester and provoke a new round of inflammation. Resolvins and protectins—and even the noble neutrophils—encourage the macrophages to chow down on the neutrophils.

As they gobble up the neutrophils and are no longer so hungry, macrophages have a change of heart. They become nicer. They release anti-inflammatory cytokines that dampen inflammation. They send out signals to cells called fibroblasts, which live in the fascia, to begin the serious repair work. Some of them start the repair work themselves.

Alas for the macrophages, they, too, have to leave the inflamed tissues for the healing cells to do their best work. The macrophages are too big to climb into neighboring blood vessels. Instead, these satiated macrophages hop a ride through the wider lymphatic vessels. The lymphatic system, which I will introduce in a moment, is essentially a parallel circulatory system. It takes particles out of the tissues that are too big to fit in the blood vessels and floats them along to lymph nodes. The lymph nodes filter out and destroy the debris, and the cleansed fluid is sent on its way to join the blood circulation flowing into the heart.

As the inflammatory macrophages and neutrophils disappear from the damaged tissues, cells and chemicals in charge of rebuilding predominate and the work of healing begins in earnest. Collagen fibers are laid down and contract, tightening the strength of the repair. For the next twelve months, the tissues will be constantly remodeled to create a repair as close to the original tissue as possible. But long before the healing is complete, inflammation should have faded away.

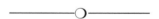

If inflammation is so wonderfully programmed to do its job and turn itself off, why was Libby so inflamed two months after her fall? In various ways, Libby had inadvertently prolonged her own suffering.

First, instead of resting her poor, painful body, Libby went back to work immediately. Her injured back and neck were too weak to tolerate the twisting and lifting demanded by her job, and she kept reinjuring them. The new injuries caused additional rounds of inflammation. More neutrophils with their destructive chemicals were drawn to the already-inflamed site, accompanied by more fluid, swelling, and pain. Had this gone on much longer, her inflammation could have become chronic.

Second, because Libby had a new baby, a toddler, and a full-time job, her stress levels were already high, and the biochemistry of chronic stress primes the body for inflammation. The injury shock of her accident added more stress. The combination of injury shock and chronic stress kept inflammatory chemicals pouring into her body.

Third, as we will see in chapter 10, Libby's fast-food diet was pouring inflammation-feeding foods into her body and starving it of the nutrients she needed to turn inflammation off.

All the inflammatory chemicals flooding Libby's tissues were like a vitamin tonic for neutrophils. It kept them alive and attracted even more of them. The explosion of destructive cells caused more tissue damage and more inflammation. These chemicals and cells needed to be flushed out of her tissues, and quickly. Libby's swollen face and neck, however, meant that the drainage routes for the fluid were backed up and sluggish. Even worse, a toxic-waste pile was growing in her damaged tissues. A vicious cycle was taking hold as her immune system tried to flush the accumulating trash away with more fluid and burn it up with destructive cells. Unfortunately, those efforts just clogged the drains even more, throwing more fuel on the inflammatory fire. The breakdown of the trash-removal system is one of the greatest triggers of continuing inflammation.

Besides helping take the shock out of Libby's nervous system, I had to help unclog the pipes that carry away the fluid and the trash. That system is called the lymphatic system, and it is the second unsung hero of health.

MEET THE LYMPHATIC SYSTEM

The lymphatic system is the body's purification and detoxification highway. It is absolutely essential to the body's capacity to control inflammation and heal from injury and infection. Named after Lympha, the Roman goddess of water, the lymphatic system is the body's second vascular system. Through it flows a vast river of fluid twice as large as the blood circulation. Beginning with tiny capillaries that envelop most of our tissues, the lymphatic system carries away excess fluid, cellular trash, and even infectious agents. Small beadlike nodules called lymph nodes filter and cleanse the fluid as it journeys from the tissues to the heart. The lymph nodes also house the immune cells that fight infection.

Since the beginning of our profession over a hundred years ago, osteopathic physicians have recognized the importance of the lymphatic system to health. Many of the techniques I and other osteopaths use are designed to promote the circulation of lymphatic fluid as it cleanses and reinvigorates injured tissues.

You may have never heard of this wondrous system. Most people know nothing about it until something goes wrong—for instance, their lymph nodes become painful after an infection or their feet swell up after they sit too long. But as you will see, the health of the lymphatic system is essential to controlling inflammation and restoring vibrant health.

We tend to think of the body as a mechanical system, but in reality the body is more a fluid system. In fact, fluid makes up between 50 and 60 percent of an adult's body weight. Our cells float in a sea of fluid—actually, an ocean of it. About a gallon of fluid circulates in the bloodstream, but five times that much surrounds the cells. Blood capillaries and their lymphatic sisters encircle the cellular ocean. Blood capillaries are full of goodies like nutrients, oxygen, and hormones. Nutrient-rich fluid leaks out of the blood vessels and into the intracellular ocean. The cells take in nutrients from the fluid and send waste products back into it.

The cellular fluids need to be flushed out and cleansed or they stagnate. The blood circulation can't reabsorb it all. The lymphatic system comes to the rescue, carrying at least three quarts of fluid a day back to the blood circulation. The lymphatics also take over the job of absorbing the large proteins and particles in the fluid that are too big for the tiny blood capillaries.

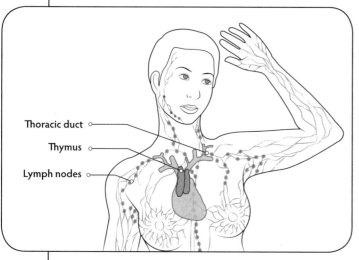

Thoracic duct

Thymus

Lymph nodes

On its journey from the tissues to the heart, lymph passes through small, beadlike nodules called lymph nodes, which filter and cleanse the fluid.

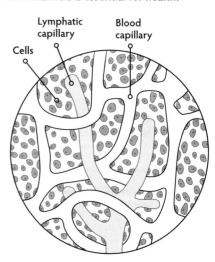

The intimate relationship of our two fluid channels is essential for health.

Lymphatic capillary

Blood capillary

Cells

As the fluid (now called lymph) journeys through the lymphatic system, it flows through filtering stations called lymph nodes, which are strung along the lymphatic vessels like pearls in a necklace. The lymph nodes are packed with nooks and crannies where specialized cells filter out and eat up the debris brought in by the lymph.

Like small tributaries flowing into a stream and then a river, the microscopic lymphatic capillaries flow into larger and larger pipes, which are lined with valves to prevent the lymph from flowing backward. The pipes merge into one of six lymphatic trunks, each one carrying lymph from a specific area of the body. Eventually, the lymph pours through large thoracic channels under the collarbones and joins the blood circulation flowing down into the heart.

Without a working lymphatic system, the body's tissues would quickly be flooded with fluid and the body would swell up like a balloon. The blood circulation, starved of fluid, would collapse. Cells would drown in a toxic stew of poisons, pathogens, and cellular garbage. Ordinary bacteria and viruses would fester in the stagnant pools and breed diseases like bronchitis and pneumonia. The lymphatics are like Cinderella, doing the unglamorous and unheralded but life-saving work of cleaning up the trash.

Unlike the circulatory system, the lymphatic system has no organ like the heart to pump it. Lymphatic circulation depends on the motion of the diaphragm, whose forceful movement sucks the fluid through the lymphatic channels. The lymphatics are also pumped by the movement of muscles, the pulsation of nearby blood vessels, gravity, and the compression of tissues by external force (like compression bandages and manual techniques that help fluid flow).

The Key to Controlling Infection

Though this book focuses on injury without infection, occasionally an injury becomes infected by bacteria or viruses. The lymphatics are even more essential to preserving life and restoring health when pathogens attack the body. The lymphatics are the transport system for the immune cells that attack infection. The lymph nodes house millions of specialized immune cells designed to destroy pathogens. These cells wait patiently there, and when the lymph brings in bacteria and viruses, the immune cells pounce. B-cells latch on to the invaders and produce antibodies that kill them outright or mark them for destruction by other cells. T-cells identify the pathogens and then go out into the body to find and destroy cells infected by the pathogens.

The lymphatic system strategically places guardian cells in regions that come in close contact with harmful organisms. The tonsils in the throat have specialized cells to kill invaders trying to enter through the mouth or nose. The body wisely puts more than half of its lymphatic tissue in the digestive system because so many pathogens and toxins try to get into the body through our food. There is so much disease-fighting lymphatic tissue in the gut that it has its own name, gut associated lymphoid tissue, or GALT, which is so important to health that it has its own Facebook fan page.

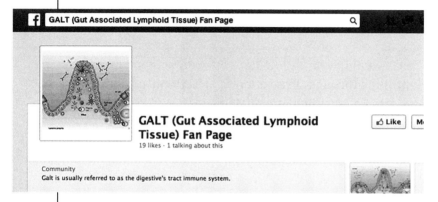

HOW THE LYMPHATICS HELP TAME INFLAMMATION

Good lymphatic flow is essential to remove the kindling of inflammation—the trash pile of dead and dying cells and the bacteria and viruses that infect the injury site and stoke inflammation's fires. The lymphatics must also take away the dangerous neutrophils and the satiated macrophages, whose presence also triggers continuing inflammation. By draining excess fluid, the lymphatics allow oxygen and healing nutrients to enter and nourish injured tissues. Inflammation will not resolve until the debris of injury is removed from the injured tissues by the lymphatics.

If the lymphatic drains are overwhelmed and/or clogged, healing nutrients have a hard time squeezing in. Destructive cells stay around too long and fuel more inflammation. The injury site teems with the powerful chemicals that turn inflammation on and keep it going. As with a stagnant river, disease and pestilence fester in the injured tissues. The healing process can be so disrupted that chronic inflammation takes hold.

Current research has discovered that lymphatic vessels are not passive drainpipes. They have a deep intelligence that helps them decide what should enter the lymphatic system and what they must reject. They are actively involved in seducing the neutrophils and macrophages to leave the inflamed tissues. Lymphatic capillaries quickly grow and expand to accommodate the increased demands created by injury. The cells of the lymphatic capillaries are even involved in the production of the chemicals that turn inflammation on and off. That's why I say that the lymphatics are truly an unsung hero of health.

How Libby and I Restored Her Health

For optimum health, the entire lymphatic system must flow freely, from the tiniest capillaries surrounding the swollen tissues to the largest vessels which join the circulation going to the heart. At any point along this road, the lymphatic highways can be impeded, constricted, or clogged. A common place for the highway to get blocked is in the upper chest, where the big lymphatic pipes have to navigate hairpin turns through dense connective tissue. Restrictions in the upper chest can turn the lymphatic channels from a four-lane highway into a crash site during rush hour. Hunching shoulders, constantly leaning forward to see a computer screen, or tightening muscles and fascia in the upper chest can narrow these pipes and back up the entire system. Libby's injuries to her upper back and shoulders, compounded by her constant twisting and hunching over a cash register, had tightened and twisted the connective tissue and muscles through which this all-important highway had to pass.

Lymphatic flow can also back up around the injury site. Since the lymphatics don't have a heart to propel the fluid, it's fairly common for the lymphatics to be clogged up here. In Libby's case, the tight fascia and spasmed muscles around her injured neck and shoulders created roadblocks for the small lymphatic channels draining from her neck and face. With the fluid in the small vessels unable to navigate through the tightened tissues, it backed up, causing Libby's swollen neck and face.

And unbeknownst to Libby, she had thrown a monkey wrench into her lymphatic system from the very beginning and had been encouraged to do so by her physician. She took NSAIDs (nonsteroidal anti-inflammatory drugs). Research is showing that almost all NSAIDs interfere with the tiny lymphatic capillaries by reducing their permeability to fluids and debris. The result can be increased swelling and pain, more inflammatory cells and debris at the injury site, more inflammation, slower and imperfect healing, and a bigger chance of inflammation becoming chronic. NSAIDs also delay the entry of the neutrophils and macrophages into the injury site. While this can decrease pain in the beginning, it ultimately disrupts the entire inflammatory process, delays regeneration and healing, and results in increased tissue fibrosis.

The first thing I did to help Libby restore her health was order her to take a week off from work. She had to give her damaged tissues time to rest and

79

heal. While this was difficult for her financially, she had been missing so much time from work because of her injury and had been feeling so sick that my instructions came as somewhat of a relief.

The next thing I did was give her a series of gentle breathing exercises like the ones in chapter 7 to help move her diaphragm. This helped stop the flood of stress hormones that were keeping her anxious and exhausted. By helping her diaphragm move more easily, she was restoring one of the lymphatic system's major pumps. As her nervous system calmed down, she was able to sleep better, which is essential for all aspects of healing.

I also told Libby to rock her baby in the rocking chair. Bouncing on the toes does wonders for pumping the lymphatics and helped reduce her swelling. Libby soon resumed her nightly walks with her children, which also helped her lymphatics flow. She began to do gentle stretches to open up her chest and the important lymphatic channels that flow through it.

I advised Libby to stop taking NSAIDs. We substituted fish-oil supplements, curcumin, and aspirin to address her pain, and they worked quite well. However, I was prepared to use traditional pain medications if they hadn't. Pain must be appropriately controlled, or it can set up a self-perpetuating pain cycle in the nervous system. At my insistence, Libby gradually dropped the fast food from her diet. This went a long way toward lowering the inflammatory burden those unhealthy foods had poured into her body. She started adding vegetables, fruit, healthy fats, and protein, eating her way back to health.

For my part, I treated the restrictions in the tissues of Libby's upper thoracic and neck region to restore motion and fluid flow and open up the lymphatic channels that drain there. I released strains in her diaphragm so her lymphatic circulation would improve. I also used one of the oldest and most effective osteopathic techniques to combat inflammation by providing her chest and abdomen with a gentle lymphatic pump. By gently rocking the tissues forward and back, I increased the flow of lymphatic fluid throughout her body.

Soon after her first visit, Libby's swelling decreased. She started to look like herself and her pain levels diminished. After two treatments and her own conscientious self-care, her inflammation and pain diminished drastically and she could more comfortably travel the road back to health.

CHRONIC INFLAMMATION

Although Libby was able to avoid it, sometimes inflammation does go out of control. Then we become victims of chronic inflammation.

Chronic inflammation, unlike the acute inflammation that mends the body, is not a healing process. It is a highly destructive disease that attacks otherwise healthy tissues. Chronic inflammation has been linked to cancer, heart disease, stroke, Alzheimer's disease, depression, arthritis, diabetes, irritable bowel disease, rheumatoid arthritis, lupus, and fibromyalgia, to name just a few. It can inflame your mood so you fight with your good-natured lover. As Andrew Weil, MD, has said, "Chronic inflammation may be the root of all degenerative disease."

Researchers are beginning to understand some of the reasons acute inflammation becomes a chronic affliction. We know that the longer inflammation lasts and its damage continues, the more danger there is that the resolving mechanisms will fail. Interfering with the natural rhythm of acute inflammation often ends up prolonging it and increases the risk of chronic inflammation. Lifestyle factors contribute to it, including obesity, diet, stress, poor sleep, and inactivity. And science's developing investigation of the lymphatics is revealing that poor lymphatic function is intimately involved in many chronic inflammatory diseases.

The subject of chronic inflammation is vast and complex—far beyond the scope of this book. There is no pill or vaccine that cures it. But giving the body the tools it needs to heal itself—removing injury shock and restoring motion to restricted areas and lymphatic pathways—are necessary first steps. Reducing the body's inflammatory burden and enhancing its health with nutritious food, exercise, stress reduction, and restful sleep are also essential. Here I'll talk about some of the major triggers of chronic inflammation. The next two chapters provide ways for you help stop the downward spiral of pain and suffering that continuing inflammation causes.

Given that inflammatory conditions have reached epidemic proportions, it's understandable that research has focused its attention on how inflammation works and how to rein in its power. Certainly, in the case of an overwhelming trauma, aggressively controlling inflammation can be a matter of life or death. But where less dramatic injuries are involved, treatments that short-circuit inflammation rather than shepherding it toward resolution have been problematic. In my opinion, the body can usually be trusted to manage its own healing with the right kind of help.

For example, efforts to block the function of the powerful neutrophils have resulted in impaired healing because the body needs their destructive chemicals to get the cleanup process started. Pharmaceuticals that delay the arrival of the big-eating macrophages can also cause serious problems.

In the normal healing process, the aggressive neutrophils die and are consumed by the husky macrophages. But if the macrophages' arrival is delayed, the neutrophils aren't disposed of efficiently. Instead of being eaten by the hungry macrophages, the neutrophils become zombies, rising from the dead

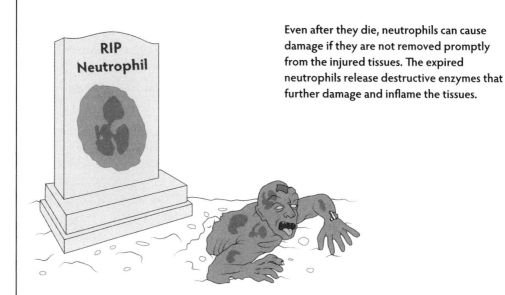

Even after they die, neutrophils can cause damage if they are not removed promptly from the injured tissues. The expired neutrophils release destructive enzymes that further damage and inflame the tissues.

to sow chaos and destruction. Technically, they undergo what's called secondary necrosis, which means they die a second time. In that zombie death, the neutrophils release harmful, destructive enzymes into the inflamed tissues. This zombie death is a very bad thing. It causes a new wave of tissue destruction, seeds more inflammation, and delays the healing process. It is even suspected of having a role in such chronic inflammatory diseases as lupus.

Delaying the arrival of the macrophages also confuses the macrophages. These particular macrophages derive their purpose in life from the dying neutrophils, which give them instructions on how to carry on the healing process. If the neutrophils have already turned into zombies, the macrophages lose their way. Instead of finishing the cleanup and orchestrating the healing process, the macrophages may start doing both at the same time, and they don't do either one well. The repairs that are made are constantly damaged, and fibrous scar tissue is laid down.

The body rebuilds injured tissues with a substance caused fibrin. In these poorly made repairs, fibrin gets laid down in chaotic meshes, binding the injured tissues into awkward, distorted scars that dam up the roadways needed to move healing nutrients into the injured region and harmful toxins out. The imperfect healing causes more damage, causing more inflammatory cells to rush in with their destructive chemicals, causing more inflammation and pain. Eventually, an endless cycle of tissue destruction and repair takes place, and inflammation never turns off.

Where once there was elastic connective tissue and responsive muscle, there is now rigid, fibrotic scar tissue. Surrounding tissues become overtaxed. Soon not only does the injured part hurt, but so does everything around it as the body is awash in inflammatory chemicals. Eventually, healthy tissue at distant sites in the body comes under attack, and conditions such as arthritis, heart disease, cancer, and diabetes explode.

By now, you've lost hope because none of this makes sense and most physicians can't give you a reasonable explanation for your suffering. They throw you into the wastebasket of fibromyalgia or ply you with anti-inflammatory drugs, which do not address the underlying cause of the problem and often make it worse.

FUELS OF CHRONIC INFLAMMATION

Identifying the fuel of chronic inflammation is the first step to eliminating it. Here are some of the major culprits:

Injury shock. Danger and trauma stimulate the fight-or-flight response of the sympathetic nervous system (SNS). One of the hormones that keeps the body ready to fight or flee is cortisol. Cortisol is also one of the body's most powerful anti-inflammatory hormones. By dampening inflammation, cortisol temporarily limits pain so the person can direct their full attention to survival. Cortisol also prevents the inflammatory response from becoming too aggressive and spinning out of control.

If the nervous system remains agitated and/or the person remains under constant psychological stress, the adrenal glands continue to produce cortisol. Eventually, the immune cells become resistant to cortisol's anti-inflammatory instructions. It's like a car losing its brakes as it's driving downhill. Unrelenting stress, either physical or psychological, eventually takes one of the body's best controllers of inflammation out of action and allows chronic inflammation to take hold.

Injury shock also has a tendency to put the diaphragm into spasm. The lymphatics need the diaphragm's pumping to keep them flowing.

Restricted motion. Misaligned joints, overstretched and tightened fascia, and injured muscles are much less resilient tissues. Even ordinary activities can overload and reinjure them. This constant reinjury can fuel a chronic inflammatory process. Tightened fascia can also impede the flow of fluids in and out of injured tissues, allowing them to stagnate.

Impaired lymphatic drainage. Poor lymphatic flow slows delivery of healing nutrients into swollen tissues. The tissues drown in a stagnant pool of toxins and debris that seed endless rounds of inflammation as the body futilely tries to remove the stagnant debris with more inflammatory cells, creating more stagnant debris in the process.

Impaired lymphatic drainage has been discovered in many chronic inflammatory conditions, including irritable bowel disease, obesity, lymphedema, and fibromyalgia. When lymphatic function is improved, many of these conditions, including psoriasis, filariasis, irritable bowel syndrome, and lymphedema have shown dramatic improvement.

Interference with the resolution stage of inflammation. The resolution of inflammation depends not only on the removal of debris and destructive cells but also on the ascendancy of the resolvins and protectins that countermand pro-inflammatory messengers and shepherd the body toward healing. Prolonging the presence of neutrophils in the tissues or delaying the work of the macrophages can interfere with resolution. And since the body manufactures resolvins and protectins from the omega-3 fatty acids provided by our diet, there is growing evidence that a body starved of these nutrients cannot marshal the forces to move inflammation toward resolution.

Lifestyle. Chronic inflammation is the twenty-first century's first plague. The toxic air we breathe, our tendency to eat inflammation-causing foods, weigh too much, not sleep enough, not exercise, and subject ourselves to constant stress are all prescriptions for a life of chronic inflammation. Even if the tissues are well aligned and the lymphatics are moving well, these good things will not completely undo the damage done on a daily basis by a toxic lifestyle.

Every day, life assaults the body with allergens, parasites, and pollution as well as the normal waste products of cells during their jobs. Adding to that burden is the typical American diet, which is full of inflammation-fueling foods that tip the balance sharply toward the building of pro-inflammatory chemicals. Even before an injury intrudes into life, the body is working overtime to deal with inflammation.

When an injury comes along, it's often the final straw. The valiant body is simply overwhelmed by the additional inflammatory chemicals piled on by the injury. Then, like the Energizer bunny, inflammation keeps going and going.

The overabundance of inflammatory chemicals spills into the bloodstream and amplifies the small inflammatory processes always going on throughout the body. Beckoned to these distant sites, immune cells attack and injure vulnerable tissues in the heart and blood vessels, the lungs, the gut, the joints, even the brain. This inflammation is often silent, burning at a low level for weeks, months, or even years until it explodes into chronic pain or a serious disease.

Remember that inflammation is basically a healing response, and the body always tries to move towards health. The next two chapters focus on the things you can do to bring it back to that healing path, including the most powerful inflammation fighter—the fuel you put in your body.

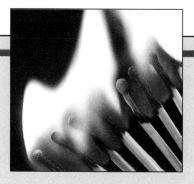

Taming Inflammation

1. Find a knowledgeable practitioner
2. Rest your injured body
3. Keep moving
4. Stay hydrated
5. Breathe!
6. Incorporate meditation, yoga, or tai chi
7. Make time for sleep
8. Use natural products for pain
9. Avoid toxins
10. Empower the lymphatics

9

Ten Ways to Tame Inflammation

Every part of inflammation, like plants turning toward the sun, moves toward healing. Harnessing the body's healing powers dramatically reduces suffering from both acute and chronic inflammation.

Inflammation is an ancient healing response. It evolved over tens of thousands of years in a species that walked and ran every day, engaged in physical tasks, slept with the natural cycles of light and dark, breathed fresh air, drank clean water, and ate a diet of free-grazing animals, wild fish, and natural grains and plants. It shouldn't come as a big surprise that the body's inflammatory burden can be drastically reduced by regular exercise, sufficient sleep, avoidance of toxins, reduction of stress, and nutritious food.

Here I list ten ways to give the body what it needs to move through inflammation to health. The eleventh—food—is so important to that journey that it gets its own chapter. Find one or two of these suggestions that can work for you.

1 Find a Knowledgeable Practitioner

While most of what I talk about you can do on your own, a skilled practitioner is sometimes essential to help the process along. A knowledgeable practitioner can help revitalize the connective tissue web in which our muscles, organs, nerves, blood, and lymphatic vessels live so fluids can flow and tissues can glide with ease. Injured and distorted tissues must be mobilized and aligned so that they are not constantly reinjured. Sometimes the work of a skilled practitioner is needed to help the nervous system restore itself to balance, a critical step in turning off the flood of chemicals that keep inflammation burning.

2 Rest Your Injured Body

In the first days after an injury, it's critical to avoid putting additional strains on injured tissues and creating even more damage and more inflammation.

If you absolutely cannot take time off from work or other responsibilities, be sure to take frequent breaks throughout the day. If you have to stand at your job, get off your feet frequently. Lying down takes stress off injured muscles and gives them a chance to relax. If you sit for long periods at your job, get up and gently stretch every half hour or so. Standing speeds up your metabolism and circulation and helps your sleeping muscles wake up.

3 Keep Moving

Even though it's important to rest an acute injury, movement is also essential for healing. Moving decreases inflammatory chemicals and promotes restorative ones. The moving of the diaphragm and contraction of skeletal muscles pumps the lymphatic channels that clear away injury's debris. Lack of muscular activity slows down lymphatic flow and independently contributes to an enhanced inflammatory burden in the body. All that stagnation worsens inflammation. Even gentle, minimal movement is important.

One of the safest ways to activate injured muscles, fascia, and joints is in water. I often suggest my patients find a pool to move in. I tell them to strap on a flotation belt or tube and simply dangle in the water. Gravity and the buoyancy of the water will slowly elongate and stretch damaged tissues without straining them.

If people are too crippled or injured to walk, either on the ground or in water, rocking in a rocking chair can help pump the lymphatics. Back in the days when health care was much less accessible, a lot of people had rocking chairs in their homes and, unbeknownst to them, helped rock themselves toward health.

Once the tissues have been aligned and more vigorous activity is possible, put twenty minutes of moderate exercise into your schedule every day. This is particularly important for people suffering from chronic inflammation. Even this modest amount of exercise can cause dramatic and system-wide reduction of inflammatory cytokines in the body. Anything that raises your heart rate will work, such as lively walking, mowing the lawn, or even gardening.

4 Stay Hydrated

Injured tissues crave water. Tissues heal faster and hold healing treatments better when they are hydrated, whether the treatments are from osteopathic care, yoga, Pilates, or massage. Sufficient water keeps injured tissues bathed in fluids and helps drain toxins from the injury site. The lymphatics need plenty of fluid so the lymph does not turn into sludge. Even when they're healthy, the cells need a lot of water.

How much water is enough? Some nutritionists recommend drinking one-half ounce for each pound of body weight each day. If you aren't accustomed to drinking water, drink two cups as soon as you get up in the morning, and space the rest out over the day. Try drinking one cup every hour.

5 Breathe!

Slow, deep breathing moves the diaphragm, which is the main pump of the lymphatic system. Anything that helps the diaphragm helps the lymphatics. When the diaphragm is not moving well, the sluggish lymphatics leave the poor injured tissues swimming in debris.

Slow, measured breathing also helps balance the autonomic nervous system and halt the flood of inflammatory chemicals that follow injury. The restorative breathing practices in chapter 7 are a good place to start.

6 Empower Your Health with Meditation, Yoga, and Tai Chi

Stress is one of the most powerful inducers of inflammation. The body doesn't distinguish between the anxiety caused by a hostile lion and the dread caused by a hostile audience you have to give a speech to. Even the thought of a stressful situation can raise the body's levels of inflammatory chemicals.

Stress in this fast-paced world is unavoidable, but you can control how you deal with it. Creating a ten-minute oasis in your day to disengage the mind can be almost miraculous in its healing powers. Yoga has an amazing ability to soothe and quiet the mind. Just ten days of a structured yoga program, according to the research, significantly decreases the chemical markers for stress and inflammation in patients with chronic disease. Tai chi and qigong, practiced regularly, are wonderful stress relievers, lowering blood pressure and cortisol levels, improving circulation, and decreasing inflammatory markers. And the practice of mindfulness meditation—which draws the mind's attention to the regular rhythm of the breath, to physical sensations, and to fleeting mental content—actually reduces the expression of inflammation-related genes.

7 Make Time for Sleep

Healing hormones, growth factors, and anti-inflammatory chemicals are replenished and released during sleep. Sleep resets the activity of the immune system, the primary driver of inflammation. Sleep is one of the most powerful anti-inflammatory tools the body has. Seven to eight hours of sleep is critical after injury; you need even more if the brain has been injured.

Lack of quality sleep jolts the sympathetic nervous system and the immune system into action as if the body were under physical attack. If you don't get sufficient sleep the body cannot heal, no matter how much good food or exercise you get.

8 Consider Natural Products for Pain Control

Pain must be controlled, or it can etch a self-perpetuating cycle into the nervous system. If pain is a problem, I often recommend curcumin—a powerful natural anti-inflammatory. My patients have reported excellent results with curcumin, and research suggests that it helps move inflammation toward resolution without interfering with it. Recent research also suggests that aspirin, in combination with omega-3 fatty acids, can be effective for inflammation-related pain.

Vitamins A and D have powerful anti-inflammatory effects. Since inflammation also depletes stores of the B vitamins, a B vitamin complex is a good addition.

High-quality fish-oil supplements provide critical omega-3 fatty acids, the building blocks of the powerful resolvins and other inflammation-quenching chemicals. Fish-oil supplements should contain at least 600 mg of DHA and EPA. Molecularly distilled fish oil, according to Andrew Weil, MD, is naturally lower in contaminants. Choose a brand that is guaranteed free of contaminants such as heavy metals and PCBs.

I generally do not recommend nonsteroidal anti-inflammatory drugs, or NSAIDs, to my patients during an inflammatory episode, because NSAIDs interfere with lymphatic drainage and ultimately with healing. Aspirin has more respect for the lymphatics and does not so severely compromise the healthy aspects of inflammation. If pain persists, pharmaceutical painkillers may be necessary as well. Pain must be effectively addressed.

9 Keep Toxins Out of Your Life

A bout of acute inflammation is the worst time to install new carpets, paint, go shopping for garden pesticides, or try a new perfume. The immune system can treat these substances as toxins. Exposure to these inflammation-provoking substances is like throwing gasoline on a fire, piling more inflammatory chemicals into the body.

10 Empower the Lymphatics

The lymphatics love movement. With no heart to pump them, the lymphatics rely on the lively dance of the diaphragm and the contraction of the skeletal muscles to push lymphatic fluid toward the heart.

I cannot emphasize enough the importance of restoring lymphatic flow to resolving inflammation. Even if you eat right, lower your stress levels, and remove distortions from the tissues, the body cannot heal unless those nutrients can be delivered to the cells and harmful substances taken away. Impaired lymphatic function constantly shows up in chronic disease conditions.

For my acutely injured patients, I recommend moving in a slow, safe way to pump the lymphatics. If someone is bedridden, they can gently and rhythmically push with their toes against a foot-board. If they are too ill to perform that motion, a friend can push gently and rhythmically on the feet until the movement causes the head to nod up and down slightly. This is one form of the lymphatic pump technique that osteopathic physicians routinely use for hospitalized patients. Of course, this should not be performed on people with severe injuries unless approved by their physician.

> ### The Miracle Doctor of India
>
> The fourth leading cause of disability in the world is a disease called lymphatic filariasis, or elephantitis, in which a parasite disrupts the flow of lymph and causes disfiguring and disabling swelling in the affected limb. It was considered incurable until Doctor S. R. Narahari, an Indian dermatologist, developed a program combining yoga, Indian manual lymphatic drainage, compression bandaging, homeopathy, and Ayurvedic and Western medicine. The result has been an astonishing reversal of the disfiguring swelling in victims of this previously hopeless condition and a return to functionality and health.

As I mentioned earlier, rocking in a rocking chair is a wonderful way to pump the lymphatics. After injuries have healed, bouncing on a small trampoline (rebounder) for five to ten minutes a few times a day is one of the best ways to promote lymphatic flow.

Yoga poses that enhance the movement of the diaphragm and the breath help pump the lymphatic channels. Postures that open the upper chest and ribs, found in chapter 18, are very helpful in unblocking the critical lymphatic drains in the upper chest. Sun salutations are a particularly effective way of opening this important area.

Also beneficial are postures that allow gravity to drain the lymphatic channels. Any inversion pose that places the feet higher than the heart, such as Legs Up the Wall (page 65), helps the lymphatics drain from the lower extremities toward the heart. Even simple forward bends effectively use gravity to stimulate the flow of lymphatic fluid and increase the rate of drainage.

And now—on to food!

The companion DVD includes a series of yoga asanas that open the lymphatic channels and enhance lymphatic flow.

10

Food Is the Best Medicine

In 2004, documentary filmmaker Morgan Spurling set out to discover what would happen to his health if he ate all his meals at a fast food restaurant for thirty days. A medical team monitored his health.

By day five, he had gained nine pounds. By day twenty-one, his liver had started to fail. His cholesterol and triglycerides had skyrocketed. He became lethargic and depressed, and his sex drive evaporated. His doctors, alarmed at the dramatic collapse of his health, asked him to stop. He refused and went the full thirty days. By the end, he had gained thirty pounds. Even though he knew the food was poisoning him, he had become addicted to it.

Thirty years before Morgan Spurling was discovering the destructive power of food, I was discovering the immense power of food to heal. When I was in my early twenties, after repeated exposures to toxic chemicals in a poorly ventilated chemistry lab, I developed uncontrollable asthma. Unable to find help with my regular physician, I reluctantly took a friend's advice and went to an acupuncturist. I was relieved to find that the needles didn't really hurt. But her pronouncement at the end of my first visit infuriated me. She demanded I immediately give up all sweets, dairy, processed and refined foods like white flour and white rice, and all meat except chicken. I was about to leave to be a camp counselor at a camp for kids with cystic fibrosis, so I asked if I could wait until I returned. "Absolutely not!" she scolded. "If you want to be my patient, you do what I tell you. If I was a Western doctor, you'd take what I say seriously."

I didn't tell her that I'd found most doctors exceedingly unhelpful with my increasing asthma and had long ago learned not to follow orders from physicians that didn't make sense to me. However, I knew from my friend that Chinese medicine had used food as medicine for thousands of years. Since I was desperate, I decided to follow her orders. I radically changed my diet.

After two months of following her food guidelines and receiving four acupuncture treatments, my health returned and I was able to successfully complete my premed training and attend medical school. I learned from her what Western doctors are increasingly coming to realize: *food is often the best medicine.*

When I started this chapter, I was excited to share my experience with the healing power of food. However, the more I read about the drastic changes in the American diet in the last forty years, and the accompanying plague of inflammatory disease—Alzheimer's disease, heart disease, diabetes, cancer, depression, and autoimmune diseases like multiple sclerosis and rheumatoid arthritis—the more alarmed I became. There is no getting around it: inflammation lives at the end of your fork. The diet most Americans choose to eat in the twenty-first century is more like Morgan Spurling's fast-food diet. It is

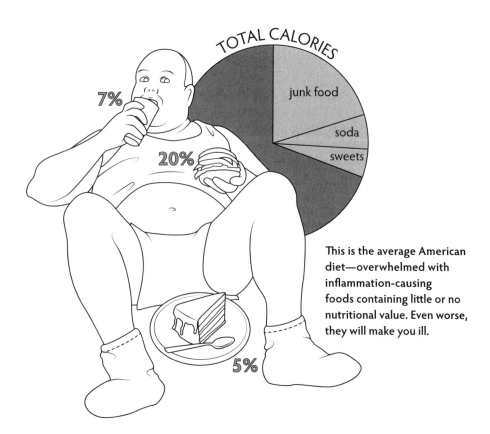

TOTAL CALORIES

7%

20%

5%

junk food

soda

sweets

This is the average American diet—overwhelmed with inflammation-causing foods containing little or no nutritional value. Even worse, they will make you ill.

poisoning us. It is inflaming us. It is killing us. Of course, it is assisted by the fact that most of us are too stressed and too sedentary to keep the lymphatics flowing vigorously enough to rid our tissues of toxins.

Injury may start the process of inflammation, but a bad diet is the gasoline that keeps it burning, spreads it everywhere, and embeds it in the tissues. The best medical care in the world will not ultimately help if every day you are feeding the inflammatory beast.

I can almost hear you groan. Diet is as deeply personal as sex and tied to just as many fierce, primitive urges. In fact, the same chemical that drives lust—dopamine—drives our food cravings. Just about everyone I know loves to eat something that is not very healthy. And for most of us, that's fine occasionally, but not every day or several times a day. I am not going to preach to you or tell you to give up everything you love. Common sense and moderation in making some dietary changes can have an immediate, profound, and positive effect on your health. I'm not going to be as dictatorial as my acupuncturist was forty years ago. Instead, I'm going to focus on three changes you can start doing today: adding healthy fats, eating healthy carbs, and consuming less sugar.

I know how hard it is to change how and what you eat when you are suffering. But pain can be the critical impetus to make necessary changes. Still, it is your choice how and when you modify your diet.

Fats: In with the Good, Out with the Bad

Fats have been unfairly targeted as the terrorists in our diet. In the 1980s, we basically regarded them like the Communist menace, dangerous and to be avoided at all costs. Some fats do belong to the evil food empire, but others are wonderfully healing and necessary.

Fats got a bad reputation because at one point, research suggested that high fat consumption caused heart attacks. That research has now been pretty well discounted. It turns out that the *type* of fat we consume has far more impact on health than the total amount of fats we eat.

We must have fats in our diet. Fats help form our hormones, are important parts of our brain, and form the membrane of our cells and the myelin covering of nerves. Without a healthy myelin sheath, nerves can't properly transmit impulses. We need healthy fats, like coconut oil, olive oil, and butter, and like the omega-3 oils in wild salmon. We need flexible fat in our cell membranes so we can let nutritive substances in and toxic substances out. A healthy diet gets at least 25 percent of its calories from fats.

Important chemical messengers that turn inflammation on and off and regulate its power are manufactured by the body from essential fatty acids. They are called essential because the body must have them to maintain health. However, the body can obtain them only from the food we eat. Foods high in omega-6 fatty acids (vegetable oils, grains, corn, factory-raised poultry, fish, and meat) tend to encourage the body to produce pro-inflammatory chemicals. Foods high in omega-3 fatty acids (cold-water fish, olive oil, walnuts, pasture-raised meat and poultry) tend to encourage the body to produce anti-inflammatory and resolving chemicals. Human beings must have both omega-6 and omega-3 fatty acids, ideally in equal proportions. A hundred years ago, the ratio of omega-6 to omega-3 fatty acids in the American diet was approximately 2 to 1. Now the pro-inflammatory omega-6 foods crush the anti-inflammatory omega-3s by a factor of 20 to 1 and sometimes even 50 to 1. The typical American diet is so overweighted with pro-inflammatory fats that when inflammation comes looking for fuel, it finds an overflowing abundance. The anti-inflammatory compounds, by comparison, are being starved.

Before I talk about the terrible things the imperialistic fats do to damage you, I need to praise the wonderfully healthy fats. Butter, especially from grass-fed cows or goats (goats are almost always grass-fed), is a great source of vitamin A and very good for you. Butter is wonderful to bake with and when added to vegetables helps the body absorb the vegetables' many nutrients and make them tastier. In fact, any healthy fat, such as ghee, olive oil, or coconut oil added to vegetables, promotes absorption of their great nutrients. Since some people are allergic to milk products, I champion coconut oil and coconut butter.

Certain fats are best at room temperature, like olive oil or butter. Others, such as coconut or avocado oil, tolerate heat much better, so it's better to use them for stir-frying or high-heat cooking.

While I'm on the subject of fats, meat has also gotten a bad rap. That's because most factory-raised beef, poultry, and fish (factory fish are fed a diet of grains, corn, soy, and other inflammatory foods) have a higher ratio of inflammatory omega-6 fats to anti-inflammatory omega-3 fats. Since cows are not able to digest corn and grains well, eating them tends to inflame their guts and may make them sick. Farmers then give them antibiotics to counter the bacterial infections caused by the corn and grains.

Pasture-raised, grass-fed beef, buffalo, and goat are totally different. They have a much better balance of omega-6 to omega-3 fats, and they are a much healthier source of protein. Free-range chicken is also much healthier than factory-raised chicken. Wild fish, particularly cold-water fish such as salmon and cod, are very high in inflammation-fighting omega-3 fats, unlike their farmed cousins, which are as inflammatory as factory-raised beef. Yes, these products are more expensive, but a little bit goes a long way. And they taste so much better. You'll be getting more healthy nutrients from them and will need to eat less and be less hungry. In the long run, you'll probably save money on food and medical care.

Now that I've talked about the more luscious choices, I'll explain why trans fats (hydrogenated fats) are so poisonous. Heating makes them even worse. Deep-fried doughnuts, chips, French fries, and chicken cooked in hydrogenated oils should no more be called food than the mercury and arsenic used by doctors in the 1800s should have been called medicine.

Partially hydrogenated fats or trans fats. These fats, such as margarine, are chemically manufactured by adding solvents and hydrogen to liquid vegetable oils so they become solid at room temperature. Trans fats are so toxic that some cities have banned restaurants from using them. Trans fats damage blood vessels and are highly inflammatory. They interfere with the body's use of anti-inflammatory omega-3 fatty acids, create insulin resistance, decrease testosterone, and dramatically increase the risk of heart disease, obesity, and diabetes.

If that wasn't bad enough, trans fats are hard, inflexible, jealous fats. When they join the cell membrane, they disrupt transport of nutrients and other substances necessary for health in and out of cells. They resist healthy

Hidden Sources of Trans Fats

- Commercial bread and rolls
- Chips, crackers, and snack foods
- Artificial cheese products
- Sauces
- Commercial salad dressings, mayonnaise, and condiments
- Fried foods
- Foods sold in the middle aisles of the grocery store
- Restaurant food and takeout
- Doughnuts, cake, and cookies

fats' attempts to knock them from their kingdom. To keep their position of power, trans fats inhibit the enzymes the body makes to incorporate good fats into our cells. Like a tyrant, they throw the good fats into the garbage so they can continue to rule. From their jealous control of our membranes, they continuously throw gasoline onto the fires of inflammation. When they join the membranes of nerves, which they like to do, they make the membranes brittle. A person whose diet is brimming with trans fats may be exposing their nervous system, including their brain, to greater risk of injury in a trauma.

The vast majority of the trans fats in your diet do not come from the stick of margarine in your refrigerator. Like the vegetable oils they are made from, they are hidden in the shortening used to make deep-fried food, in restaurant foods, commercial baked goods, cereals, and processed foods. How can you tell? The ingredient label will include "partially hydrogenated" in its list. Items that say they have zero grams trans fats can still contain them, so read the ingredient list. If hydrogenated oil or vegetable shortening is included, don't buy it. If you have foods in your cupboard with hydrogenated fats, throw them out.

Polyunsaturated vegetable oils (canola, cottonseed, soybean, peanut, safflower, corn, and sunflower oils), used in many restaurants and processed foods, are high in inflammation-fueling omega-6 fatty acids. Vegetable oils were touted for many years for their "heart healthy" properties, but they are in fact one of the prime offenders in heart disease and inflammation. Practically every processed food contains at least one of them. Like trans fats, these oils are hidden in processed foods, fried foods, and restaurant food. People are also doused with them indirectly when they eat meat and poultry raised on corn and soybeans. Virtually unknown a hundred years ago, they now make up 30 percent of our calories, and along with them has come the dramatic rise in inflammation-based chronic disease.

Stop Eating Inflammatory Carbohydrates

The calories in the American diet primarily come from carbs, mostly consisting of rice and things made from flour—pasta, bread, buns, crackers, cookies, pastries, bagels, and such. Most of these foods are made from white rice and white flour, which are created by processing all the natural goodness out of the whole grain. These low-quality fuels are stripped of most of their natural mineral, fiber, and vitamin content. Calories from denatured carbs with little nutrition left in them frustrate and annoy the body. The body craves vitamins, minerals, and fiber so it can go about its business of healing your injuries and helping you feel energetic and wonderful.

The nutritional emptiness of these foods is just one problem. These carbs are simple carbohydrates—meaning that when you eat them, the body rapidly turns them into glucose. The sudden rise in glucose causes a rapid increase in insulin production. Excess insulin is a main provocateur of inflammatory chemicals in the body.

Since insulin is so important for regulating inflammation, let's look at it for a moment. Insulin is a hormone produced by the pancreas. Insulin regulates how the body deals with its main fuel: glucose. Insulin is the key that unlocks the doors of the cells so that glucose can enter and be stored for fuel. When glucose levels go up in the blood, the pancreas releases more insulin so

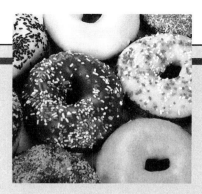

The Truth About Fats

Here's my advice: Stay away from fried foods and processed foods. In your own cooking, substitute good oils like olive oil, avocado oil, and coconut oil for these inflammation-producing products. The occasional use of safflower, peanut, sunflower, or sesame oil for your stir-fry is fine as long as you are vigilant about the other, hidden sources of these fats. Try to choose ones that are from organically grown seed and made without harsh chemical solvents.

Corn, soy, cotton, and canola oil are commonly made from genetically modified plants. Over tens of thousands of years, we have developed the enzymes to digest traditional foods. Genetically modified foods seem to have structures that our guts cannot readily identify, break down, and appropriately use. I also believe that genetically modified orgnisms (GMOs) can cause inflammation in the gut, which can lead to "leaky gut" syndrome, a situation where foreign products get into the lymphatic and blood channels and cause systemic inflammation and pain. In the course of my more than thirty years of practice, I have come to believe that many of my patients' guts, especially those of children, have become inflamed by the newly created chemicals of GMOs. Unfortunately, there is no way to know whether a product contains GMOs. Unless it's otherwise labeled, assume that it does.

the cells can take up more glucose. If there is more glucose in the blood than the cells can take up, the liver helps out. The liver grabs up the extra glucose and stores it in fat cells. Fat cells are like little inflammation factories, spewing forth inflammatory chemicals. If this keeps up too long, as in Morgan Spurling's case, the person can end up with a fatty liver, a dangerous situation for this important organ.

Some things like high-fructose corn syrup, cortisol, and too much insulin lock the doors of the cells, causing something called insulin resistance. These stubborn insulin-resistant cells refuse to let the insulin unlock their doors to let in glucose. The fearful pancreas releases even more insulin, trying to unlock the doors, which causes yet more inflammation. The excess glucose roaming around in the blood desperately knocks at the door of the liver. The generous liver takes in the wayward glucose and turns it into fat, and more inflammation results. If someone keeps eating foods day after day that keep their insulin levels too high, the poor pancreas eventually will wear itself out trying to produce all that extra insulin. Type 2 diabetes can be the result.

Each carbohydrate has its own rate that it turns into glucose, which is called the carb's glycemic index, or glycemic load. Certain carbs cause the worst glucose spikes. Simple carbs such as white flour impose a large glycemic load on the insulin system.

To help get inflammation under control, I recommend replacing low-grade carbs with better ones. Brown rice is better than white rice. Products made with whole grains are healthier than ones made from white flour. Notice I said whole grains, not just whole wheat. Whole wheat is usually white flour with a tan. Look for breads made from stone-ground wheat, which keeps the goodness of the grain intact.

While some whole grains still pack a pretty hefty glycemic punch, overall they are better for you than the empty carbs that plague the American diet. There is evidence that despite their relatively high glycemic load, whole grains help control insulin production. When it comes to these insulin spikes, less is better.

Cut Back on Sugary Desserts

Alas, sugar—table sugar, sucrose, dextrose, and maltose—is highly inflammatory for the same reason that denatured carbs are. Table sugar, being half glucose, causes insulin levels to go up, which provokes inflammation. Foods rich in sugar can be so seductive, delicious, and addictive that even the best of us are willing to trade a little bit of ill health for the comfort they give us. But don't be fooled by the boost of energy sugar gives you—it's fool's gold.

If you are addicted to sugary treats, try the advice I gave my daughter. She was hooked on her daily chocolate. I told her not to give it up entirely. I suggested she eat half of her treat in the afternoon and half in the evening and then slowly move toward eating only the half after lunch. I also told her it was very important to take some good-quality supplements like chromium, zinc, and a multiple B-vitamin, to replace the nutrients that sugar was using up. These nutrients are important in glucose regulation. She found that taking the supplements hugely decreased her sugar cravings, and instead of becoming a daily indulgence, it became a special occasion treat that she looked forward to.

Although sugar is not great for you, I vastly prefer foods made with sugar to those containing high-fructose corn syrup (HFCS). This is a source of great contention among nutritionists. My own view, after reviewing the research, is that HFCS is much more damaging to the body than sugar. Not only is it massively inflammatory in its own right, but compared to ordinary table sugar it increases belly fat and raises the risk of liver disease and insulin resistance, which are independent risk factors for inflammation. Soft drinks are full of the stuff.

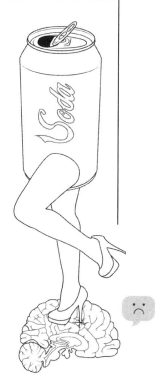

Toxic food like deep-fried food, trans fats, and high-fructose corn syrup stomp on you with stiletto heels before sending you to your grave.

Many breakfast cereals, condiments like ketchup, and commercial sweets have HFCS as well. The average American consumes sixty-two pounds of this toxic substance every year. Because consumers are realizing how dangerous HFCS is, the food industry has decided to rename it corn sugar. But corn sugar is HFCS by another name. Read the labels. Try to avoid the stuff, particularly in beverages. That comes next.

Cut Back on Sweetened Drinks and Sodas

Soda and sugary drinks get their very own section because Americans drink so much of this zero-quality fuel. There is something so refreshing about drinking a cold soda on a hot day. But there's nothing charming about drinking two gigantic sodas every day, at least if you value your health.

Soda is basically high-fructose corn syrup, water, and flavoring, so you might as well be drinking liquid inflammation. In 2004, soda made up 7 percent of the typical American's calories. Now it's the single biggest daily source of calories for Americans, and over 16 percent of daily calories for teenagers. Besides being inflammatory, soda is linked to osteoporosis (particularly in teenage girls), high blood pressure, diabetes, high cholesterol, and coronary heart disease.

Diet sodas don't get off the hook, either. Studies show they are just as inflammatory, put you at additional risk for developing diabetes, and are bad for your kidneys. The mold inhibitors in diet soda can damage your DNA and cause allergic reactions such as asthma and hives. If you're drinking diet soda to lose or maintain weight, forget it. For a number of reasons, diet soda actually makes you gain weight. You're better off drinking sweetened soda.

Let me tell you how Al got off his addiction to cola. Al knew the large bottle of soda he drank every day was really bad for him, but it gave him energy, and he was addicted. I advised him to do a few things. First, I told him to switch to cola made with sugar. Costco, some beverage stores, and some health food stores sell colas made with sugar. Then, I suggested that every time he opened a bottle of soda, he pour four ounces into a glass and toss it down the sink. Every time he drank a soda, he agreed to drink two large glasses of water along with it. Last, I told him to take supplements containing chromium, zinc, and B-vitamins to help reduce the sugar cravings.

Very gradually, Al got his soda down to every other day, then every three days. Eventually, he really looked forward to his twice-a-week soda. After about nine months, he didn't like the taste of it anymore and was able to stop.

Learn Which Foods Are Right for You

Some foods, like trans fats and high-fructose corn syrup, are bad for everyone. Then there are foods that may be fine for me but bad for someone else. Some perfectly wonderful, highly nutritious foods can inflame a person and make them feel awful if that person happens to be allergic to them. In fact, that's what an allergic reaction is: an inflammatory reaction to food the body doesn't like.

The flood of conflicting advice about what foods to eat is overwhelming. I think that sometimes when health-seeking people at last discover the foods that were making them sick, they are so overjoyed that they turn their discovery into a dogma for everyone else. A friend of mine became so confused at all the conflicting information about the best diet that she made a chart. The chart revealed that a food one diet claims is essential for health, another diet insists is equivalent to poison.

Take orange juice. "Wonderful," says one diet. "High in vitamin C. Much better than soda." "Terrible for your pancreas—too sweet," says another. "Only drink orange juice squeezed from the whole fruit," says a third. "Stop drinking juice. Eat the whole fruit instead," says a fourth. "Eat only organic oranges," a fifth says. "Eat only locally grown organic oranges in season," says a sixth. "Never eat raw fruit, heat it up first," says a seventh. And finally, "Citrus fruits cause arthritis—don't eat oranges at all," says number eight.

"Just forget it," says my friend. "The only thing you can safely eat is organic dirt."

Each of those conflicting pieces of advice has a kernel of truth for different people, but turning a helpful suggestion into a rule makes most people give up looking at their diet altogether. Switching from drinking soda to drinking orange juice would be a great first step in changing an unhealthy eating habit. For other people, orange juice is too sweet. Oranges are a great food for some people. Other people are allergic to citrus fruits. We are all different.

How do you get beyond the dogma and figure out what's right for you? Here are a few suggestions:

Look at your genetic heritage and see what foods your original culture used. For example, many Asian, Mediterranean, and African people don't tolerate dairy products from cows. It's the Northern Europeans—the Swedes, British, Irish, and Germans—who usually have the best enzymes to absorb cow's milk.

Eat Right For Your Type. This book discusses the effects of genetic heritage on our ability to absorb nutrients. I found that with my blood type O, I do better with meat, walnuts, figs, and blackberries, and I crave them. Scientists have learned that different genes turn on and off throughout our lives. Trauma and other factors influence this process. I hated dairy until I was fifty, and ate very little. This dislike probably reflected the influence of my mother's Jewish genes. Jews, like most Mediterranean folks, usually don't digest cow dairy well. Then, at fifty, I suddenly liked dairy and it started agreeing with me. Did my new delight in dairy come from decades of avoiding it? Or had my mother's Jewish genes turned off and my father's Swedish genes turned on, allowing me to better digest diary? I don't know. Since many of us are a mixture of races, it can take trial and error to figure out how our heritage affects us at different times of our lives.

Blood type eating should not become another dogma, for we are much more complicated than our blood type. Despite their blood types, people can have or develop food allergies; food sensitivities to wheat, eggs, gluten, tomatoes, corn, soy, peanuts, and shellfish are some of the most common. I suspect that when we eat a genetically modified product, the toxicity created by the GMO causes our gut to become sensitized to other foods we consume along with the GMO product. As with all my recommendations, listen to your body. Once you get used to listening to your body's prompts, you will be wiser than any dogma.

Individual allergies to individual products should be diagnosed and addressed. There are blood tests that can diagnose quite a few but not all food allergies. If you suspect serious food allergies, an elimination diet is the most accurate way to assess your situation.

THE HEALING-FROM-INJURY DIET

Let's remember why you picked up this book. You're in pain and/or have been injured. Your injured cells are crying out in pain and need healing nutrients. It's not my intention to set out a list of dietary rules that take all the pleasure out of eating and make mealtime a burden and a chore. I'll simply suggest some guidelines to follow as you eat your way back to health:

Add lots of fresh vegetables and fruits in a rainbow of colors to your diet. Your mom was right: eating fruits and vegetables is a recipe for health. They are powerhouses of the vitamins that quench inflammation, the minerals that help repair damaged tissues, and the antioxidants that protect us from free radicals. Science is just beginning to discover how these foods heal, but you don't have to wait. We know already that fruits and vegetables heal and protect against the ravages of inflammation.

Different colors have different concentrations of nutrients; generally, the darker the color, the more power-packed they are. Blues, reds, and purples contain antioxidant anthocyanins. White, orange, and yellow fruits and vegetables also have antioxidants, minerals, and vitamin A and C, and green fruits and vegetables are inflammation fighters. My advice: eat the rainbow.

Cook with adventure! Nature has provided a cornucopia of inflammation fighters in the form of herbs and spices. Spice up your cooking with these flavorful and delightful additions to health. Spices and herbs gently impact a broader range of inflammatory compounds than pharmaceuticals and, instead of simply suppressing symptoms, they create health—and make food delicious.

Turmeric, garlic, and ginger—all wonderful in chicken and vegetable dishes—have well-studied anti-inflammatory properties. Curcumin, the yellow pigment in turmeric, vigorously nudges inflammation towards resolution without disrupting or short-circuiting the inflammatory process. Cinnamon, a staple of cooking in the Far East, has particularly potent anti-inflammatory effects in the gut. Oregano, bay leaves, ground cloves, chili peppers, rosemary, thyme, and sage have joined the list of spices that quench inflammation's fires.

Sources of Omega-6 and Omega-3 Rich Foods

Omega-6 Rich Foods	Omega-3 Rich Foods
• Canola, cottonseed, soybean, peanut, safflower, corn, and sunflower oils • Hydrogenated oils • Foods fried in the above oils • Mayonnaise and dressings made with the above oils	• Extra-virgin olive oil • Avocado oil • Coconut oil
• Factory-farmed chicken	• Organically raised free-range chicken
• Farmed fish	• HIGH | Wild cold-water fish: wild salmon, anchovies, cod, whitefish, pacific sardine, bluefin tuna, Atlantic herring, mackerel, rainbow trout • MODERATE | Mussels, wild eastern oyster, halibut, pollock, crab, shrimp, scallops
• Grain-fed beef	• Pasture-raised beef
• Turkey • Pork	• Goat
• Eggs	• Omega-3-enriched eggs
• Most nuts and seeds	• Walnuts • Flax seeds
• Corn • Grains (wheat, rice)	• Black beans, kidney beans • Wild rice
• Processed foods (pastries, chips, cookies, and doughnuts)	• Leafy green vegetables

Battered bones and joints need minerals. Fruits and vegetables are full of minerals. If your digestion is "off," I recommend partially cooked fruit and vegetables. I've found most of my ill and injured patients do better with cooked vegetables and slightly warmed fruit than with raw foods. Nutritive soups, such as turkey or chicken soup made with the bones, can be very nourishing. Lots of healthy minerals can be gained by using bone broths in cooking.

If you've just been injured, add protein. A lot of it! Injury damages the structures of your body made out of protein—like muscles and joints. Pour in the protein to rebuild damaged tissue. Eating fish, buffalo, lamb, and grass-fed beef and goat are the easiest way for most people to absorb protein. Meat has iron and complete essential amino acids. Chicken, turkey, and fish help provide protein, but not as much as the red meats. You need a lot of amino acids to rebuild all the damaged tissues. If you don't eat meat, you'll have to work extra hard to incorporate other sources of protein.

Eat healthy fats. The omega-3 oils in our diet are probably the most powerful ingredient of the healing-from-injury diet. Omega-3s are the building blocks of the resolvins, protectins, and maresins that actively orchestrate the end of inflammation. Omega-3s can reverse the progression of such inflammatory conditions as lupus, multiple sclerosis, childhood asthma, and inflammatory bowel disease. Adding omega-3s to your anti-inflammatory diet is a must to achieve optimum health.

At least 25 percent of our calories should come from healthy fats like coconut oil, olive oil, butter, and nuts and seeds. We need a balance of pro-inflammatory omega-6 and anti-inflammatory omega-3 rich foods in our diet, ideally in a ratio of 1 to 1.

Eat fermented foods like yogurt or sauerkraut or drinks like kombucha to help heal the injured gut, promote good digestion, and help get more nutrients to the injured parts of your body. Often, if a patient becomes allergic to just about every food after an injury, the problem is an inflamed, unhappy gut and not the food.

Drink water—eight to ten glasses of purified or filtered fluid per day. Water helps the lymphatics flush out toxic debris, hydrates injured tissues, and keeps spinal discs happy. If you have kidney problems, speak to your physician first.

Add probiotics and digestive enzymes to your meals to help your gut absorb nutrients. Probiotics are probably the primary supplement that helps your gut heal and combat inflammation. Many nutritionists recommend daily probiotics for anyone battling inflammation as well as for anyone over forty. Many of us have lost critical protective bacteria in our gut and therefore need regular supplementation, especially those who have had several courses of antibiotics. Luckily, there are good probiotics that don't have to be refrigerated. I recommend switching brands regularly so as not to overpopulate one strain of probiotic over others.

Use a green powder like spirulina or chlorella, which provide a lot of nutrition, if you were recently injured or are fighting chronic inflammation. Mix them up with water or chew the tablets. One of my patients told me these powerful green products taste little better than dirt, so she doesn't eat them. Luckily, she likes lots of leafy green vegetables, so she's keeping her body happy with other greens. I like the taste of spirulina and am not as virtuous about leafy vegetables. See if you can find a green food you like.

It goes without saying that you should *cut down on or eliminate the inflammatory foods* I talked about in the beginning of the chapter: foods made with trans fats and vegetable oils, excess sugar, empty carbs, and soda.

Avoid alcohol. I recommend that, after trauma, you temporarily avoid drinking alcohol. The liver has to work pretty hard to break alcohol down, and you want it to focus its attention on detoxifying the by-products of injury and producing the nutrients necessary for health. Furthermore, alcohol is hard on neurological tissue. With any kind of neurological or brain injury, including almost all car crashes, alcohol should be avoided for several weeks or months. I am not an alcohol purist. I enjoy an occasional margarita or Rob Roy, but after my minor rear-end collision, I avoided both.

How to Eat

Graze. Eating a little bit of food frequently is easier on your body than gulping down a mammoth meal. Grazing helps you absorb critical healing nutrients. Overeating can cause inflammation as more stuff goes into the gut than the body can safely process.

Eat in a relaxed fashion, with your nervous system as calm as possible. You don't want to fuel up your sympathetic nervous system and suppress your nutritive, parasympathetic nervous system. Sit down at home or in a restaurant, not in your car! Eat slowly, without distractions. You'll absorb a lot more nutrients that way. Think of yourself as being Italian—or any nationality that exuberantly cherishes eating.

Chew well. Digestion begins in the mouth. You need your powerful teeth to crush up the fabric of food and thoroughly mix it with the digestive chemicals lacing your saliva. After an accident slams your body, your liver and pancreas may not be able to produce the full array of enzymes necessary to help you absorb your food. Help your gut by doing your share of mouth work. If I'm alone, I eat slower and chew longer if I listen to music or read. See what works for you.

Since we have been discussing a very personal part of your life, you are probably feeling annoyed about the task ahead of you. That's understandable. I know absorbing all these dos and don'ts seems like a lot, especially when, after an injury or living with chronic pain, you feel like a refugee from your own body. Unless you are extremely ill, you are usually better off if you make these changes gradually. Gradual change is both psychologically and practically easier. Do what you can. You are in charge, and if you follow even some of these guidelines, you will reap amazing rewards. As you make these changes and begin feeling better, you'll be inspired to make more changes. Since eating nutritious, organic food is more satisfying, you'll find you'll need less of it, will feel less hungry, and, if you're carrying extra weight, will usually lose weight without effort. When we don't eat nourishing foods, our cells call out with hunger, hoping that we'll provide them with missing nutrients. We end up consuming lots of only slightly nourishing foods in our desperate search for the right nutrients, getting fatter in the process.

You will also find that as you eat healthier foods, healthy foods start to taste more delicious and damaging substances start to taste awful. Eating becomes yet another place where awareness and follow-through reap tremendous benefits.

Be of cheer. Eating should be a joyous event, and a little bit of attention to it often provides thrilling benefits.

III.

Restore Motion, Restore Health

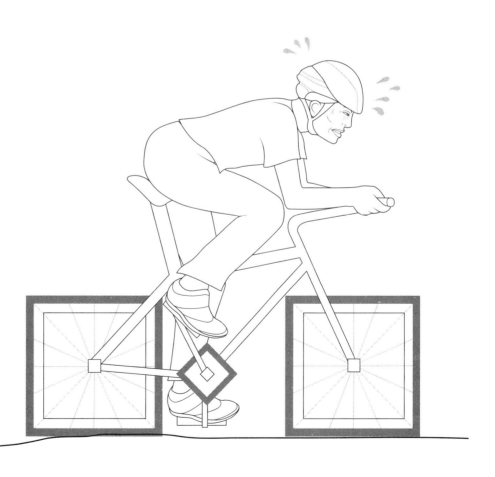

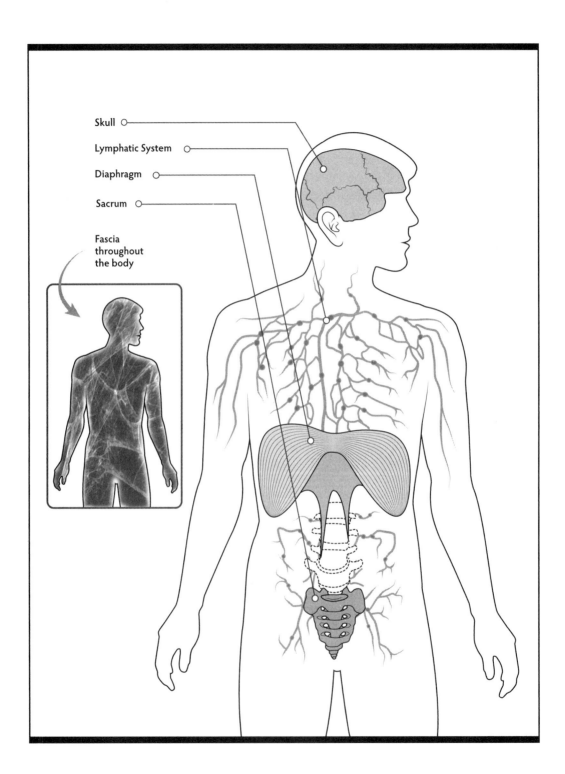

Skull

Lymphatic System

Diaphragm

Sacrum

Fascia throughout the body

11

The Five Unsung Heroes of Health

Life is motion. Every fluid, every cell, every organ, joint, and bone moves, pulsates, or ebbs and flows. These fierce rhythmic motions heal us, but sometimes they need help. That's why, in order to fully revitalize a person healing from trauma, motion must be restored to stagnant and restricted tissues.

We know that the heart must beat fully and the lungs expand freely for vibrant health. But the free motion of other organs is also crucial. The gut must pulsate as it removes nutrients from the bowel and funnels the goodies into the blood. The liver must rock to turn nutrients into hormones as it processes toxins to make them less poisonous. And the most essential organ of all, the brain, must beat six to fourteen times a minute, enlivening the whole nervous system.

Just as essential for health are the waves of fluid that permeate the body. These include the free flow of cerebral spinal fluid within the spinal cord and brain, the flow of blood and lymphatic fluid throughout their respective circulatory systems, and the other currents that surge through all cells.

In my many years of practice, I have come to realize that trauma can compromise any of these motions. Restoring motion, both simple and profound, is the third essential component of healing from trauma.

Given the body's vast interconnectedness, a problem in one part or system of the body can have distant repercussions. A twisted ankle can result in headaches and menstrual cramps as the body twists and turns to compensate for the injured joint. An area whose tissues are compressed can become a monkey wrench in the body's complex mechanics, causing the body to scream with pain at a point quite distant from the primary injury.

This section describes ways to answer the body's many calls for help. Although the parts of the body always operate together in a kinetic chain of motion, restrictions in certain areas have more dire consequences. There are five critical areas that, being heroes when they move vibrantly, tend to be the biggest culprits of ill health when they don't. I call them the five unsung heroes of health.

When I treat, I pay special attention to these five structural elements: the diaphragm, the lymphatic system, the sacrum, the fascia, and the skull. Most practitioners tend to focus on the more immediate symptoms of trauma and overlook these heroes. But I have found that when these often-ignored heroes are treated, healing proceeds much more quickly.

THE DIAPHRAGM: Affecting Every System in the Body

I've already introduced the first hero, the diaphragm. In the chapter on the breath, I highlighted the diaphragm's critical role in breathing and calming an agitated nervous system. In the section on inflammation, I celebrated its role in pumping the vital lymphatic system. Because the diaphragm connects to so many systems and organs, it is one of the most important keys to both health and recovery from injury and illness. Without a fully functioning diaphragm, you can suffer from constipation, reflux (GERD) and other digestive problems, high blood pressure, heart disease, asthma, bronchitis and other breathing problems, fibromyalgia, depression, anxiety, infections, fatigue, neck and back pain, and problems with healing.

How does one muscle manage to be so important? The mighty diaphragm is not only anchored to the rib cage, breastbone, and spine. Its fibers also fan out to the heart above and the liver below and weave into the beginning of the stomach. Openings in the diaphragm allow passage to the esophagus, the great vessels of the heart, and the miraculous lymphatic channels. When the diaphragm is working well, every contraction moves the rib cage, tractions the low back, massages the liver and adrenal glands, keeps stomach acid contained, helps pump the blood, circulates the lymphatic fluid, assists fluid flow into and out of cells, and moves the other systems to which it is so intimately connected. Throughout the book, I talk about the diaphragm and its crucial role in health.

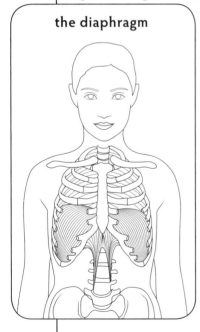

the diaphragm

THE LYMPHATIC SYSTEM:
The Key to Controlling Inflammation

In the section on inflammation, I showed how the second unsung hero, the lymphatic system, creates the body's immune channels and toxin-removal system, which is key to controlling inflammation (see chapter 8). In the section on brain injury, we'll see how the brain's system for clearing toxins, including the potentially damaging proteins that cause Alzheimer's disease, is intimately tied to the lymphatic system.

Like so much of the body, the lymphatics depend on the heroic diaphragm to flow freely. Restricting the movement of the lymphatics can lead to inflammation, pain, infection, and ill health.

THE SACRUM: Foundation of the Body

The third unsung hero, the sacrum, is a complex of bone at the end of the spinal column. The sacrum is in charge of everything from reproduction to digestion. It supports the pelvis and upper body and rocks in rhythm with the pulsations of the brain. It moves even more when we walk as it distributes the forces generated by our movement. It pumps the spinal discs and lumbar fascia, preserves the health of the spine, and keeps the low back free of pain.

Since nerves to the sex organs come through the sacrum, a restricted sacrum can cause problems with fertility, erections, and menstruation. The central nervous system ends in front of the coccyx bone at the tip of the sacrum. Since the sacrum is connected to the brain by the dural membrane, free sacral mobility is essential for neurological health. Injury to the sacrum can cause everything from headaches and sexual dysfunction to low-back pain and lumbar-disc herniations. Restore the sacrum to its proper position, and *voila!*—your life has lovely juice again.

I talk about the sacrum in the chapters on the back, the pelvis, and sexual healing.

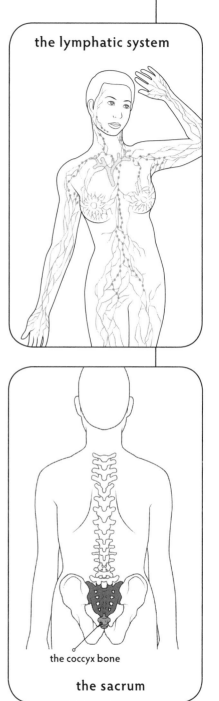

the lymphatic system

the coccyx bone

the sacrum

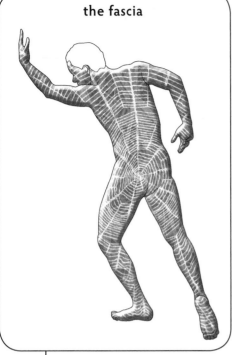

the fascia

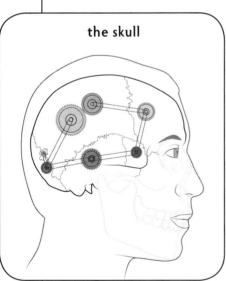

the skull

THE FASCIA: Making the Free Motion of the Body Possible

Moist fascia unites the body as it falls like a living curtain from the skull. Like the Russian dolls that fit inside each other, fascia creates three progressively smaller layers throughout the body. Living, pulsating fascia is part of the body's vibrant paradise, which constantly and rhythmically tries to restore motion to tissues and reinvigorate fluid flow restricted by injury and disease. Like a living spider web, the fascia embraces every nerve, muscle fiber, blood and lymphatic vessel, tethers the organs to their homes, and enables the very movement of life itself. Our fourth unsung hero is in fact the dominant internal structure of the body.

When the fascia becomes twisted or tightened, it can cause significant problems in any of the systems it entwines. It becomes a dam holding back needed fluid flow. It can be a culprit in everything from pericarditis (swelling around the heart) to low-back pain. I talk more about fascia and its critical role in the chapters on the back and chest.

THE SKULL: Orchestrating the Healing Response

The fifth unsung hero, the skull, is composed of twenty-two bones that minutely flex at joints called sutures, allowing for the expansion and contraction of the brain. The intricate and subtle motion of the cranial bones is critical for everything from accurate vision to brain health.

I think of the skull like a three-dimensional Swiss watch with intricately interconnecting gears. As with any complex mechanism, a glitch in one area can cause profound consequences elsewhere. A blow to the face, for example, can compress the facial sinuses and stop their effective discharge of fluid, causing terrible sinusitis.

A fall on the back of the head can jam the occipito-mastoid suture in the back, causing ear infections, digestive problems, vision disturbance, headaches, and vertigo. A blow to the head can cause problems with thinking, memory, and mood and impede critical fluid flow in and out of the brain. It can damage the delicate pituitary gland, resulting in weight gain and loss, menstrual problems, hormonal disruption, and depression.

Because of the complexity and profound effects of head injury, I devote five chapters to head and brain injury and to the nervous system's role in pain.

Freeing the Body's Fluid Waves

Fluid waves bathe the cells and ensure that every bit of the body is immersed in rhythmic, pulsating flows. The heart beats fifty to eighty times a minute, sending pulsations of blood through the body. The brain beats six to fourteen times a minute, sending surges of cerebral spinal fluid throughout the nervous system. Scientists in Russia have documented a slower wave that courses through the body approximately three times a minute. These rhythms keep all tissues and cells in motion.

Medicine often thinks of the body as the atomized parts depicted in the illustrations of anatomy books. Yet the living body is more like a Fred Astaire movie, perpetually in an interconnected, interrelated dance. Practitioners trained in manual medicine feel this living, pulsating quality of the tissues as well as each kind of fluid flow. We can then distinguish areas where these flows hit a wall of restriction. One of our main jobs is to gently remove these restrictions so that fluid flows easily and fully throughout the body.

I suspect that my childhood spent bodysurfing in the Atlantic Ocean

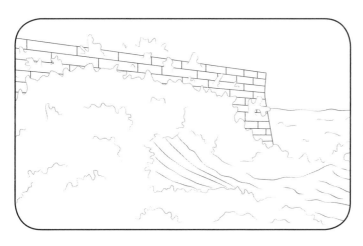

Practitioners of manual medicine can feel the body's complex fluid waves. They gently remove restrictions so the fluid flows more easily and fully throughout the body.

waves helped me develop the sensitivity to feel the currents in the human body. Interestingly enough, just as the planet's surface is 70 percent fluid, so, too, are our bodies. But even people without a feel for the ocean's currents can learn to feel these rhythms and learn to sense impediments to motion and remove them.

In this section and the next, I will talk about how restoring motion to the spine, pelvis, chest, skull, and brain promotes health on every level. Although I break up the body into distinct parts, never forget that the body is a dynamic unit. The real source of your suffering may come from far away and from a seemingly unrelated injury.

Some problems you'll be able to fix yourself with the information I give you. Other times you'll need the help of a trained practitioner. But once you make sense of what's really wrong, you'll have a much better idea of how to help your anatomy regain its natural motion. Reclaim your living, moving anatomy and recreate your destiny!

12

Healing Back Pain

The human spine is ingeniously engineered to hold us upright as we move through the world. From its origin in the neck to its foundation in the sacrum, the spine undulates like a Slinky toy to dissipate the forces created by our movement. The spine achieves flexibility through its brilliant anatomy of shock-absorbing curves, cushioning discs, and precisely angled joints. Yet we are neither a snake nor a worm, and the upright spine also has the seemingly impossible task of

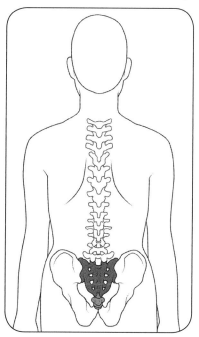

being strong and stable so we can lift a box, run a marathon, or fend off a tackle in a football game. To achieve strength and stability, the spine's powerful muscles, thick fascia, and ligaments lash it to the foundation of the sacrum and the rest of the pelvis.

The sacrum is a wedged-shaped triangular bone at the end of the spine that receives the weight of the upper body and distributes it to the pelvis and powerful lower extremities. In essence, the sacrum is the keystone of the body as it wedges itself into the pelvis and provides a supportive system for everything above and below it. For the spine and back to be pain-free, the sacrum must sit balanced in its pelvic home, joined at the optimum angle with the spine on top of it, and rocking gently back and forth with the undulations of the spine. When the sacrum is unbalanced or out of alignment, the spine above it suffers.

The marriage of the sacrum and lumbar spine is indeed a troubled one. When their union falters, low-back pain erupts. Despite all the powerful ligaments, muscles, and fascia working to steady it, the lumbar spine's attachment to the sacrum tends to be an unstable structure. Why is this? Lucy made it so. Not Lucille Ball, but a distant relative in Africa, the original Lucy. Three million years ago when Lucy stood up and walked, she changed human history. This regal posture freed up Lucy's hands—and eventually our hands—to play the flute, catch a basketball, or toss a stone. Since the brain devotes so many billions of neurons to moving the hands and fingers, scientists believe that once the upright pelvis freed the hands from being feet, our fingers' complex motions forced our brains to grow into their mammoth size.

However, being forced to walk on two feet instead of four put many more demands on the place where the spine and the sacrum meet. Instead of being supported like a tabletop on four legs, the upright spine had to balance on two. The sacrum had to change its position to be in just the right spot for the lower lumbar vertebrae to link snuggly to it. That makes us much more vulnerable to low-back pain than our four-footed friends. The angle where the upright spine and the sacrum meet has relatively little margin for error. Tip it forward or backward too much, and back pain explodes.

And if any of the elements that maintain this structure falter—bones, muscles, fascia, ligaments, or discs—that, too, can create back pain. All these structures must work together as a team, one for all and all for one. Like a team of gymnasts balanced in a moving pyramid upon one another, when one locks up all can falter or fall. Let's meet this amazing team of synchronized athletes.

BUILDING BLOCKS OF THE SPINE

The Vertabrae. The spinal column is made up of bony rings called vertebrae, which are stacked on top of each other like cleverly balanced blocks. There are seven vertebrae in the cervical region, twelve in the chest, or thoracic, region, and five in the lumbar, or low back.

The vertebrae are set at subtle angles that together create a graceful set of

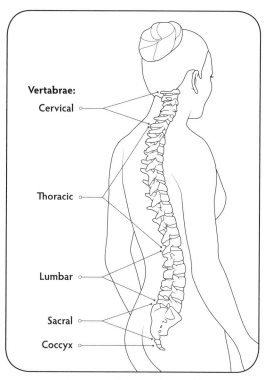

Vertabrae:

Cervical

Thoracic

Lumbar

Sacral

Coccyx

The curves of the spine act like springs in a coil, distributing mechanical forces as the body moves.

four curves. These spinal curves act like springs in a coil to distribute mechanical forces as we move, allowing us to walk, dance, and run without pain. If the curves get too large or too flat, the spine's muscles, fascia, tendons, and ligaments have to work a lot harder to keep us upright and balanced, and the result is often neck and back pain.

This column of twenty-four movable vertebrae rests on the sacrum, which gives the spine a stable yet flexible base. The sacrum is made up of five large vertebrae that fuse as we grow older. At the end of the sacrum, four (usually) fused vertebrae make up the tailbone or coccyx.

Although each vertebra of the spinal column is unique, they share certain features. All but the first two cervical vertebrae have a drum-shaped body in front that bears the body's weight. Behind the drum is a bony ring with a hole in the center through which the spinal cord passes. Several finger-like processes protrude from each vertebra. The bumps you can feel in your back are called the spinous processes. Two bony projections called the transverse processes flare out on either side. Together, these three bony outcroppings serve as attachment points for the muscles and connective tissue (fascia) that move the spine. Little ligaments and muscles attach to the spinous processes and tie each vertebra to the ones above and below it.

Facet Joints. The facets are bony outcroppings on the top and bottom of the vertebrae. The facets of adjacent vertebrae form joints that direct and limit the motion of the spine. The facets are angled differently in each area of the spine to allow different kinds of motion. In the neck, the facets create the flexibility that allows the head to turn from side to side and nod forward and back. In the chest, the facet joints and the ribs don't allow much spinal movement. In the low back, the facets keep the back from twisting or side-bending very much,

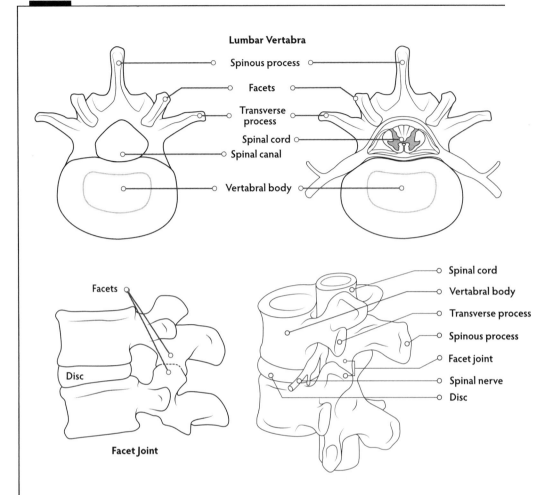

Lumbar Vertabra

Spinous process

Facets

Transverse process

Spinal cord

Spinal canal

Vertebral body

Facets

Disc

Facet Joint

Spinal cord

Vertebral body

Transverse process

Spinous process

Facet joint

Spinal nerve

Disc

but allow quite a bit of forward bending. Each facet joint has a cap of smooth cartilage—part of a fluid-filled capsule that lets each bone glide easily over its partner.

When the facets are pushed out of alignment by muscle spasm or trauma, they no longer glide over each other easily. If trauma compresses a facet joint, the healthy gap between the bones disappears, and instead of juicy lubrication separating the two parts of the joint, the bones start grinding away the cartilaginous lining. In time, the joint becomes inflamed, painful, and/or arthritic. Facet joints are rich in nerve fibers and, once misaligned or inflamed, can cause pain not only at the injured joint itself but also in the places the nerves exiting from the facet joint talk to. Inflamed or locked facet joints are one of the major sources of back pain.

The Discs. Shock-absorbing gelatinous discs separate the vertebrae, give the facets room to glide nicely over each other, and help create a generous canal for nerve roots to pass through. Discs also act like cushions to absorb force and contribute to the spine's slinky movement. Too much pressure on a disc can cause it to balloon out to the side and put pressure on the nerve roots exiting the spine, which can cause agonizing pain. A bulging disc can start a chain reaction of destruction. As the disc loses height, the facets move closer together and can start grinding on each other. The joints

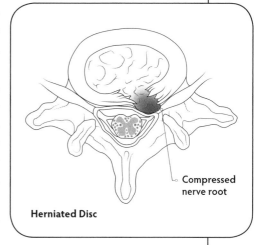

Compressed nerve root

Herniated Disc

become inflamed and painful. The nearby nerve roots can be compressed. In one of the most painful scenarios, a disc can burst (herniate), leaking out acidic gel that burns the nearby nerves.

The Spinal Cord and Spinal Nerves. The spinal cord is a tofu-like collection of nerves that originates in the brain and runs down through holes in the vertebrae to the lower back. As the spinal cord travels down the spine, thirty-one pairs of spinal nerves pass through holes in front of the facet joints, fanning out to the entire body. A thick layer of connective tissue called dura covers and protects the nerves. These nerves convey messages between the brain and all areas of the body. Pressure on these nerves from a jammed facet joint, a bulging disc, or a twisted vertebra can cause pain where the nerve exits the spinal cord. Pain, weakness, or numbness can also be experienced in the place the nerve goes to, such as the leg (sciatica).

FIVE CULPRITS IN LOW-BACK PAIN

All the components of the spine must move and work as a team: that simple principle guides my work when I treat patients with intractable back pain. Every part of the spine—bones, muscles, ligaments, tendons, blood vessels, nerves, and fascia—must remain moist and move freely so the spine can undulate as a unit from the base of the skull to the tailbone.

As with a good team, every player in the spine has a role and every player must do their part. If one part of the spine is injured, other team members have to pick up the load. If one of those team members is overworked, it may cry out in pain, but it's not necessarily the main cause of the problem. The pain may instead be a message that the suffering part is compensating for an injury elsewhere and is being forced to do a job it was not designed for. To relieve the problem, I have to find and fix the root cause.

I can't cover the many causes of back pain in one chapter. My focus is on five structural problems that show up over and over after trauma. These five problems limit the spine's healthy motion and cause most of the difficult problems I see but respond happily to treatment. Though traumas large and small can cause them, everyday habits such as improper sitting, driving too much, hunching over a computer, and not exercising can be culprits as well.

1 A Distorted Sacrum

Fixing the sacrum is often the key to fixing low-back pain. The sacrum and the spine are connected to each other as bedrock and pillar, waltzing together to allow us to dance, leap, and run. The sacrum sits between the two large hipbones. Together these three bones form the pelvic ring. When a person stands, the sacrum wedges into grooves in the back of the hipbones so the ring can support the weight of the upper body. The places where the sacrum and the hipbones meet are called the sacroiliac joints. (The back of each hipbone is called the ilium.)

The last vertebra of the lumbar spine sits on the sacrum's broad base, cushioned by a large disc, and their connection unites the spine and the pelvis in a single functional unit. The entire structure—spinal column, sacrum, and hipbones— form the central axis of the body. If the sacrum becomes twisted or misaligned in its pelvic home, the weight of the structures above it will press down unevenly, causing low-back pain and even herniated discs. When the sacrum is twisted or unstable, the back is unstable. Much of my work in relieving low-

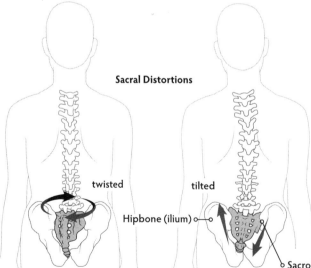

Sacral Distortions

twisted   tilted

Hipbone (ilium) o—o

Sacroiliac joint

When the sacrum is rotated or tilted, nearby structures become distorted, the spine destabilized, muscles and fascia tightened, and discs and nerves pinched.

back pain involves freeing up the motion of the sacrum and making sure its connection to the lower lumbar vertebrae is flexible and balanced.

The sacrum and pelvis must provide a steady yet flexible base for the body while still accommodating walking. That's asking a lot of it. The sacrum also has to support the reproductive and elimination organs and house an abundance of nerves. The more demands placed on this finely tuned structure, the more easily it can become compromised. Given all these demands, it sometimes seems that the hardworking sacrum would rather be vacationing in Greece, where it can bask in the sun. Sometimes you have to coax your sacrum to come back home and get back to work, rocking ever so slightly back and forth between the hipbones.

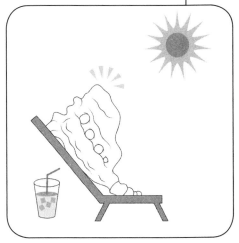

Sometimes it seems like the hard-working sacrum would rather be vacationing than holding up the rest of your body!

When the sacrum runs away from home, generally it doesn't get as far as Greece. When trauma pushes the sacrum away from its home between the hipbones, the low back suffers. Here are some of the common problems this can cause:

- If the sacrum becomes rotated—with one side forward and the other side back—it can no longer move easily or provide the stable base on which the spine depends. A rotated sacrum places painful stress on the sacroiliac joints. A sharp or burning pain in the crack of the buttocks tends to reflect the grinding of the sacroiliac (SI) joint. The twist can also catch up nerves coming through the sacrum to the pelvis and legs. The sacrum can twist as a result of a fall on the back or buttocks, a car crash, or a repetitive habit such as a cashier twisting between the groceries and the cash register.

- When one corner of the sacrum is pushed up—common in car crashes when the braking foot shoves the leg and pelvis upward, or from stepping off a curb into a pothole—the protruding edge can injure the disc above it, causing searing pain in the low back, pelvis, or leg. A raised sacral corner also tilts the lumbar spine into an imbalanced, untenable position. As the spine twists and tips to accommodate the unbalanced sacrum, facet joints, ligaments, discs, and fascia struggle to hold up the spine. In the process, they can become strained, torn, or weakened. This imbalance can result in pain in the lower abdomen, pelvis, or low back or even down the leg.

123

- Sometimes the sacrum simply becomes jammed between the hipbones and loses much of its rocking motion. A fall on the buttocks is a common cause. A car crash typically launches the pelvis up two inches and then slams it back down, locking the SI joints. When the sacrum doesn't rock, it can't distribute force efficiently, and the spine above the sacrum has to absorb the additional strain. If there is a weak place in the spine that can't cope with the extra effort, muscle spasm or a bulging disc can result. If you have surgery on the bulging disc but don't unlock the sacrum, the forces of daily living or another trauma will go to another weak spot and compromise the disc there.

- Lumbar discs require the rocking motion of the sacrum to pump fluid into them and keep them plump. When the sacrum loses mobility, over time the discs tend to dry out, weaken, and shrink. The facets move closer together and grind on each other. The passageways for the nerves exiting the spinal cord become narrower, and sometimes the nerves can become pinched. All this can cause burning, throbbing, searing, stabbing, or aching pain locally and in the area the nerves go to. The connective tissue (fascia) that provides stability to the back also depends on sacral pumping to be juiced up and moist. A stagnant sacrum leads to tightened fascia, which can cause pain anywhere in the back, hips, legs, torso, or neck.

2 A Poorly Moving Diaphragm

The second culprit in chronic back pain—and in herniated discs—is a poorly moving diaphragm. The diaphragm, like the sacrum, is intimately involved in the health of the back. Because the diaphragm is anchored to the first three lumbar vertebrae, the movement of the diaphragm tractions the spine and pumps fluid into the upper spinal discs. The diaphragm's fibers interweave with the powerful muscles that stabilize the spine and link it to the pelvis— the psoas and the quadratus lumborum muscles. Together, these muscles help stabilize the entire central structure of the body. Recently, researchers actually measured the movement of the diaphragm in patients with chronic low-back pain and confirmed what I have found for thirty years: people with chronic low-back problems have a poorly moving diaphragm.

When both the diaphragm and the sacrum are restricted, the problem is even worse. Together, they create a vise that squeezes the lumbar discs. Think of the Slinky toy. If the Slinky is held on each end (diaphragm and sacrum) and then wiggled, the forces ripple fiercely throughout the middle of the Slinky.

That's what happens to the lumbar spine when the diaphragm above and the sacrum below are not moving. Even the ordinary forces of daily life will batter the spine in between the vise, causing severe back pain and putting enormous pressure on the discs. That's why I say the lumbar spine pays for the sins of the diaphragm above it and the sacrum below. Okay, the sacrum in sunny Greece is not really sinning, nor is the ever-vigilant diaphragm ever truly lazy. But the image will help you remember: address the sacrum below and the diaphragm above to heal the back.

————————◯————————

FELIPE. Four years ago, Felipe stumbled into my office, bent over in agony. He reported that weeks earlier, he had been lifting heavy boxes in his garage when he experienced a sudden and severe searing pain that ran down his left leg and made it almost impossible to walk. He was bent forward and leaning to the right to take pressure off the screaming nerve.

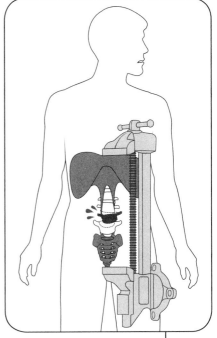

When the diaphragm and the sacrum are restricted, they create a vise that squeezes the structures between them.

His MRI study revealed a severely herniated (broken) disc on the left side between his sacrum and his last lumbar vertabra, known as the 5th lumbar disc. The acid gel oozing out of the disc not only pressed on the nerve root to his left leg but also burned it, causing excruciating pain. He came to me in desperation. Surgery was scheduled in two weeks, and he hoped to avoid going under the knife.

I took his history and gave him homeopathic *Colocynth* for his pain and disc protrusion. On examination, I found his sacrum was basically frozen. Due to its anatomical connection to the base of the skull, the sacrum should have been rocking back and forth six-plus times a minute in coordination with the pulsations of the skull and brain. Not only did the sacrum not move and the surrounding tissue feel as dead as dried wood, but the sacrum was also tilted up on the left, compressing the lumbar disc above it.

Why would picking up a box cause a disc to herniate? The quality of Felipe's tissues held a clue. The dryness and toughness of the tissues suggested blood flow and movement had been restricted for quite a while. In other words, his sacrum had been out of position for a long time. The chronic malpositioning

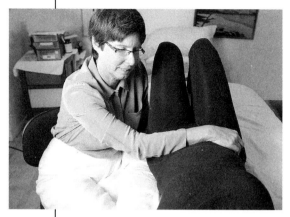

By gently clothes-pinning the hipbones inward with my arm and hand, I create more room for the sacrum to slip back into place.

of the sacrum had probably weakened the disc above it. When Felipe picked up the heavy box, the additional pressure on it was too much and the vulnerable disc blew apart. When there has not been a direct, forceful trauma to the spine from a fall, collision, or car accident, I find that most disc problems are the end result of many microtraumas in conjunction with chronic malpositioning of the sacrum.

To treat Felipe, I placed my left hand under his sacrum. With my right hand and forearm, I clothes-pinned his hipbones. Pulling the hipbones together in front created more room in back for the sacrum to slip down into place. I imperceptibly rocked the sacrum with my left hand and gently coaxed it downward.

Slowly, Felipe's sacrum moved farther away from his lumbar disc. It now moved rhythmically, three times a minute. Progress. I then worked to relax the back muscles, which had been in constant spasm since the disc had herniated. By gently putting pressure on the body of the muscle and bringing its ends toward each other, I was able to remind the muscle how to relax. I also stretched out the muscles' contracted fascial wrappers, taking out the twists that had resulted from his weeks of bending to the side in a mostly futile attempt to keep pressure off the injured nerve.

Finally, I addressed the spasm in Felipe's diaphragm. Like most people with lumbar-disc problems, Felipe's spasmed diaphragm and the rigid and partly tilted sacrum had created a vise that squeezed the discs in between. In Felipe's case, the vise was strong enough to cause a herniated disc.

After Felipe struggled to climb off the treatment table, he felt a little better and stood up straighter. Three days later, he returned. His pain had markedly diminished, he had less diaphragmatic and lumbar spasm, and his sacrum moved better. I repeated much of what I'd previously done.

Suffice it to say that Felipe canceled his surgery. Within a week and a half, he felt 60 percent better. The disc herniation eventually resolved, once the compression from above and below it was released. He was pain-free after three months, aided by physical therapy and appropriate exercises. An MRI taken a year later found no evidence of a disc herniation.

I've treated many patients with bulging and/or herniated discs, and rarely has surgery been necessary. Almost every time I treat a lumbar-disc problem, the sacrum and diaphragm are restricted. Even when the patient does not have a disc problem, the sacrum plays a role in low-back pain, with the diaphragm often tagging along. Treating both can markedly diminish most severe back pain.

3 Excessive Curve in the Lower Back

ROSE was a highly successful exotic dancer in San Francisco. One night, while walking offstage in four-inch heels, her low back suddenly gave way. She was in agony and could barely make it down the steps. She came to see me the next morning so that I could attend to this problem quickly.

The healthy spine has a slight backward curve (lordosis) where the lumbar spine and the sacrum meet, called the lumbosacral angle. When the sacrum tips too far forward and the angle gets too large, it's a recipe for disaster. Anything that makes the butt stick out more increases the lumbosacral angle. When stylish gals like Rose get their fashion fix with high heels, they have lovely curves, but they also markedly increase their lumbosacral angle. Other situations

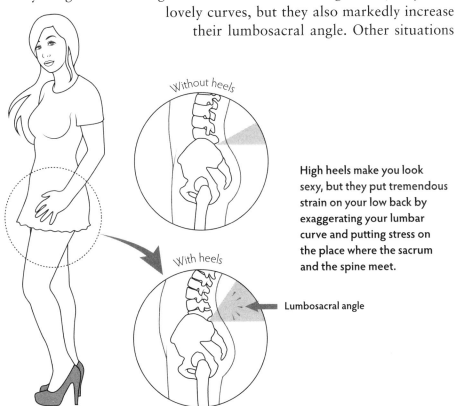

Without heels

With heels

High heels make you look sexy, but they put tremendous strain on your low back by exaggerating your lumbar curve and putting stress on the place where the sacrum and the spine meet.

Lumbosacral angle

like a pregnant belly, significant weight gain, or weak abdominal muscles can increase this angle as well.

As the lumbosacral angle grows larger, the fascia, muscles, and ligaments connecting the lumbar spine to the sacrum have to work much harder to stabilize an increasingly unstable structure. Ligaments and fascia get overstretched and weakened. Muscles go into spasm, valiantly trying to help the failing fascia and ligaments.

Without strong deep abdominal muscles to help stabilize this collapsing structure, the angle becomes even steeper, further straining the muscles, ligaments, and fascia. All that backward bending of the lower lumbar vertebrae presses on the back of the discs, causing them to bulge.

In Rose's case, repeated dancing in four-inch heels bent the top of the sacrum too far forward and the lower lumbar vertebrae too far back. Her lumbosacral angle had gotten way too large, and the sacrum had lost its lovely rocking motion. Using techniques similar to the ones I used with Felipe, I coaxed the sacrum into a better position and helped it rock again. I also restored the lumbar vertebrae that sat on top of it to a more normal position. I did this by heeding the advice of one of my mentors, Muriel Chapman, DO, who advised me, "Always remember to treat the front of the back." By using the connections between the abdomen's muscles and fascia and the muscles and fascia of the spine, I was able to relax the muscles holding the vertebra in the wrong position.

My treatment helped decrease Rose's lumbosacral angle and eased her low-back problem. Then it was up to her. I forbade her from wearing heels for a week. I sent her to a physical therapist to help strengthen her abdominal muscles and a yoga instructor to help keep her sacrum moving freely.

4 Locked Facet Joints

In order to support the 70-plus pounds above it, the large lumbar vertebrae and their facet joints are designed for stability. The lumbar facets allow the spine to bend forward, yet limit sidebending and rotation (twisting). In this way, the lower back sacrifices flexibility for stability.

The lumbar facets' dislike of sidebending or twisting explains why people who are twisted or bent sideways at the time of an impact are much more likely to suffer disc and lumbar spine damage. I commonly find facet injuries when the patient was twisting to reach something in the back seat at the moment their car was struck. This is also why people throw out their backs when they twist around to lift something. The facets are not designed for this movement. When forced to do it, they tend to lock together.

Acute facet pain tends to be sharp, stabbing, searing, or aching at the specific joint. A twisted or locked facet joint can also squeeze the nerve root exiting the canal formed by the joint. The resulting pain can be felt anywhere along the nerve's pathway. In the low back, facet-joint injury can cause pain that radiates down the buttocks and into the back of the leg. Patients may receive injections into the facet joint to relieve the pain, but if the facet joint is not mobilized and unlocked, the problem will generally recur.

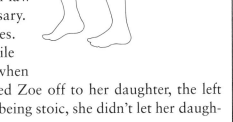

Locked facet joint

GLORIA was thrilled to be taking care of her one-year-old granddaughter for the weekend while her daughter and son-in-law went away to celebrate their anniversary. Gloria and little Zoe were good buddies. Zoe loved riding on Gloria's left hip while Gloria did her chores. Unfortunately, when Monday came around and Gloria handed Zoe off to her daughter, the left side of Gloria's back was killing her. But being stoic, she didn't let her daughter know and kissed Zoe good-bye.

She hobbled in to my office later that week, pointing to a specific spot in her low back, and said, "I feel like someone's stabbing me here." She described her weekend of hitching up her left hip to hold her grandchild.

"Does it hurt more when you twist?" I asked.

"Oh, that's terrible," she replied.

A jammed facet joint generally hurts more with twisting or backward bending. I suspected she had locked a facet joint in her low back.

My physical exam confirmed my suspicions. I put my fingers along two of her lumbar vertebrae and bent her to the side. She bent easily to the left, but her spine wouldn't budge when I bent her to the right. The facet joints between the vertebrae had glued themselves together on the left side.

Manual medicine has a number of ways to unstick locked facet joints. When the problem is fairly recent, it's much easier to fix. In Gloria's case, the fascia binding the vertebrae together had not lost its flexibility or hardened into a distorted shape. Many joints, including facets, can be unlocked with a method resembling twisting open a stuck jar lid. First, I slightly compress the stuck parts so that they can move more freely on each other, and then I unwind. This approach worked with Gloria.

I also made sure Gloria's diaphragm and sacrum were moving well. She climbed off the table feeling 50 percent better. Once motion was restored to the joint, her body did the rest of the work. By the end of the week, all her symptoms had melted away.

5 Compromised Fascia

Compromised fascia is the fifth potential culprit in low-back pain and a critical element in resolving it. We think of muscles and bones as the structures that hold the body together, but that view is not completely accurate. The muscles and bones—and everything else inside the body, for that matter—would be flopping about and crashing into each other if they were not insulated and held in place by something else. That something is fascia, a moist, pulsating, stretchy, gossamer connective tissue web that wraps the inside and outside of all our parts, including our muscles and bones, and links them together. Fascia extends from the top of the head to the bottom of the feet and surrounds every blood vessel, lymphatic vessel, nerve, and organ. In fact, fascia is more of the body's skeleton than the bony skeleton is.

For a moment, imagine there is a magic camera flying around inside your body and projecting out a three-dimensional image of your fascia. Spinning before you, you would see an intricate web of strands that looks exactly like . . . you. You

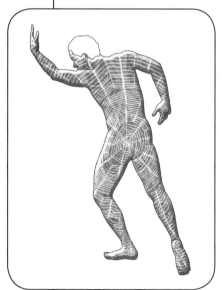

would see your body wrapped in a garment of fascia, with every wrinkle in your skin and every muscle outlined. As you go deeper and deeper, the spaces where the organs live would come into view, shaped like your unique organs. You would fly through tiny channels where nerves, blood vessels, and lymphatic paths weave in and out. You would see, down to the smallest detail, even individual cells. If you raised your arm and watched your fascial body react, you would see the entire web of fascia change its shape: moving, stretching, contracting, and reforming in an interconnected wave from outside to inside, from head to toe.

Fascia allows structures to move and glide over each other without friction. Fascia links the organs to their homes in the body and to one another. Fascia functions like an affectionate mother—giving organs and vessels free play to enjoy their functions but reining them in if they stray too far. It has an intimate role in regulating fluid flow at the cellular level, communicates with the immune system, and is a key player in both inflammation and healing. The complex feedback mechanisms between the brain and the fascia enable effortless graceful motion. It's primarily through the fascia that the body realigns itself as we move.

> *"The fascia is the place to look for cause of disease and the place to consult and begin the action of remedies in all diseases."*
>
> —Andrew Taylor Still, 1899
> Founder of osteopathic medicine

Because it is stiffer than muscle tissue and expands and contracts independently of muscles, fascia protects muscles from overstretching, acting like the guy wires of a suspension bridge to provide the harmonious tension that keeps the body upright and moving.

Like the lymphatics and other heroes of health, fascia has been mostly ignored by medicine. It was long considered packing material around the really important stuff—the bones, muscles, and organs. But every cell and system of the body relies on the fascia.

Not surprisingly, some of the strongest fascia in the body is found in the back. A large, dense, diamond-shaped fascial sheath called the thoracolumbar fascia runs from the pelvis to the mid-back. The thoracolumbar (TL) fascia is a primary stabilizer of the low back. Its three layers surround and unite the back's major structures, including the diaphragm, the vertebrae, the large muscles, and the sacrum. It transmits and distributes the forces generated by the large back muscles—in fact, virtually all movement of the torso is transferred through it.

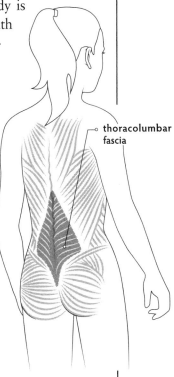

thoracolumbar fascia

To stay healthy, the TL fascia needs to move. If the surrounding tissues become lazy and lose their motion, the TL fascia tends to gets sticky and tough. When the diaphragm and the sacrum tighten and create a vise for the spine, the TL fascia that surrounds them contracts. If motion is not restored to these structures, the fascia will eventually stiffen and help maintain the vise. As the TL fascia slowly dries out and stiffens, it shrink-wraps the muscles, making it harder for the muscles to contract and relax. Problems with the fascia can cause diffuse, non-specific back pain that doesn't seem to stay fixed in any one place. And because the TL fascia is

Avoiding Surgery

Numerous studies have shown the effectiveness of osteopathic manipulative therapy for chronic low-back pain. The latest study done in 2013, involving 455 adults with chronic low-back pain, showed that six osteopathic treatments significantly reduced their pain levels and enabled them to decrease their prescription usage.

connected to the back, neck, shoulders, pelvis, and abdomen, its problems can be felt anywhere in this vast connective tissue web. If you have been suffering aching or gnawing pain in any of those regions that does not respond to stretching or other forms of treatment, consider the health of your fascia.

The lumbar fascia can also be injured directly by trauma, which can twist, rip, and/ or tear it. Fascial tears can turn into fibrotic scars that will further compromise the fascia's resiliency and the structural balance of the low back. The resulting decrease in blood flow through the tightened tissues prevents needed oxygen and nutrients from reaching the fascia. Since fascia is laced with ten times more pain fibers than muscle, injured fascia tends to ache, burn, throb, sear, or sting. Constricted fascia also tends to squeeze the blood and lymphatic vessels needed to supply nutrients and remove debris from muscles. Over time, this can contribute to painful inflammation. Fascial restrictions can take some time to develop, but the longer they remain in place, the harder it becomes to restore the fascia to its original mobility and the more painful the back tends to get.

Fascial health depends not only on movement but also on its staying moist. Moistness depends on proper fluid absorption and good rhythmic movement. Here's where people have a lot of power over their health: moving every day and drinking sufficient water. Slowly stretching the muscles through wide arcs of motion helps the fascia. Swimming, tai chi, and the twisting poses in yoga are excellent for stretching tightened fascia.

The manual therapy employed to release restricted fascia also needs to be slow and precise. Wise practitioners understand how the fascial planes are laid down, so they can feel fascial restrictions and address them. Fascial release techniques are among the most powerful and effective tools of manual medicine for decreasing pain and restoring function.

I am also excited by a new treatment therapy addressing the lubrication and mobility of fascia called M.E.L.T., created by movement therapist Sue Hitzmann. M.E.L.T. utilizes small balls, soft rollers, and various movement techniques to moisten and restore vibrancy to fascia. I am recommending M.E.L.T. to some of my patients as a fun and effective way of restoring mobility to restricted fascia.

When Surgery Is Necessary

Some back problems cannot be resolved without surgery. The two main kinds I've seen are described below:

Foot drop. If a person cannot fully lift a foot while walking, they have foot drop, which may indicate a serious compression on a nerve by a disc or bone. It may require surgery to prevent the condition from becoming permanent.

Spinal stenosis. When bone grows inside the vertebra and squeezes the spinal cord, the condition, called spinal stenosis, may warrant surgery.

My mother had this problem. She had the classic symptoms, including pain in both feet made worse by walking. As the discs in her low back shrank with age, the leathery ligaments binding the vertebrae together became slack. The vertebrae began to wobble, and the bones tried to grow together to stabilize them. Bones are rather clumsy at this, and they often grow inward. That's what they did with my mom, squeezing her spinal cord and creating agony in the nerves to her feet.

Spinal stenosis surgery to open up the spinal canal tends to be pretty successful. I aligned her spine prior to the operation and gave her homeopathic remedies like *Arnica* afterward to promote healing. She was thrilled to recover her ability to walk without pain, and she thereafter referred to her "gold-plated back" with a smile.

Red Flags

The following conditions in the low back demand immediate medical attention:

- Sudden, severe back pain can result from a number of serious conditions, including a life-threatening abdominal aneurysm, appendicitis, an ectopic pregancy, infection or abscess in the chest or abdomen, or a blood clot or bowel obstruction.

- Back pain that is worse at night and unrelieved by rest can be from an aneurysm or an infection, or a symptom of cancer in the spine.

- Back pain that does not respond to treatment can be a symptom of prostate, testicular, uterine, or ovarian cancer.

WHAT YOU CAN DO

Once I have addressed the structural problems contributing to a patient's back pain, I send them to a physical therapist, yoga teacher, Pilates instructor, or other movement therapist for an individualized strengthening and stretching program. Since everyone is different, there is no one-size-fits-all program for healing the back. However, sometimes very simple things can work wonders. In chapter 18, you will find movement tools for healing back pain, and I list a few others below.

Know that these healing practices, though exceedingly helpful, cannot completely compensate for the damage done by hours of slouching over a computer, carrying a heavy backpack, or wearing worn-out shoes. Your back will heal even faster if you can recognize and change the everyday habits that keep your back aching. Here are the most common culprits I have found:

- Carrying a child on the hip
- Wearing shoes that are worn out or flimsy
- Sitting on a wallet, especially while driving a car or truck
- Prolonged sitting (this places tremendous pressure on the lumbar discs)
- Working at desk/keyboard that is too high or too low
- Sitting in a car seat not shaped for your body
- Carrying a heavy backpack or purse
- Wearing high heels
- Sitting in a soft or uneven sofa or chair
- Sitting on the same foot (twisting the sacrum)
- Swinging a golf club incorrectly (with golf, you're always twisting the same way, so that's already potentially compromising)

Five Healing Habits

Stay hydrated. No matter what modality you choose to help your back pain (and pretty much everything else), drinking enough water can help tremendously. Researchers have discovered that patients who are fully hydrated benefit much more from manual medicine treatments. Spinal discs do a much better job when they are fully plumped up with water. Muscles and fascia are also very thirsty tissues. Dehydration makes fascia less stretchy and more prone to injury and inflammation. Since the muscles are wrapped in fascia, this inflexible fascia shrink wraps the muscles, making it harder for them to contract and weakening them.

How much water is enough? As I mentioned in the section on inflammation, some nutritionists recommend at least half a person's body weight in ounces per day. A 120-pound person should drink at least five cups (60 ounces) of water. I keep a big jug of water on my desk.

Move! The body needs movement to push the fluids into the tissues. Even gentle walking is helpful. If you sit at a computer all day, take a short break—even just one minute—every half hour. Stand up while you answer the phone or do other tasks. If it's possible, a few times a day, lie on the floor with your legs up on a chair—it allows the discs to plump up a bit.

I often recommend that my patients with lingering back problems do aquatic therapy. For those with lumbar compression, I suggest wearing a float around the waist, attaching weights to the ankles, and hanging vertically in the water. This gentle traction will slowly release compression on the discs.

Breathe! Getting the diaphragm moving is critical to keeping the vertebrae separated, tractioning the spine, and pumping the spinal discs. The breathing practices in chapter 7 are particularly helpful for restoring the diaphragm's full motion.

Keep trim. Losing some extra pounds literally can take a load off your entire spinal structure. I realize it's not easy to do, particularly if pain is limiting exercise, but exercise in water and gentle walking every day for thirty minutes can contribute to controlling weight.

Sleep comfortably. A comfortable, supportive mattress can help back pain immensely. If your mattress is saggy or unsupportive, think about replacing it. If your mattress is fine and you still wake up with an aching back, try sleeping on your side with a pillow between your knees. This takes the strain off your sacroiliac ligaments and puts your pelvis into a much more balanced position. Sleeping on your back with a wedge under your knees also can be helpful (see photos page 321).

Back pain can be extremely frightening, but realizing that it has treatable causes should strip away much of its fearsome power. As you gradually regain control of your body's foundation, you will move toward diminishing and even eliminating your back pain. Please also read the next chapter on the pelvis so you can see other ways that the critical unsung hero, the sacrum, contributes to low-back health.

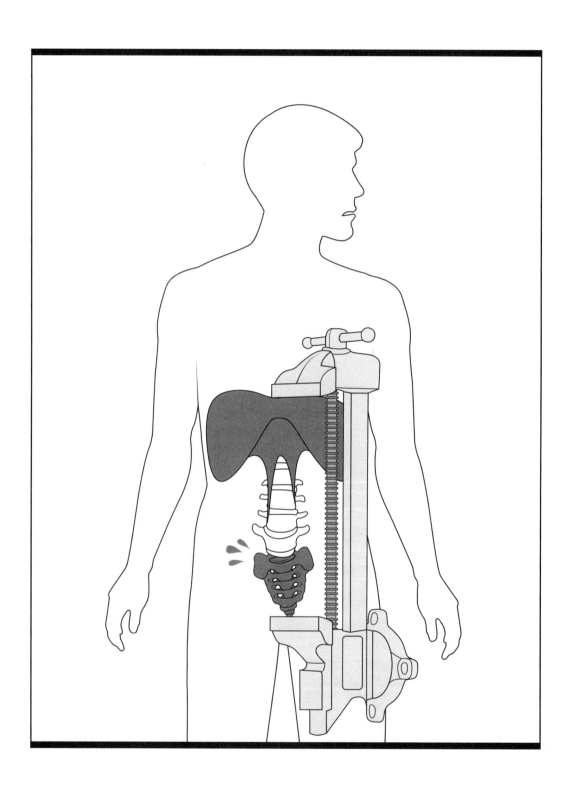

13

The Pelvis and Sacrum

The human body has over two hundred bones, but only one is called sacred. That bone is the sacrum (from the Latin word meaning "sacred bone"), the triangular-shaped bone that lives at the base of the spine. If the sacrum were an astrological sign, it would be Pisces—working in the background but, like water, essential for everything.

The free motion of the sacrum is key not only to a pain-free spine but also to sexual health, a vibrant brain and nervous system, and flourishing digestion. The sacrum's many roles in health are the focus of this chapter.

The sacrum and the hipbones make up the pelvic ring. The sacrum has grooves and ridges on each side that wedge into corresponding notches in the back of the hipbones. Tough yet pliable ligaments bind the bones of the pelvis together. These ligaments allow the sacrum to rock forward and back between the hipbones as we walk, dance, or run.

If the sacrum becomes twisted or misaligned in its pelvic home, the weight of the structures above it will press down unevenly. In addition to causing low-back pain and herniated discs, a misaligned sacrum can cause sexual, neurological, and digestive difficulties.

Because of the sacrum's intimate connection to the brain and the nervous system, osteopathic medicine has always given the health of the sacrum great prominence. The

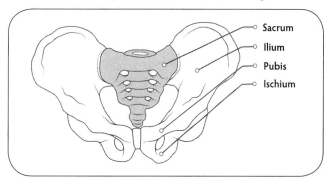

Sacrum
Ilium
Pubis
Ischium

Symptoms of a Jammed Sacrum

- Back pain
- Headaches
- Sciatica
- Insomnia
- Neck pain
- Bladder infections
- Infertility
- Difficult labor and delivery
- Painful periods

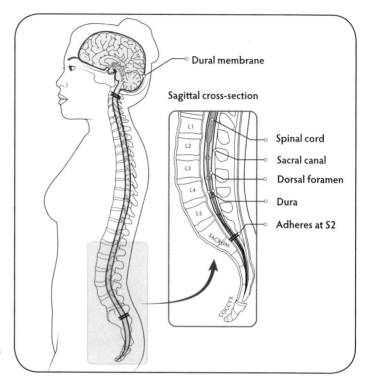

Dural membrane

Sagittal cross-section

L1
L2
L3
L4
L5

SACRUM

COCCYX

Spinal cord

Sacral canal

Dorsal foramen

Dura

Adheres at S2

Because of the dural connection between the skull and the sacrum, what happens to one affects the other.

dural membranes that wrap the brain attach to the top two vertebrae in the neck, drape the spinal cord, and then anchor themselves to the inside of the sacrum. As the healthy skull and brain expand and contract, the sacrum rocks back and forth in rhythm with these pulsations. The link between brain and sacrum is so profound that what happens to the sacrum has a direct impact on the brain, and vice versa. Osteopaths use the connection between cranium and sacrum to treat many problems, including headaches, neck pain, reproductive problems, and digestive dysfunction.

The sacrum also affects the fight-or-flight sympathetic nervous system (SNS). From its origins high in the spine, the SNS courses down in front of the sacrum and ends in a critical bundle of nerves in front of the coccyx called the ganglion impar. The nerves of the ganglion impar can be stretched, pinched, or irritated if the sacrum is not positioned correctly. This problem can result in severe perineal pain, leg pain, sexual-performance problems, digestive upset, and the hyperirritability of the sympathetic nervous system I call injury shock.

The next three cases show the kinds of nervous system problems that a twisted sacrum can cause.

RACHEL came to me in excruciating pain. For more than two months, blinding headaches kept her cocooned in bed. The MRIs, CT scans, and EEG were all negative. Powerful drugs kept her pain under control but left her drowsy and unable to concentrate in class. Rachel's mother knew something was very wrong, but she didn't know where to turn for help. One of my patients who knew her suggested that she take Rachel to see me.

The nineteen-year-old girl described her plight to me. Every day, headaches wrapped themselves around her head and squeezed and tugged on her eyes. As always, I asked, "What do you think caused this?" It is amazing how often people sense the true cause of their suffering.

"I've never felt right since I slid into the goalpost during soccer season," she said. Her mom added, "She did hurt her ankle, but that healed fine."

I performed a complete musculoskeletal exam, starting with her feet. Her ankle ligaments had regained strength, but her ankle bones (talus and calcaneus) felt welded together, indicating that she had slammed the goalpost with considerable force. As I suspected, the force had been transmitted up her right leg, shoving her thighbone into her pelvis. This pushed her right hip up half an inch higher than the left, twisting her sacrum and rotating it to the left.

Why did this cause Rachel's headaches? The brain's membranes (the dura) fasten to the vertebrae in the neck and eventually to the inside of the sacrum. Anything that pulls or twists the sacrum pulls on the dura, which in turn tugs on the neck, the skull, and the brain. Rachel's twisted sacrum was constantly yanking on her upper neck and head, pulling them down. I suspected that this also pinched nerves in her skull and neck, as well as compromised blood flow into her head. Each of these problems can create agonizing headaches. Given the structural problems I found when I examined the base of her head, I felt that both the nerves and blood vessels had been com-

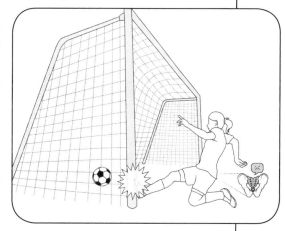

Rachel's collision with the goalpost twisted her sacrum. That pulled on the dural membrane attached to her sacrum, neck, and skull, causing her headaches.

promised. Like the pelvis, her head was shoved up on the right and pulled down on the left.

I loosened the pelvic and low-back muscle spasm that was keeping the right side of her pelvis pulled up. Then I repositioned her sacrum. I gently pulled Rachel's right leg back down. I released some muscle spasm at the base of her skull and evened out her head, using cranial techniques I describe in chapter 20. Since Rachel was young and basically healthy, her body responded quickly. When she stood up from my table, the headache had diminished by 80 percent. Within forty-eight hours, her headaches were gone, never to return. Because she felt fine, she did not return to see me. I called a year later, and her mother told me she was still headache-free and doing well in college.

JEFFREY. After a hard tackle in a weekend football game, my weekend warrior patient Jeffrey ended up with severe sciatica. The thirty-eight-year-old had suffered stabbing pains down his left leg ever since he was tackled from behind and landed hard on his hip. His neurological tests and MRI confirmed that his lumbar spine was fine. When I asked him where his pain started, he pointed to the side of the crack in his buttocks. "I had a burning, grinding pain there. Now it's a gnawing pain that hurts me most when I try to get out of bed or out of my car."

I examined him. His sacrum was twisted between his hipbones, with the left side rotated up and slightly forward. This malposition jammed the sacrum into the hipbone (ilium) on each side. This compression is known as a sacroiliac restriction. This sacroiliac problem squeezed the cartilage and nerves between the joint and caused the typical burning and grinding pain near Jeffrey's buttocks' crack.

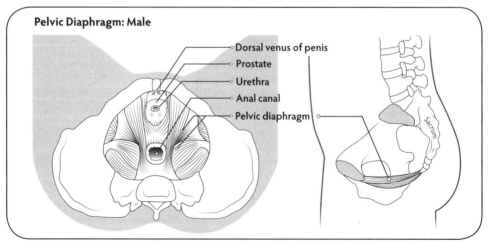

The pelvic diaphragm is a group of paired muscles and connective tissue that runs between the pelvis and the coccyx. Problems with the pelvic diaphragm can cause vascular congestion, contributing to pelvic and leg pain and sexual dysfunction.

Because twisting further grinds this joint together, the sacroiliac pain worsened when Jeffrey twisted to get out of bed or step from his car.

The pain down Jeffrey's leg came from other pelvic problems. Twists in the pelvis bind up the pelvic fascia and cause muscle spasms there, especially the piriformis muscle in the buttock. The piriformis muscle has a knack for catching up and squeezing the nearby sciatic nerve to the leg, causing leg pain.

Over the next four treatments, I repositioned the sacrum and relieved the piriformis spasm so I could stretch the bound-up pelvic fascia. This reduced the pain down his leg by 50 percent. Of course, I treated (realigned) the rest of his body as well.

On the fifth visit, because Jeffrey still had some buttock and leg pain, I realized something else needed to be done. I needed to treat the muscular pelvic diaphragm at the bottom of his pelvis. The pelvic diaphragm is a group of paired muscles and connective tissue that runs between the pelvis and the coccyx, containing holes for the anus and the urethra, the prostate in men, and the vagina in women.

Unless this diaphragm pumps fully, vascular congestion can build up and put pressure on nerves and muscles. In Jeffrey's case, the extra fluid kept pressure on his sciatic nerve. Problems with the pelvic diaphragm in women can contribute to menstrual pain or pain with intercourse. A weak pelvic diaphragm is a relatively common problem. Both men and women can strengthen this area with Kegel exercises, which I describe in chapter 18 (page 215). Sexual intercourse also tends to tone this area for both men and women.

After I got his pelvic diaphragm pumping well, 90 percent of Jeff's sciatic pain was removed. In time, all his pain disappeared.

CYNTHIA couldn't get a good night of sleep. Just as she sank into a nice, luxurious state, she awoke with a start. She became so sleep deprived she wanted to throw her four-year-old son out the window. "I know I won't toss him away, but I hate how I feel."

I went through her history. Six months earlier, her car had been hit from behind while she had her foot on the brake. After a month, her neck had healed fairly well. She had some aching hip pain and gnawing low-back pain for a couple of months, but they both went away. Then, two weeks before she came to see me, she stumbled off a curb. That misstep sent a jolt up her leg, and that night she couldn't sleep.

On examination, I found that her right hipbone was shoved up and rotated backward. Her sacrum was high on the right, and crooked. Instead of her sacrum moving six times a minute, its rocking between her hipbones had dropped to three times per minute. I told her what I'd found.

"Could that have happened stepping off a curb?" she asked.

"Probably not," I said. "This much distortion usually comes from a pretty significant trauma. Your pelvis was probably pushed backward during the car accident. Then, when you stumbled off the curb and rotated your pelvis a bit more, your sacroiliac joint could no longer compensate. Given the many bundles of nerves around your sacrum, all this tugging agitated your nervous system."

I suspected that the twisted sacrum caught up sympathetic nerve fibers that end at the front of the coccyx bone, the ganglion impar. Constant tugging on the ganglion had pushed the SNS into its fight-or-flight mode. I gently coaxed the sacrum back home, released tension on the ganglion, and rotated the hip slightly. Cynthia later reported to me that she slept like a baby that night and never had further sleep problems.

THE SACRUM AND REPRODUCTIVE HEALTH

The sacrum's role in reproduction probably is why it's called the sacred bone. If you have created children or enjoyed the fun of sex, please thank your sacrum. The nutritive parasympathetic nervous system (PNS) goes out through the holes in the sacrum and supplies nerve impulses to the descending colon, bladder, penis and testes, and vagina and clitoris. The sacrum is curved to cuddle the lower bowel, rectum, bladder, and sex organs. In chapter 14, I talk about the importance of a happy sacrum in sex. Here I briefly mention its role in reproductive health.

ELENA started having horrible menstrual periods right after someone pulled a chair out from under her and she landed hard on her bottom. "I would shoot heroin to get rid of this agony," she said, bent over double.

"Luckily, you won't have to," I told her.

I had her lie down on the treatment table. I found that the accident had shoved her sacrum upward. The uterus is attached to the sacrum by a pair of uterosacral ligaments, so the trauma that displaced the sacrum also pulled on the uterus. Both distortions compromised the blood supply and nerves to the uterus, causing her terrible menstrual cramps.

Over several visits, I repositioned her sacrum, treated her lumbar spine, diaphragm, and cranium, and further rebalanced her pelvis. Her next period, though painful, was 30 percent better. Her second period felt 75 percent better. As often happens, the last 25 percent of improvement took as long as the first 75 percent. After five months, her periods were pain-free.

Far more than painful periods are at stake when trauma compromises the sacrum. I have found that a restricted sacrum can contribute to infertility and uterine hemorrhage during menses. During menstruation, the excess uterine lining sloughs off, no longer needed to accept and nurture a fertilized egg. The amount of blood and tissue released depends partly on hormones. It also depends on the uterus to fully close off the generous supply of blood vessels that had provided a nurturing bed for the fertilized egg. I have found that when a patient has excessive bleeding, often both the sacrum and the uterus are twisted. Repositioning both can resolve that problem.

CARLOTTA. Early in my practice, the wife of one of my colleagues was hemorrhaging so profusely during her periods that her OB-GYN scheduled a hysterectomy. When I examined Carlotta, I found that both her sacrum and her uterus were rotated to the left and twisted. She could remember no trauma to her pelvis. Perhaps her three pregnancies had caused a pelvic distortion. This is not uncommon for several reasons. During pregnancy, the expanding uterus typically rotates to the left to get out of the way of the liver. This can pull on the utero-

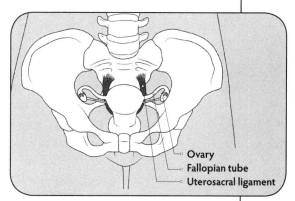

Ovary
Fallopian tube
Uterosacral ligament

The sacrum and uterus are tied together by a pair of ligaments. A distorted sacrum can distort the uterus, contributing to painful periods and even infertility.

sacral ligaments that attach the uterus to the sacrum and twist the sacrum. Sometimes the sacral rotation does not resolve after delivery.

A rotated sacrum can also distort the uterus. If a woman has the misfortune of delivering on a surgery table with her feet in stirrups, rotating the legs outward to remove them from the stirrups can jam the sacrum. She would do better if her legs were internally rotated (so the knees move closer together) when removed from the stirrups. If compromised, the sacrum can distort the shape of the uterus. I suspect that sometimes a distorted uterus can no longer properly clamp down on and seal up the blood vessels that open up with menstruation.

To treat Carlotta, I rotated her sacrum back between the hipbones, rebalanced her sacrum, and, using a vaginal approach, untwisted and repositioned her uterus. After two treatments, all hemorrhaging ceased and she was able to keep her uterus.

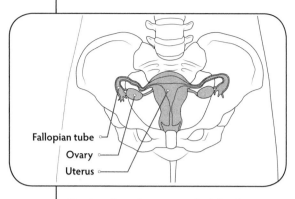

Fallopian tube
Ovary
Uterus

Uterine distortions can make it hard for the fallopian tube to catch the egg when it is released from the ovary.

Anatomy helps explain the anecdotal evidence that manual medicine treatments can help promote fertility. The fallopian tubes funnel out from the top of the uterus on each side, and at the end of the tubes, sea-anemone-like fingers reach toward the nearby ovaries so they can catch the monthly release of an egg. Twist the uterus, and the fingers may not quite reach the released egg. Then the egg cannot be transported to the uterus to be fertilized.

I speculate also that the proper fluttering of these fingers on the ovary may aid the ovary's job of releasing hormones in a full and balanced manner. I have certainly found that a contentedly rocking, happy sacrum seems to contribute to hormonal health.

Nineteenth-century medicine misinterpreted the uterus's role in hormonal balance to create the doctrine of hysteria. When women behaved in ways deemed inappropriate, medicine decided it was the fault of a misbehaving uterus. In some cases, physicians claimed that the obstreperous uterus would detach itself from its pelvic moorings and wander through the body, creating all sorts of mischief. When it wandered up into the neck to choke women, they were thought to scream out in uncontrollable ways. Removing the uterus became a medically respectable way of treating hysteria—hence the name hysterectomy. Fortunately, modern medicine has a much better understanding of the uterus's actual talents and failings.

After treating more than a hundred pregnant women, I have repeatedly found their pregnancies are much easier if they receive osteopathic treatment. I have also found that their deliveries are generally two to four hours shorter as well as less painful. Of course, making sure the sacrum moves freely between the hipbones is an essential aspect of their treatment. This, too, makes anatomical sense. Healthy mobility of the sacrum generally adds two to three millimeters of room in the pelvis. The baby has that much extra room to slide through.

THE SACRUM AND DIGESTIVE HEALTH

The parasympathetic nervous system, which controls gastrointestinal motility, lives in the sacrum and passes its nerves through holes in that bone. Problems with the sacrum's position and motion tend to have a profound effect on digestive

Many people don't realize that the pelvis and the gastrointestinal system are intimately related. Attention to the sacrum can have a profound effect on digestive problems.

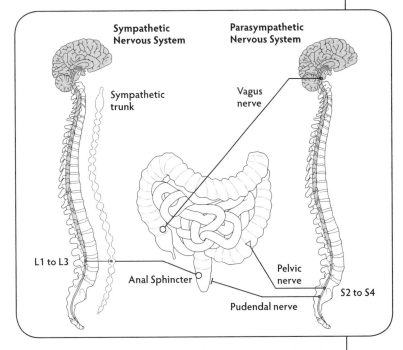

health. Many times, when someone has come in to see me for some musculoskeletal problem, they only mention in passing they've had digestive problems for years. They don't realize that the pelvis and the gastrointestinal system are intimately related. The movement of waste through the large intestine is orchestrated mostly by nerves coming from the sacrum. Attention to the sacrum and pelvis is one of the ways osteopathy can have a profound effect on digestive problems, addressing everything from irritable bowel problems to constipation and abdominal pain. Sacral problems are often reflected in the large intestines. When sacral and lumbar issues are treated, problems in the lower gut often clear up.

Osteopathic care is especially invaluable after abdominal surgery. Even if the intestines are treated with reverence, abdominal surgery tends to irritate the gut so that the autonomous nervous system gets very upset. Feeling under attack, the gut goes into hibernation and gut motion (peristalsis) stops. If the postoperative slowing and shutting down of the gut (known as ileus) lasts more than forty-eight hours, it is considered pathological. Ileus shows up as constipation and the inability to pass gas. Both of these can be quite painful. Osteopathic manual medicine's success in preventing postoperative ileus (POI) has been confirmed in research studies dating back to 1965.

In 2009, a retrospective analysis of 331 patients with POI found that patients who received osteopathic manipulative therapy (OMT) recovered from ileus much more quickly, and the length of their hospital stay was approximately 2.8 days less. A more recent 2011 study performed in a Brooklyn hospital had even more dramatic results. The patients had all undergone major gastrointestinal operations (small or large bowel restrictions, or gastric resection or repair). Bowel function returned approximately one and a half days sooner for the group receiving OMT and their hospital stay averaged five days less. These remarkable results were achieved after a single fifteen to thirty-five minute treatment with OMT within forty-eight hours of surgery.

When I worked in hospitals, I was frequently called in following abdominal surgery to help wake up the patient's gut and get it moving again. I recently visited a friend who had just undergone major abdominal surgery. To nurture the gut and help her parasympathetic nervous system wake up, I put my hand under her sacrum. Like those of so many other patients I have treated after similar surgeries, her sacrum had lost most of its motion. I ever so gently encouraged the sacrum's motion. Within minutes, her gut started to gurgle. The gastrointestinal system had begun its slow and steady march back to function. The profound effectiveness of OMT in such postoperative cases is important not only for patient comfort but also because OMT markedly diminishes the likelihood of the potentially dangerous consequences of surgery: infection, poor wound healing, and dangerous drug reactions.

I have found that once the sacrum or pelvis is significantly restricted, you will usually need the help of a skilled practitioner of manual medicine to assist in recovery. Even after thirty years of practice, I am constantly amazed at what miracles of healing occur when I pay proper attention to the sacrum. Consequently, I almost always start my treatments there.

There is much that you can do to help restore motion and balance to your pelvis and sacrum. If the imbalance is not severe or long-standing, pelvic and sacral motion and alignment often can be helped by yoga, Pilates, and physical therapy. In chapter 18, I include some helpful exercises and practices to restore motion to the sacrum. But perhaps the best way to pump life back into the sacrum and pelvis is sexual healing, which comes next.

14

Sexual Healing

Sex gives us some of our greatest joy and yet creates our deepest despair. Pain and injury can have a dastardly role in making our sexual life miserable by interfering with any of the numerous parts that take us from desire through arousal into the thrilling land of orgasm. Or we can just hurt too much to want to bother. To make matters worse, pain and injury often make people feel less attractive and less deserving of sexual attention.

I am not a sex therapist and don't presume to give advice when the frustrating tentacles of unfulfilled desire clutch at your heart. But if you are having difficulties or just lack of desire caused by pain or injury, I can offer some simple solutions. Throughout this book I emphasize people's right—indeed, their responsibility—to provide themselves pleasure to accelerate their healing. I have profound respect for sex's ability to promote healing, so I encourage sexual pleasure, whether provided by yourself or by a lover. Sexual pleasure promotes luscious fluid flow, helps calm an irritated nervous system, diminishes chronic pain cycles, helps restore motion to jammed areas, and floods the body with healing chemicals. When sex involves an attentive partner, it can bring back some of the intimacy that pain steals away. This chapter will help people understand why an injury not only causes a headache but also smacks away desire, and what to do about it.

First, I discuss the three stages of sexual response and which parts of our being contribute to each stage's success. I'll talk about the ways trauma and pain undermine each stage. After that I offer suggestions on how to avoid pain and promote satisfaction, as well as a few other delightful hints. I include advice for heterosexual and gay couples alike as well as for people to pleasure themselves.

STAGE 1: Desire

While desire is a multifaceted interplay of body and mind, the brain is the main orchestrator. Pleasurable brain chemicals like oxytocin, norepinephrine, and vasopressin are released the second we see someone we find attractive. The brain also releases dopamine, the gotta-have-it chemical of desire. Dopamine not only lights up desire but also propels us across a crowded room. Like all of the body's chemicals, dopamine does not limit itself to one function; it also stimulates arousal and lubrication.

When we fall in love, the brain releases chemicals that resemble the endorphin rush of cocaine. No wonder some people become addicted to falling in love and hop from person to person. I don't recommend that way of pleasuring yourself—no more than I recommend a cocaine habit. I mention the power of these brain chemicals to emphasize that the brain is our most important sex organ. Fantasy can take some people all the way from desire through arousal to orgasm by enlisting these magnificent brain chemicals. People can have very satisfying sex in their dreams.

Delicious hormones play a critical role in desire. In women, the kick of progesterone produced by the ovaries during ovulation can send desire through the roof. Estrogen keeps the reproductive system responsive and fertile. Desire in women is also stoked by testosterone, which plays a role in both female and male arousal and orgasm.

The male testes produce the male sex hormones called androgens, of which testosterone is the most abundant. Testosterone is essential not only for desire but also for performance. All these sex hormones are fats (steroids) created primarily from cholesterol—provided by the liver. Once again, the liver is critical, and it's time cholesterol gets some of the respect it deserves.

Bladder
Symphysis pubis
Vas deferens
Seminal vesicle
Ejaculatory duct
Prostate gland
Anus
Urethra
Glans penis
Epididymis
Testis

The male reproductive system.

Many parts of the brain have fingers in this sexually tantalizing piece of desire. However, a little love triangle called the hypothalamic-pituitary-gonadal axis (HPGA) is probably the most essential. The hypothalamus sits right above the pituitary gland in the brain and feeds hormones and nervous impulses into the pituitary that tell it how to act.

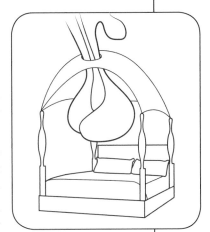

And act it does! The pituitary produces or influences the production of every other hormone in the body. It regulates desire by secreting hormones that tell the testes and ovaries how much testosterone, estrogen, and progesterone to produce. The posterior of the pituitary secretes oxytocin, one of the brain's love drugs, which also helps female lubrication, performance, and satisfaction, including the rhythmic contraction of the uterus in orgasm.

This magical pituitary gland swings back and forth in the exact center of the skull. It hangs from a stalk of tissue over a bony outcropping called the sella turcica (Turk's saddle). To me, the sella turcica looks like a four-poster bed with a canopy over it. (How fitting for the master gland of sex to hang over a bed.) This canopy is made up of connective tissue called meninges and has a hole in the middle for the stalk of the pituitary. A freely moving, happy pituitary gland is necessary for every aspect of good sex, from desire to orgasm. When the pituitary is bouncing off of bent bedposts or its swing is off-kilter as a result of trauma, bye-bye to the hormones of lust.

STAGE 2: Arousal

Once we have desire, second base is arousal. Arousal is also an interplay of body and mind, though feelings of arousal generally depend on specific nerve pathways from our erogenous zones to the brain. We need a dynamic balance between the sympathetic and parasympathetic nervous systems to bring us through arousal and performance to climax.

In females, stimulation of the clitoris (for many women, the most exquisitely powerful promoter of desire and arousal), the vulva, the vagina—especially the entrance (introitis)—and the rest of the perineal region (the bits around the genitals and anus) enthuse females with desire and arousal. We feel these tantalizing sensations thanks to the brain and the neurological pathways of pleasure. Nerves from these areas funnel through the sacrum to a large network of nerves called the sacral plexus. The sacral plexus rushes pleasure signals to the spinal cord and

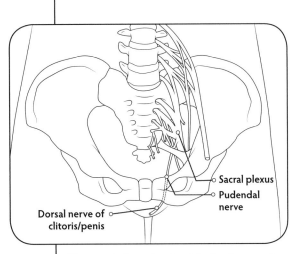

Sacral plexus
Pudendal nerve
Dorsal nerve of clitoris/penis

The sacral plexus is critical for both arousal and orgasm. The dorsal nerve of the clitoris or penis originates from the sacral plexus.

up to the brain, where the brain's pleasure centers send instructions back down the same pathway. These instructions tell the parasympathetic nervous system (PNS)—ironically, the rest-and-digest system—to dilate the blood vessels in clitoral erectile tissue. Signals from the PNS also cause the entrance of the vagina (introitus) to narrow, which, if it is enjoying the penis's strokes, provides the penis with more pleasure. The PNS instructs the lubricating Bartholin's glands (strange that they are named after a man) to secrete mucus into the entrance of the vagina to provide vaginal lubrication.

Breast and nipple stimulation can also transmit sexual pleasure through the thoracic nerves in the midback into the spinal cord and the brain. Attention to the breasts can induce sensations that run the gamut from desire and arousal to orgasm.

Similarly in men, the PNS signals coming from the sacral portion of the spinal cord cause the penis to fill with blood and become erect. (I was so disappointed to learn at sixteen that this is called a hard-on. When I had first heard the phrase several years earlier, I had heard it as "heart-on." I think having a heart-on is much more poetic.)

The tip of the penis, like the clitoris, is generally the most exquisitely sensitive tissue. Stimulation of the skin around or inside the anus, the scrotum, and the perineal region can also stimulate desire and arousal. These sensations travel the same sacral and neurological pathways as in women. And according to my gay male friends, the recipient of rectal penetration can experience orgasm.

If any part of this pleasure highway is damaged or compromised—the nerve fibers going to or from the genital regions, the sacrum, the spinal cord, or the brain—arousal and orgasm can find themselves alone and frustrated, exiled in their own barren wasteland, never to be enjoyed.

STAGE 3: Orgasm

Now, the sympathetic nervous system (SNS) gets a turn. The SNS nerves originate in the thoracic and lumbar parts of the spinal cord. In women, continued stimulation of the clitoris and/or vagina initiates an SNS reflex that feeds into

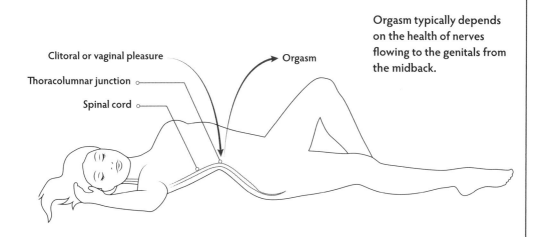

Clitoral or vaginal pleasure

Thoracolumnar junction

Spinal cord

Orgasm

Orgasm typically depends on the health of nerves flowing to the genitals from the midback.

the midback area, and then bounces back to the genitals to help create orgasm. At the same time, the pleasured brain releases oxytocin from the pituitary gland to increase the uterus's joyous, rhythmic contraction. The PNS, not wanting to be left out, causes the blood vessels at the vaginal entrance to swell, further contracting the entrance. The brain responds to all this stimulus by temporarily increasing whole-body muscle tension—tension that soon leads to the most marvelous release, then relaxation and peace.

The male orgasm depends on a similar interplay between the PNS and SNS. Triggered by the lovely squeezing of the penis by a vagina, rectum, or hand, the reflex centers of the spinal cord emit sympathetic impulses that leave the spinal cord from the thoracic and lumbar junction and pass to the genitalia. This expels sperm into the urethra inside the penis, creating pleasurable sensations that speed to the sacral spinal cord and excite rhythmic contraction in the penis, resulting in ejaculation.

While orgasm is certainly not just a spinal reflex, it helps to have that neural circuit functioning well. Unfortunately, the sympathetic nerves exit the spinal cord at the thoracic-lumbar junction, a region where the spine switches its curve. That makes the area especially susceptible to injury. When injury happens, sexual satisfaction can go down the drain.

THE THIEVES OF DESIRE

Successful and pleasurable sex depends on the health of every part of this pleasure circuit. Trauma can damage any part of this circuit—the brain, sacrum, low back, spinal nerves—or just cause enough pain to stop desire or performance in its tracks. I'll talk about the ways trauma can interfere with our sexual pleasure and how osteopathy can help heal these problems and restore sexual function. Later, I'll talk about the things you and your partner can do to heal sexuality and enhance sexual pleasure.

Hormonal Disruption and Depression

Hormonal disruption is one of the thieves of desire. Because the brain holds the controls to so much of our sexual pleasure, it's not surprising that brain injury can stamp out desire. Traumatic brain injury compromises the function of the pituitary gland almost half the time, and that can cause production of sex hormones to plummet. In women, failure of the pituitary to do its job can interfere with desire, arousal, vaginal lubrication, and orgasm. In men, a dysfunctional pituitary can interfere with desire and his ability to have or maintain an erection. The pituitary's failure to sufficiently stimulate the thyroid gland can also lead to such tremendous fatigue that sex becomes an annoying bother.

I will talk in more detail in the section on brain injury about how easily trauma can slam the tender pituitary gland against the posts of the four-poster bed over which it swings. Trauma can also bend these bedposts (the clinoid processes), leaving the poor pituitary to swing unevenly as it moves from side to side with the pulsations of the brain. An off-kilter or battered pituitary can slack off on the production of the hormones of sex, including progesterone, testosterone, estrogen, and oxytocin, leaving us too uninterested to bother with sex. Disruption of these hormones, of course, can also lead to other problems: vaginal dryness, erectile problems, and problems with orgasm.

Fortunately, the posts of the pituitary's bed can sometimes be straightened by a practitioner well versed in appropriate cranial treatment. In the chapter on treating traumatic brain injury, I discuss how I use the dural membranes that attach to the bedposts to fix them. This can help the patient regain some, if not all, of their pituitary function and sexual prowess.

Hormones produced by the thyroid, at the direction of the pituitary, regulate the body's energy production. If the pituitary's unhappiness has affected the production

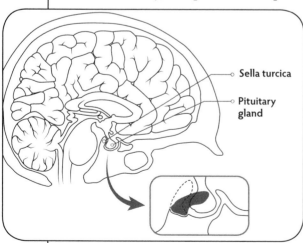

Sella turcica

Pituitary gland

A bent clinoid process can stop sex in its tracks.

of thyroid hormones, straightening out the bedposts can help relieve the extreme fatigue that often accompanies traumatic brain injury. Of course, the thyroid gland might be slacking off on hormone production for other reasons. Sitting exposed on the front of the windpipe, it's vulnerable to neck trauma. If lab tests show that the pituitary is fine but the patient is still tremendously fatigued, the head and neck may need some manual treatment to restore the thyroid's vitality.

While cranial osteopathic work can do wonders to restore hormonal function, it may also be important to work with a neurologist and an endocrinologist who understand the relationship of brain injury to hormonal problems and the possible need for hormonal supplementation.

Depression is not just a thief of desire; it can deeply wound the spirit and soul. More than half the victims of traumatic brain injury suffer from depression a year later. Even among patients who sustained a seemingly minor physical trauma, 18 percent will still suffer from major depression twelve months later.

We don't know all the reasons that depression is so common and lingers on after injury, but increasingly, depression is being regarded as one of many diseases linked to inflammation. Inflammation disrupts the chemicals in the brain associated with the regulation of mood, including the neurotransmitters dopamine, serotonin, and noradrenaline. Since inflammation is the body's way of healing from injury, that would explain why depression is so common after trauma. It would also explain why the same things that can reduce inflammation—such as reducing injury shock, eating an anti-inflammatory diet, exercise, and meditation—can have a powerful, curative effect on depression. Practices that free up the diaphragm and the breath, such as manual medicine, yoga, or swimming, can help resolve depression. Reducing chronically high levels of cortisol by removing injury shock can also help. Losing weight, acupuncture, and tai chi are just some of the ways in which a person can effectively take charge of this part of their healing.

Depression has been thought of primarily as a problem with brain chemistry—too much of this, not enough of that—so the standard treatment has been drugs that alter the brain's chemicals. I certainly believe that antidepressants can be the right choice for some people. But some of these drugs, such as Prozac, Zoloft, and other selective serotonin reuptake inhibitors (SSRI), may depress sexual desire. Besides pharmaceuticals, it is also important to consider approaches like the ones I've mentioned, which have been shown to bring significant relief of depression. Psychotherapy also can be helpful.

I wish I had a magic wand or a single treatment that could take away all my patients' suffering from this terrible, debilitating condition. There is no denying that it takes the joy out of sex—and of life—for far too many people. I have found that treating the diaphragm and restoring motion to injured areas, particularly in the skull, have the most profound effect in relieving depression. I have treated quite a few patients with posttraumatic depression who showed startling improvement when treated with a combination of homeopathy and cranial osteopathy.

Once you've stoked up desire, which generally means that the brain is doing pretty well, the rest will usually take off on its own. But when desire isn't enough to thrust the body forward toward orgasm, then the neurological pathways of sex may have been waylaid somewhere along the way. Trauma anywhere in the spine can interfere with the neural circuits between the genitals and the brain. Here are some of the usual suspects.

Pelvic Pain and Dysfunction

The first place where the pleasure circuit can be compromised is the magnificent pelvis, which lets us not only walk but also reproduce and enjoy sex. The pelvis is made up of three bones, the big innominate or hipbones, which wrap from front to back, and the sacrum, the triangle-shaped bone that wedges between them. Misalignment of the sacrum in the pelvis is common after many kinds of trauma and can cause pelvic pain, pain with intercourse, and problems with the nerves to and from the genitals.

For women, a well-aligned sacrum is essential in order to comfortably spread their legs. When the misalignment of the sacrum causes pelvic pain, sex becomes very uninviting. Women are more susceptible to pelvic problems because their pelvic ligaments tend to be looser and the sacrum shorter and wider in order to facilitate pregnancy and childbirth. If the sacrum has been rotated to one side, the ligaments on the other side typically become over-stretched and complain loudly. This sacroiliac pain tends to be a burning pain that runs up and down on the side of the buttocks' crack. Twisting increases the burning sensation, so the gyrations of sex can be quite painful and further strain these ligaments.

The main pathways of pleasurable feelings are the tangle of nerves that run either through holes in the sacrum or pass nearby it. Sacral distortions can hold these nerves hostage so they can't initiate sex's wonderful sensations. If you feel passion, but then the penis doesn't rise enthusiastically, or the vagina fails to lubricate or the clitoris to engorge, nerves to this area might be compromised by a twist in the sacrum.

The sacrum can be brought back into proper position through manual therapy, as I talk about in the chapters on back pain and sacral health. In two or three weeks, once the sacroiliac ligaments are mended, some gentle sex can get fluid to the region and help it heal.

Fluid Congestion

Trauma has a tendency to cause fluid congestion in the pelvis. The abdomen and pelvis are ripe with lymphatic channels that remove excess fluid and cellular debris, but they can easily become overwhelmed and clogged after trauma.

As I discussed in the previous chapter, the wise pelvis has created its own mini-diaphragm to help pump away fluids. This pelvic diaphragm is a sheath of muscle and fascia slung between the penis and rectum or between the vagina and rectum and anchored to the tailbone (coccyx). Since the coccyx is at the end of the sacrum, twists in the sacrum twist the coccyx and with it the pelvic diaphragm, weakening the diaphragm's ability to pump. The resulting fluid buildup can cause prostate problems in men and menstrual cramps and painful intercourse in women.

The sacrum needs to be properly aligned for the pump to function and for the sacral nerves that are the key to pleasure to transmit properly. Kegel exercises (see page 215) can help both men and women to strengthen and empower their pelvic diaphragm. Sex itself is a wonderful way to pump the pelvic diaphragm.

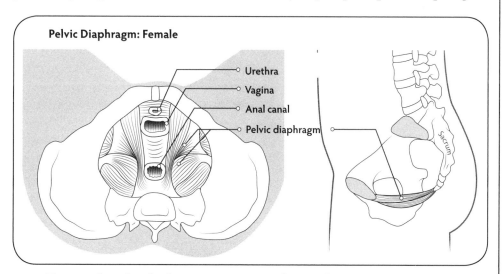

Pelvic Diaphragm: Female

- Urethra
- Vagina
- Anal canal
- Pelvic diaphragm

The muscular pelvic diaphragm promotes not only reproductive health and pleasure but also the health of the low back.

Cauda Equina Syndrome

If the penis won't rise or there's numbness around the penis, scrotum, vagina, and/or clitoris, it may signal a serious problem called cauda equina syndrome. This is a rare condition in which a disc or bony fragment presses on nerves to the pelvis. Other serious symptoms can include leaking of urine or the bowels.

If this happens, see your doctor or go **to the emergency room immediately!** It can require emergency surgery.

Low-Back Pain

Back pain can ruin your sex life. Even if the mind is willing, the prospect of suffering debilitating pain can put the kibosh on your most intimate moments. But there is no need for you to suffer needlessly from back pain. Because it's such a common affliction, I've included a whole chapter on it. Most of the time, even chronic back pain can be relieved with proper treatment and care. Restoring the free movement of the sacrum, the pelvic diaphragm, and the abdominal diaphragm is critical to restoring the back to health.

Problems with Orgasm

If you have moved through desire and arousal but cannot reach orgasm, there may not be enough juice coming down from the critical spinal nerves in the lower thoracic region to bring the body to climax. Injury or pressure on the spinal nerves that usually fire the reflexes of genital orgasm can make orgasm a distant memory.

Orgasm is as complicated as sex is. It's certainly not just about spinal reflexes—women and men can have orgasms without any genital stimulation at all, and the body has provided an alternate pleasure pathway through the vagus nerve that completely bypasses the spinal cord. That is why people with spinal cord injury can still experience orgasm.

I talked about the treatment for spinal nerve problems in the back-pain chapter. Releasing muscle spasm, freeing the diaphragm, aligning the sacrum, and making sure the spine moves freely can take the pressure off these sexy nerves. There's no magic in this, though it may seem magical afterward.

An Unhappy Liver

> *"I warrant you, sir; the white cold virgin snow upon my heart*
> *abates the ardour of my liver."*
> Ferdinand, in The Tempest, *Act IV, Scene I*

Listen to Shakespeare: an excellent liver is essential for passion. I know you're probably chomping at the bit to get to practical suggestions, but as Shakespeare did, I have to give the liver its due.

Most of the cholesterol needed to make sex hormones is formed in the liver. The liver takes the big master hormone pregnenolone and decides whether it gets modified into progesterone, testosterone, or estrogen. It also breaks down unneeded sex hormones and regulates the hormonal balance necessary for full and vibrant sexual function. The liver can have a role in one of the main problems of female fulfillment—a dry vagina created by insufficient estrogen.

Stress causes the diversion of pregnonelone to cortisol at the expense of testosterone, estrogen, and progesterone. Since testosterone and progesterone are drivers of desire, and estrogen is necessary for female lubrication, stress can cause the liver to diminish the hormones of lust. The forces of trauma can toss this heavy organ about, causing it to twist around its attachments to the diaphragm, the abdomen, and other digestive organs. In turn, the twisted and now-congested liver pulls on the diaphragm, causing the diaphragm to go into spasm, shortening breath. The spasming diaphragm then further pulls on the liver.

My job as an osteopathic physician is to lead the liver back home and tuck it back in its bed, where it snuggles up against the diaphragm. Once the liver is nicely in place, the person feels better and the liver can better put together the necessary hormones. Sexual desire increases. Pleasure increases. Orgasms get richer—and your liver can burn with passion again, like Ferdinand's in *The Tempest*.

STEPS TO SEXUAL HEALING

You now know numerous reasons that trauma can chase sex drive away and understand why, in the case of sex and trauma, anatomy is destiny.

If someone gets their full sex drive back soon, that's a good sign. My male patients tell me that their sex drive comes back pretty quickly. Women generally need more time. Well, I'm sorry, but spreading your legs and making that juicy space available is physically harder for women. And since women's hormones are infinitely more complicated than men's, women's hormones are much easier to upset and harder to fix.

There is much you can do to regain your sexual desire and performance, however. As I said earlier, most of this chapter provides suggestions that apply to heterosexual and gay couples alike. If you are single, please modify them. Being single, you still have a right and responsibility to provide yourself sexual pleasure. Your body relishes touch, which you can provide yourself.

If you have a partner, intimacy interrupts the isolation of illness and pain. Even if you don't feel desire, try touch. Kind touch itself heals; kind touch sends in endorphins, soothes the crying nervous system. Touch commandeers the spinal pathways that transmit pain, often muffling the pain signals' attempts to reach the brain. Injury tends to make you feel broken. Attentive, caring touch reassures your body and mends together the broken bits. Tenderness coaxes hope into your tissues. Kind embrace removes isolation and makes you feel connected and cared for.

So bathe your body in touch, luxuriate in tenderness, and awaken desire, which will help kick in anti-inflammatory hormones (progesterone, growth hormone, testosterone). If you are better able to hear and respect your sexual feelings, this will help you acknowledge other good feelings and you will be better able to provide your body with the tools of healing.

This all sounds very good, but there is also another reality that can make sexual healing very difficult. Many people have grown up feeling ashamed of sexual feelings and desires. Others have had brutal or disastrous sexual experiences. For others, sexual activity is linked with painful rejection.

I encourage you to use this recovery process from injury and pain as an opportunity for a fresh start. Here are some guidelines for your journey:

Acknowledge your feelings. What do you feel, and what do you want? Both may differ from what you experienced before.

Communicate clearly and patiently what you want. Encourage your partner to touch you, hold you, caress, and stroke you. Tell them what feels good. Whether the touch feels magnificent or too rough, communicate your reaction.

Women can have problems asking for what they need if they feel they don't have the right to experience pleasure. Assert your right to enjoyment. Guys often have a lot of trouble asking for what they need because they feel they've got to be in charge. These can happen even in gay relationships. Gentlemen, you've got to tell your partner what you want. Take it as an excuse to tell your partner secret desires you've not articulated before. If you want your penis or balls licked, tell your partner. You get to ask for a blow job. Most of the time, a blow job will be a lot easier on you than intercourse.

Be selfish. Absorb the physical kindness. Take time for yourself. This is not greedy—it's necessary. It's especially important because most women need fifteen to thirty minutes of gentle, rhythmic clitoral stimulation before they are ready to achieve orgasm.

Accept lack of desire for the time being. You can still relish touch. Your body may be marshaling all its energy to rebuild injured cells. Encourage sex (and have your partner do so), but do not demand. For many of us, kind, reassuring touch stimulates desire.

Give your partner the main work to do. The person with the greatest injury dictates position. The injured person usually does best lying on their back with good neck support and support under their arms. But a heavy person on top could smash together sore bits, so the injured person may do best lying on their side while hugging their partner or a pillow.

For some women, heterosexual intercourse is easier and more pleasurable when they lie on their side in the spoon position and the man enters the vagina from behind. This position doesn't require her to spread her legs as much and risk further straining her sacroiliac joints. An injured woman may find receiving oral sex not only pleasurable but also much easier on her body if she's lying on her back.

View the injury as a chance to explore pleasurable and comfortable positions. Injury can break the ice of shyness and help couples develop new and stimulating practices. For example, a woman might find herself comfortable sitting astride her male partner on his back with his penis full mast. The woman can lower herself down, maintaining control of her movements. But please avoid extensions (backward bending) of the lower back and neck, particularly flexion-extension injuries (also called whiplash), as that can further insult areas injured by trauma. Unless your knees hurt, you should be able to have some good fun in that position. Try other varieties of sitting. Have the man sit on a chair. Sit on his lap, either facing him (quite a bit harder on the sacroiliac joints) or facing away (easier on the sacroiliacs).

Avoid arching the neck and low back. If you are the one lying on top for intercourse, this puts your low back into an arch or extension. For most victims of car accidents, this will hurt. Similarly, arching of the neck with intercourse or oral sex can strain the poor neck. Wearing a cervical collar may protect you, especially if you tend to get a bit carried away. (Maybe we can start a new fetish: brightly colored cervical collars.)

Don't stress about going for the gold. Orgasms are great if they happen, but getting there might take more work than the bruised body can manage. Do not fret too much, but if you are having new sexual difficulties, do report this fact to your physician right away—for instance, if you're used to having orgasms and now can't. Inability to orgasm may be another sign of the cauda equina syndrome, which I mentioned earlier.

But let's assume you have no serious medical or neurological problem. If the orgasm doesn't oblige, accept the pleasure and don't push for orgasm. Your pelvic muscles may not want all that clenching and squeezing. The hormones may not have fully recovered. The nerves to the genitals may have gotten slammed and may need time to recover.

Address vaginal dryness. Women who never had vaginal dryness suddenly can have trouble with dryness after trauma. You can buy a product like Emerita feminine personal moisturizer (produced by Emerson Ecologic) as a lubricant. But dryness also can be an indication of hormone imbalance or a sign of allergies. If the inside of the nose is raw and inflamed, often the vagina is, too. Your nose screams at you when it's burning and raw, but you tend not to notice a dry vagina unless you're trying to have sex. Taking antihistamines may stop the nose from running, but they can further dry out the raw vagina and make penetration intolerable.

If a woman has persistent vaginal dryness or sexual dysfunction after an accident, I strongly recommend she undergo testing of her thyroid and sex hormones, including estrogen, progesterone, and testosterone. Imbalance or decrease of any of these hormones can affect sexual function and often be remedied with supplemental hormones in the form of estriol cream applied directly to the vagina.

Choose oral sex. As you are healing, oral sex can be just what the doctor ordered, so lie back and enjoy it. If you've never asked for oral sex before, give it a try. This applies to women as well. If your partner isn't very good at it, this is a great time to ask him or her to explore with a gentle touch and tongue the clitoris and vagina. And luckily, vaginal dryness isn't an issue with oral sex.

However, no performing oral sex with a bum neck. Anyone who's been in an accident shouldn't provide their partner with oral sex until their neck heals. With a bad neck, the extension you have to put your neck into for oral sex is bad. Later, when your cervical spine gets better, protect your neck by putting a pillow on the floor at the foot of the bed and kneeling on it. Then bring your lover down to the edge of the bed. That puts your injured neck at a better angle. This slight cervical flexion (forward bending) is a better position.

Be thoughtful about birth control and pregnancy. Heterosexual couples may need to readjust their birth control usage. If possible, please have the non-injured party use the birth control. A diaphragm that worked before an injury may not fit tightly any more in the distorted pelvis, meaning intercourse could now result in pregnancy. Or the diaphragm that was comfortable before suddenly becomes painful. Be sure to get the diaphragm or cervical cap rechecked. And please don't start birth control pills right after an accident—don't force your injured body to adjust to strange chemicals.

I also advise new victims of an accident to avoid getting pregnant until they receive proper treatment. Maintaining a pregnancy—or having an abortion—are both very hard on an injured body. I have seen women with a seriously injured pelvis have trouble maintaining a pregnancy. I've seen very difficult births for both the mother and the baby after the mother's pelvis has been distorted by an accident. If you are already pregnant when you are in an accident, try to get your pelvis balanced by a gentle and qualified practitioner of manual medicine before giving birth.

Anal sex may be a problem if there is a sacral injury. Please try to avoid it until the sacrum and nerves passing through it recover. Of course, the partner receiving rectal penetration, whether male or female, must always prepare first with a rectal douche to empty the rectum of stool. Otherwise, anal intercourse can lead to serious trauma to the lower intestine, including possible rupture and death.

Experiment with sexual aids. Sex toys can help restimulate sexual desire. Vibrators or a water nozzle on the clitoris can improve sexual pleasure and may help reignite sexual appetite. Both women and men may be helped by pornography or sexual aids. If you are on your own or have a sexually unavailable partner, providing sexual pleasure for yourself can be very healing, but injury may have compromised your ability to give yourself pleasure. If you used to be able to satisfy yourself but now masturbation hurts your wrist, neck, or back, a sexual aid may come in handy. As I recommend repeatedly throughout the book, learn to listen to and respect your feelings and desires. Try to express them in a safe and healthy way; tender and/or passionate sex is one of the most profoundly empowering ways.

Talk with a therapist. Just as proper anatomical alignment and function can be helpful in fulfillment and optimal pleasure, a good psychotherapist can also help people address psychological issues that restrict sexual pleasure. There is a whole specialty within the therapy field that focuses on these very personal issues.

Sex is a wonderful and healing part of life that injury can steal away. Sexual pleasure helps the body regain its healing trajectory. Please do not be ashamed; learn to luxuriate in your body and the gifts it can give you.

15

Restoring Motion to the Chest

Patients who have mysterious health problems with the neck, shoulders, lungs, or heart do not usually connect those symptoms to chest trauma. Yet a stagnant chest can open the floodgates of disease and pain, unleashing allergies, bronchitis and pneumonia in the lungs, palpitations in the heart, and severe pain in the neck and back. It can also trigger anxiety, fatigue, and depression in the mind.

Because of its massive size, the chest is often injured in trauma. In fact, it's hard to imagine a fall or a car accident that does not in some way involve the chest. Chest trauma can be extremely serious and must often be immediately evaluated by appropriate medical personnel. My focus is not on acute trauma but on the residual consequences of that trauma.

In earlier chapters, I discussed how trauma involving the chest can lock the body into injury shock. In this chapter, I talk about how loss of motion to the ribs, lungs, heart, and diaphragm can cause many other problems. Once you understand how the parts of this marvelous structure work together, you will have a clearer understanding of how an unhappy chest can affect your health. There is much you can do to restore motion and health to the chest's critical structures. Whether you work to fix these problems yourself or need the assistance of a trained practitioner, knowing the cause of your symptoms is essential to knowing what questions to ask and what steps to take to heal them.

When people think about chest injury, they think of the ribs and lungs, and sometimes the heart. Rarely does the diaphragm cross their radar. Yet if I could only address one structure in the body, it would be the diaphragm. I introduced this amazing hero in the section on injury shock, where I discussed

Symptoms Associated with Lack of Motion in the Chest

- Anxiety
- Back and neck pain
- Bronchitis and flu
- Breast lumps
- Depression
- Fatigue
- Immune problems
- Painful breathing
- Arrhythmias
- Heart palpitations
- High blood pressure
- Pericarditis
- Constipation
- Pneumonia
- Allergies
- Chest pain

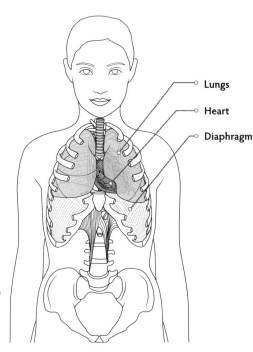

Lungs

Heart

Diaphragm

The diaphragm is intimately tied to the lungs, the lymphatic system, and the heart, and its enthusiastic pumping keeps them vibrant and healthy.

its importance in restoring calm to the nervous system. In the lumbar chapter, I showed how the diaphragm is essential for the health of the spine. Here I focus on the way the diaphragm maintains the health of the lungs and heart.

It is said that Native Americans regard the diaphragm as the boundary between heaven and earth. It divides the chest from the abdomen, with the organs of spirit—the heart, lungs, and brain—above it and the organs of earth—digestion, reproduction, and excretion—below it. But the diaphragm is more than a boundary or partition. It is the body's vital pump.

The chest does not simply contain the heart and lungs. The chest's organs, muscles, fluids, bones, nerves, and fascia move together and assist each other in an intricate ballet orchestrated by the diaphragm. The lung's protective covering spreads out over the diaphragm's surface, and the thick wrapper surrounding the heart also adheres to the surface. The constant pulsations of the diaphragm tug and release these organs, massaging and invigorating them. The heart's great vessels pierce the diaphragm on their way to and from the lower organs, and the diaphragm's expansions and contractions help propel the circulating blood and promote lower blood pressure. The diaphragm's muscular attention to the lymphatics pushes their fluids and nutrients toward the heart. And, of course, its pumping expands and lifts the entire ribcage.

A blow to the chest or back can disrupt the diaphragm's motion and the motion of all the organs attached to it. These structures can also be harmed by twisting or rotational forces that spin them on their axes. Spinning forces generated by falls, bicycle crashes, car accidents, or football tackles toss the organs and their surrounding fascia into distorted positions and crimp nerves, blood supply, and lymphatic flow. These twists and compressions can cause the health problems I listed on the previous page, including heart arrhythmias, bronchitis, and immune problems.

The diaphragm and all the structures of the chest love to move. To them, vigorous motion is like winning the lottery. They soak up anything that assists their movement, whether that is yoga, manual medicine, Pilates, rocking in a rocking chair, or bouncing on a rebounder (a small trampoline). They thrill when we walk, swim, and jog. Because practitioners can put their hands right on them, the chest and diaphragm respond to manual medicine as a puppy does to its attentive mother.

EMILY. Moira was driving her four-year-old daughter, Emily, to school when a white van weaving through freeway traffic struck their car at 80 miles per hour. Moira's sedan spun out of control and plunged off an embankment.

An ambulance took Moira and Emily to the emergency room. Little Emily was severely shaken up, but because she had been tightly strapped into her five-point-harness child seat, she had been spared from more severe injury.

Within days of the accident, Emily developed a persistent cough that rattled her small frame day and night. Even her intermittent sleep didn't provide rest, as night terrors filled her dreams. As the cough turned into bronchitis, her mom took Emily to yet another doctor. Two rounds of antibiotics could not control Emily's devastating wet cough, which brought up thick green mucus. She had also developed terrible constipation, with painful abdominal swelling. Only after taking a laxative did she move her bowels.

A month after the accident, Emily's desperate mom brought her in to see me. When I examined Emily, she was still in injury shock. Her breathing was rapid and shallow and her chest barely expanded with each breath. The forces of the spinning car had pushed her into her forward restraints, jamming the front of her ribs into her sternum. Her traumatized, spasmed diaphragm hardly moved.

I could also feel that the back of her ribs had been shoved forcefully into her spine. That irritated the hubs of the sympathetic nervous system (SNS) lying

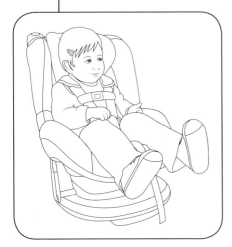

The restraints of Emily's car seat saved her life, but the compression of her ribs and diaphragm caused respiratory, immune, and digestive problems.

along the ribs, worsening the fight-or-flight response in her nervous system. The constant bath of stress hormones had overwhelmed Emily's restorative parasympathetic nervous system (PNS). Without the PNS to promote peristalsis (gut movement), her stool had backed up and become hard. She was profoundly constipated, and when she couldn't eliminate toxins, her body was forced to reabsorb some of them, which in turn further inflamed her body, making both her gut and lung inflammation worse.

Emily's poorly moving diaphragm caused stagnation in her lymphatic channels. As we saw in the chapter on inflammation, the vast lymphatic system removes toxins, cellular waste products, and excess fluid from the tissues. The lymphatics also are essential in the transport of white blood cells and the creation of antibodies that fight infection. The lymphatic system's circulation relies on body movement and the vigorous pumping of the diaphragm. When the diaphragm is not moving properly, lymphatic flow slows down.

Because of Emily's poorly moving diaphragm, her lymphatic circulation was sluggish. Fluid had stagnated in her lungs, breeding a host of bacteria that turned into chronic bronchitis. Once the infection started, the compromised lymphatics couldn't deliver enough of the immune cells that attack infection to the lungs.

My first job was to restore the diaphragm's powerful motions to assist Emily's sluggish lymphatics. I also needed to free up her jammed ribs and help wake up her restorative PNS so she could breathe more easily.

First, I coaxed Emily's diaphragm to relax and pulled her stuck ribs away from her spine. Releasing the ribs' compression on the spine and untwisting the binding fascia there helped her crippled lungs expand and took pressure off the sympathetic chain ganglion that had kept her body in injury shock. Once the SNS stopped screaming "ALERT!" the PNS started to wake from hibernation and began to coax her gut into action.

To invigorate her sluggish lymphatic flow, I applied a gentle yet powerful lymphatic pump to Emily's chest and belly. The slow, repetitive compression and release techniques helped loosen the mucus in Emily's lungs and aided the movement of lymph, which helped drain the clumps of infection. As the lymphatic system increased its flow, it recruited infection-fighting cells from many locations to attack the bacteria assaulting her lungs. My pumping also assisted the diaphragm's massage of the liver and adrenal glands, speeding up the flow of antibodies and hormones, and helped the movement of food and waste through her digestive system.

I also restored motion to Emily's sacrum to help calm the sympathetic nervous system and encourage gut motion. I gave her a high dose of homeopathic *Aconitum* and *Arnica* to address her shock and trauma.

Emily climbed off the treatment table taking much deeper breaths. That evening, she coughed up gobs of green mucus, then fell into a deep, peaceful sleep that lasted ten hours. After that first treatment, she slept undisturbed by nightmares. Her peaceful sleep showed that I'd removed much of the shock of the trauma and had begun to restore balance to her autonomic nervous system. Twenty-four hours after the treatment, she no longer had a cough. Though not yet at their optimal expansion, the ribs, diaphragm, and lungs had regained much of their motion, and

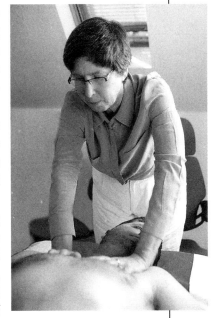

I use the lymphatic pump technique to increase the flow of lymphatic fluid, immune cells, and infection-fighting antibodies throughout the body.

the lymphatic channels in the lungs were flowing more freely. Most of the inflammation in her chest had eased. Two days later, Emily's bronchitis had completely resolved.

Magical as her treatment seemed, I knew that after such extensive trauma, Emily would need more care. Though her constipation improved somewhat with her treatment, it didn't totally resolve. I later gave her homeopathic *Papaver* to address her fear and constipation. That remedy markedly diminished her sense of fear and helped resolve her constipation. I continued to treat other traumatic influences of the collision. The dangerous bronchitis and tormenting nightmares never returned.

———————○———————

Emily's virulent bronchitis was not surprising to me. Chest injuries can cause many breathing problems.

The lungs fill up all the nooks and crannies in the chest not taken up by the heart. Being mostly filled with air, the lungs are the body's lightest organ.

The 1918 Spanish Flu

Before the advent of penicillin, osteopathic physicians kept flu patients who developed pneumonia alive using lymphatic pump techniques similar to the ones I applied to Emily. During the 1918 flu epidemic, a much greater percentage of patients survived under the care of osteopathic physicians (DOs) than did the patients of allopathic doctors (MDs). Contemporary studies have shown that the same lymphatic-pump techniques used successfully almost a hundred years ago can have dramatic healing effects on the course of recovery from pneumonia. Of course, I'm thrilled that we have antibiotics in our tool chest now, but they are not always enough.

A healthy lung looks like a big pink sponge because of its rich blood supply. The lungs have no muscle tissue. It is the pumping of the diaphragm and the expansion of the ribs that pulls air into them.

Every day, the lungs suffer a constant toxic assault of viruses, bacteria, air pollution, mold, dust, and allergens. To deal with this assault, the body produces three quarts of mucus a day to wash toxins from the sinuses and lungs. The body needs full, deep breathing to effectively scrub the respiratory pathways clean.

As with Emily, when trauma impedes the movement of the diaphragm, the ribs, and the lymphatics, the chest loses the power to flush this toxic mucus stew out of the lungs. This stew becomes a welcoming Petri dish that breeds viruses and bacteria and can result in bronchitis and even pneumonia that is resistant to treatment until motion is restored to the ribs and the diaphragm. The lack of motion also handcuffs the lungs' ability to wash away the normal irritants of daily life—dust and other small particles—and can cause an allergic response as well. This is why after chest trauma, people who have never had respiratory problems can develop asthma, bronchitis, or some form of difficult breathing. Of course, people who have lung problems before the injury often get a lot worse.

CHEST TRAUMA AND HEART PROBLEMS

KAREN, a stately, dark-haired beauty, walked into my office and stood still and startled, like a deer caught in headlights. No wonder. Karen had been to numerous medical practitioners, and most of them had added to her terrible pain. Along with her neck and back pain, her thinking was fuzzy, and she was suffering from severe bouts of anxiety. The heart palpitations that came without warning terrified her and made the pain much worse. She was desperate but fearful that I, too, would compound her injury and add to her unrelenting suffering.

Three months earlier, a much larger car going 45 miles per hour crashed into the back of Karen's Maxima. Her seat belt had sprung loose from its clasp, causing Karen to slam into the steering wheel. Karen was rushed to the emergency room where the physicians X-rayed her from head to toe. She wept from the excruciating chest pain as she told the emergency room physician that something in her chest must be broken. The radiologist reported that the X-rays showed no injury. She was sent home with a pat on the head and told to take aspirin.

Three days later, almost incoherent from the pain, she returned to the emergency room, where once again she was treated like an hysterical woman and sent home. Fortunately, a friend referred her to an excellent orthopedic physician, who ordered more X-rays. His diagnosis was immediate: Karen had fractured her sternum, the heavy breastbone that protects the heart and lungs and to which the ribs attach. The physician gave her appropriate pain medication.

But the damage had been done. The weeks of unrelenting pain had kept her body in injury shock. Despite the strong medication, she was not able to break the cycle of pain. Even though she was exhausted, she could not relax. Sleeping was difficult because whenever she lay down, her heart palpitations worsened, something her doctors could make no sense of. She felt as if her body was on a perpetual infusion of caffeine. Even worse, her episodes of heart palpitations seemed to be increasing, accompanied by intense feelings of terror. No one had a diagnosis for her.

When I put my hands on Karen, I could feel that she was still in injury shock and that her fractured sternum was healing in a distorted position, with the top part somewhat sheared to the right. Her diaphragm was also in spasm and pulled to the right.

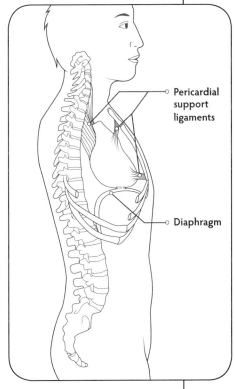

Pericardial
support
ligaments

Diaphragm

The heart and its great vessels are connected by fascia to the sternum, the diaphragm, and the spine—all the way up to the neck. Accidents can twist these tethers, displace the heart in the chest cavity, and cause mysterious arrythmias and anxiety.

169

Because the heart's covering, the pericardium, attaches to the diaphragm and to the sternum, their rightward tilt had dragged Karen's heart toward the right side of her chest. The malposition was so extreme that when Karen lay down, her heart would slide partway down the vertebral ridge toward the right. I could feel this very process with my hands, just as I could feel the palpitations build as the heart was pulled down.

Right behind the breastbone lie two groups of nerves, the cardiac plexus and sympathetic fibers from the vagus nerve. These nerves can speed up the heart when they are irritated. I suspected that one or both of these groups of nerves were strained whenever the heart slid to the right. When they were tugged on, these nerves fired, causing the heartbeat to accelerate and causing palpitations. Given these sudden, repeated episodes of palpitations, it was no wonder Karen was a nervous wreck.

Over the next six weeks, I gently repositioned the sternum until it lined up more properly in her chest. To do this, I had to stretch and untwist the fascia connecting the heart to the sternum and the diaphragm. Layers of fascia link to each other, so I could use the fascial drapes flowing from under the collarbone to manipulate the twisted fascia. Manual treatment can be extremely effective in helping fascia regain its position and flexibility. Once the fascia regains a significant amount of that flexibility, the body, with its currents of fluid and waves of motion, can usually finish the correction.

With the tension on the critical nerves to the heart eased, Karen's nervous system calmed down, her palpitations ceased, and her pain and anxiety resolved. Karen was then able to recover. Certainly, her body would have kept working to try to bring these structures home, but she needed manual medicine to successfully and fully resolve the problem.

SAMUEL. Samuel, my dear eighty-eight-year-old friend, tripped on a curb and fell on his side, bruising his chest. Being a proud man who in his eighties had more energy than I had in my thirties, he just mentioned his tumble to me in passing. I had long given up offering to treat him, as he always refused. He took care of everyone around him, not the other way around. On this visit to California, though, he reported feeling more tired than usual.

When he returned to New York, he saw his physician. Testing revealed Samuel had pericarditis, inflammation of the covering of the heart. The inflamed and swollen pericardium was squeezing the heart within it, causing his fatigue. The cardiologist put Samuel on steroids, which temporarily reduced the swelling.

His physician daughter, knowing the value of osteopathic care and thinking that his bruised and restricted rib cage contributed to his pericarditis, encouraged him to see a local specialist in osteopathic manual medicine, but he refused. I suspect it was his stubborn, I'll-take-care-of-it-myself nature.

The steroids helped Samuel for a while. Then the swelling came back, weakening his elderly heart, which no longer had the strength to pump against the restriction of the rib cage and its own swollen covering. He had a heart attack and died.

Looking back, I believe that the fall had most likely bruised the pericardium, causing inflammation and swelling between its two lubricated layers. As most falls involve twisting as well, I suspect that both the diaphragm and the pericardium were twisted, making Samuel's situation more perilous. The twisted pericardium created roadblocks to the normal flow of fluid between its two layers. The buildup of waste products caused inflammation, which the cortisone partly controlled. But the cortisone could not address the fascial and diaphragmatic twists that prevented proper fluid drainage. The swelling eventually increased again around his heart, and it killed him.

Would restoring motion to his restricted ribs and diaphragm, and freeing up the twists in his pericardium, have saved Samuel's life? I believe it would have. My experience treating patients with pericarditis and other cardiac problems has shown me that often I can improve cardiac function by directly releasing strains in the diaphragm and sternum that pull on the heart. That's certainly part of what I did with Karen. I wish I had flown east and insisted on treating Samuel. But something I could have figured out for a patient escaped me when the person was a beloved friend.

Fortunately, most people's trauma is not as severe as Karen or Emily's, or

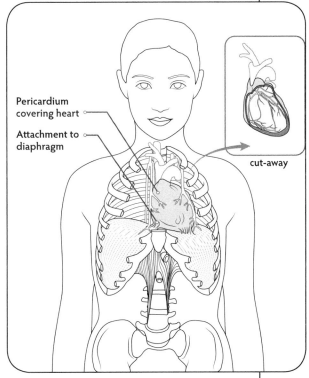

Pericardium covering heart

Attachment to diaphragm

cut-away

The diaphragm and the heart are so intimately connected by fascia that the diaphragm is sometimes called the second heart.

have as devastating a consequence as Samuel's. Yet these stories illustrate the far-reaching and often surprising effects trauma can have on the heart and lungs. I have treated dozens of patients with severe chest pain, heart palpitations, and arrthymias after they have been cleared by cardiologists of any diagnosable heart pathology. Once I spend several sessions restoring mobility to their ribs, chest, diaphragm, torso, and neck and remove strains from the heart's attachments, their heart's rhythm normalizes and most of their pain disappears.

TRAUMA TO THE NECK AND RIB CAGE

The rib cage jealously protects the heart and lungs while remaining flexible enough to allow the heart to beat and the lungs to expand. With its 150 joints and all the demands placed on it, it's not surprising the rib cage can cause problems and pain like Caroline experienced.

CAROLINE was a ferocious athlete, working toward her black belt in jiu-jitsu, a martial art that involves throwing and grappling one's opponent. Caroline regularly found herself in her physician's office after particularly grueling sessions, suffering from shortness of breath and sharp chest pains. Her cardiac tests and her X-rays for lung problems were negative. After a final panicked visit to her doctor, where a thorough cardiac workup turned up nothing, she decided to see me.

When I examined Caroline, I found that her second, third, and fourth ribs had been twisted in back where they meet the spine. This forced them to dip in the front and caused their knife-like edges to press on the vulnerable intercostal nerves running right below the ribs. These nerves enter the spinal cord right next to the nerves coming from the heart. Due to a process called facilitation, or cross talk, the spinal cord thinks that the chest pain is coming from upset heart nerves, not the intercostal nerves under the ribs. The cross talk can make the person experience the rib displacement as a squeezing of the heart. Facilitation can work the other way around, too, making an organ problem feel like a musculoskeletal problem. This is one of the reasons a heart attack can feel like shoulder, jaw, or arm pain. Of course, all chest pain must be carefully evaluated, as Caroline's was, for serious cardiac and lung problems.

All of Caroline's throwing, grappling, and landing hard on the mats had distorted her ribs and overstretched the ligaments that bind the ribs in the back to the vertebrae. The fascia that runs between the ribs was also overstretched. I reset the bones in their proper places and forbade Caroline from practicing jiu-jitsu until the ligaments and fascia healed and regained their strength. Having a relatively stingy blood supply and very slow metabolic activity, fascia heals slowly. Ligaments, which are a denser and more organized form of fascia, also take a long time to heal, usually many more weeks than patients and healthcare practitioners are ready to give them. Ligaments would certainly appreciate a minimum of four to six weeks to heal.

Caroline took the time to heal. Two or three times a year, she returned for a treatment to keep her disorderly ribs in place and prevent chest pain.

Symptoms of Restricted Ribs

• A twisted rib can cause an aching pain at the joint or a sharp pain where the rib strikes the nerve underneath it.
• A twist in the upper ribs can cause neck pain.
• A twist in the lowest rib (called the floating rib) can cause a dull, aching pain in the midback.

More subtle symptoms:
• Breathing takes more effort and is not as deep.
• You are short of breath or mysteriously anxious.
• You repeatedly come down with a cough, the flu, bronchitis, or another respiratory infection.
• You become tired and fatigued for no apparent reason.

A word of caution: always get a physician to evaluate chest pain for cardiac or lung problems.

WHAT YOU CAN DO

The ribs and diaphragm are the keys to the health of the chest. Since the diaphragm's pumping helps lift and widen the ribs, any movement that frees the diaphragm will help expand the ribs. A free-moving diaphragm and flexible rib cage also benefit the lungs and heart. Chapter 7 has a program for helping restore the diaphragm to full motion.

Yoga can be wonderful for expanding the chest and rib cage and helping restore proper rib position. Some beneficial poses that open the chest are demonstrated in chapter 18.

Exercise. While exercise in many forms is beneficial to promoting chest health, swimming is amazing for its ability to help the chest expand and reposition wayward ribs. When one of my ribs is out of place, swimming freestyle will often fix it. Swimming also builds up back muscles that help pull the torso backward, compensating for all the leaning forward we do as we read, drive, or work on a computer. The deep breathing of swimming helps the diaphragm expand as well.

If the pain is coming from a twisted rib in the upper back, try these techniques to get it back in place:

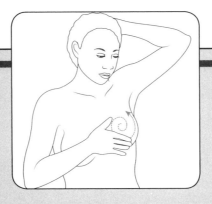

Breast Lumps and Trauma

I've seen breast lumps develop in women after chest trauma. I suspect that in car crashes, the impact from the shoulder harness compresses the fragile lymphatic vessels and nodes that course over the chest and drain the breasts. Trauma-induced breast lumps will dissolve in one to two months after the twists are removed from the ribs and chest, the diaphragm is released, and lymphatic congestion addressed. A dose of the homeopathic remedy **Conium maculatum** can be helpful for breast trauma.

Of course, for all breast lumps, the person must consult a physician and get an accurate diagnosis, as they might not have noticed a potentially dangerous lump before their chest hurt. This includes men, too. (Though it is rare, men can have breast cancer.) Knowing that chest trauma can cause temporary lumps, however, reduces patients' anxiety should they find a lump following injury to the chest.

There is a Japanese form of self-massage I was once taught that I believe promotes lymphatic drainage and breast health. If done regularly, it can also function as part of a breast exam, something we women are often reluctant to do.

Start with a gentle massage around the nipples, slowly making larger circles until they cover the whole breast and end by massaging the armpit. Some Japanese women do this daily and believe it can prevent breast cancer. If a woman does this slowly, carefully covering the whole breast and surrounding areas, she should be able to detect most lumps while focusing attention primarily on health, rather than disease. This is certainly a more enjoyable experience.

Use your doorjamb. My first osteopathic mentor, Muriel Chapman, DO, taught me a method she used on herself: lean against a doorjamb and rub the upper back against the edge of the frame. This can help relax spasmed thoracic muscles. The jamb acts like a helping hand to move the rib back into place. Sometimes it helps to twist against the jamb as well. Try it if you have a rib problem. It feels good, if nothing else, and once you've practiced it for a while it can become quite effective.

A foam roller, a M.E.L.T. roller, or a rolled-up blanket can also be helpful in opening up the chest and getting the ribs back in place. Acting like you're making snow angels with your arms while lying flat on the roller or the blanket can sometimes help reseat ribs into a better position. This exercise is demonstrated on page 219.

When motion is restored to the structures of the chest, an amazing thing happens: neck pain often goes away. Neck pain and how to fix it is the subject of the next chapter.

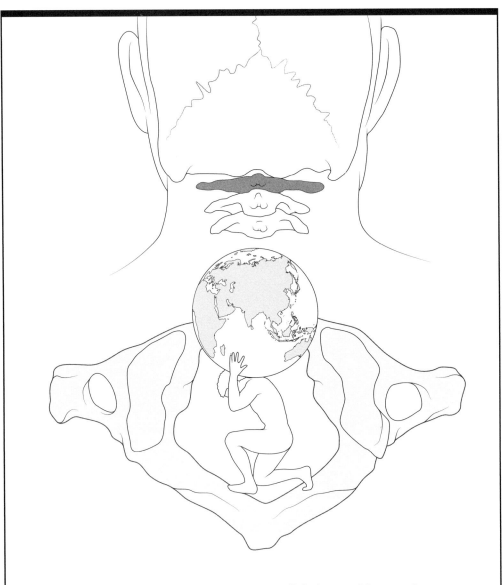

The first cervical vertebra is unique among all the bones of the spine. It is called the atlas because, like the Greek Titan, Atlas, who carried the world on his shoulders, the atlas bone bears the heavy weight of the head. The proper alignment of this small bone can dramatically influence the health not only of the neck but also of the head, brain, nervous system, and back.

16

Recovering from Neck Injury

The body gives the neck two daunting, often contradictory tasks. The neck must accommodate the demands of the massive chest. At the same time, the heavy head insists that the neck move freely so the eyes can scan for predators. To be able to answer each master, the neck is designed for flexibility. But this very flexibility makes the neck exceedingly vulnerable to injury, especially when a trauma such as a car accident takes the head in one direction and the torso in another.

Another characteristic of the neck makes it ripe for insult. The neck is the body's superhighway, with most of the body's essential systems linked to or passing through it. Injury to the neck not only can cause pain but can also dampen or stop breathing, compromise the heart, restrict blood flow to the brain, and close off the channels that drain the brain's toxic debris. Digestion, immune function, blood pressure, and fluid balance depend on the neck, as do all the nerves that journey from the brain to the rest of the body.

I cannot cover all the neck's remarkable dimensions in one chapter. Instead, I focus on some relatively simple ways to heal the neck after trauma. These methods depend on understanding that both the head and the chest have their talons lodged deep into the neck. Therefore, I always make sure to restore motion to the neck's two masters before I work directly on the neck. Second, injury shock and neck trauma are intimately linked. Neck injury will not respond well to treatment until injury shock has been significantly diminished.

In chapter 12, I discussed the basic structure of the spine. The small cervical vertebrae are fairly similar to their large colleagues in the low back. However, the neck's facet joints are less steeply angled, to allow more rotation

Symptoms of a Neck Injury

- Cognitive problems
- Fatigue
- Problems with hearing
- Ear infections
- Weakness and numbness in the arms or legs
- Difficulty breathing
- Headaches
- Forearm and wrist pain
- Shoulder pain
- Neck pain
- Upper-back pain
- Sinus problems
- Dizziness
- Memory problems

When to Go for Immediate Medical Care

- Neck pain following a violent injury, including motor vehicle accidents or sports injuries, should always be evaluated to rule out spinal cord injury.
- Shooting pain radiating to shoulder or arm, numbness or loss of strength in arms or hands, leg weakness or difficulty walking, or bowel or bladder problems can indicate ruptured disc(s) or spinal nerve root or cord compression.
- Neck pain that is worse at night or occurring with a fever or weight loss may indicate an infection or other serious condition.
- Throbbing neck pain may be related to heart problems.
- Neck pain preceding or accompanying a headache can indicate a stroke.

and side-bending, giving the neck its vaunted flexibility. The narrow canals the nerve roots transverse as they leave the spine are longer and knobbier in the neck. That means neck trauma can slam nerve roots against the canal's bony protrusions, increasing pain, dysfunction, and injury shock.

To better illustrate how trauma attacks the neck, I introduce Keiko and her son Martin.

KEIKO, a very fit fifty-two-year-old, was waiting at a stoplight in her sedan, admiring the red stripes in a teenager's purple Mohawk as he danced across the crosswalk. Her grown son, Martin, sitting in the passenger seat, was admiring his own haircut in the mirror on the sun visor.

"Watch out!" he shouted, too late, as he saw the SUV behind them about to slam into their car. The collision launched Keiko's purse from the armrest into the dashboard and threw both Martin and Keiko into their restraining seat belts.

Feeling shaky and disoriented, Keiko got out of her car. She was relieved that she hadn't hit the boy with the Mohawk; she saw only a tiny dent on her bumper.

Her neck ached when she tried to look around, and she kept rubbing her left shoulder because it was sore. Her son yelled at the other driver who had been texting before colliding with them. Keiko sent Martin back to the car while she exchanged infor-

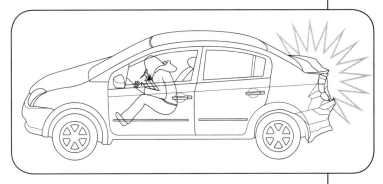

mation with the apologetic driver of the SUV. But since neither car had sustained much damage, neither woman considered the accident a big deal.

For Martin, the crash was not a big deal. He resembles the volunteers used in most vehicle crash tests: a healthy male in his early twenties, with no history of prior neck injury. Like the volunteers, he was both looking straight ahead at the time of the collision and anticipating the crash. His neck and right shoulder ached for a few days after the accident, but three weeks later he had no obvious symptoms.

Keiko, however, was not so fortunate. The next day, her upper back and neck ached and she felt vaguely nauseated. As the CEO of a software company, she didn't feel she could take time off and was back to work as usual.

Four days later, she woke up feeling much worse. Her neck throbbed and she had searing pain at the base of her skull and up into her head. She had difficulty turning her neck. Her upper back burned, and her neck was swollen and sore to the touch—even her jaw ached when she ate her breakfast bagel. She was exhausted despite eight hours of sleep and a little short of breath.

As the days went by, other symptoms appeared. She awoke one morning with a splitting headache and her right hand laced with pins and needles. Then her left arm began to ache and would suddenly get weak, causing her to drop silverware. Her right shoulder blade ached all day. She became dizzy when she attempted to exercise. She found herself grabbing onto desks and cabinets as she tried to catch her balance. She was accustomed to being calm in a crisis, but now even a small obstacle made her feel anxious. It was several weeks before she acknowledged that her condition was not improving. Along with her headaches, neck pain, and anxiety, she was making mistakes at work and becoming exceedingly forgetful, frequently losing her keys and once leaving her wallet on the counter at the grocery store.

One month after the accident, she came to see me. Despite her rather alarming symptoms, Keiko told me, "I couldn't be hurt. My car was hardly damaged."

After years of treating people who have been in car accidents, I knew that for her to do the things she needed to do to fully recover, she would have to acknowledge how serious her injuries had been. If I quoted the decades of research about the extensive damage that low-speed collisions can inflict on the victims, I wouldn't convince her. Instead I said, "If I hit your head with a hammer and crushed your skull, do you really think I could defend my actions in court by holding up the hammer and saying, 'Look, not even a scratch. Your head can't be hurt!' Cars are big and hard and designed to survive a crash without much damage. We aren't."

Keiko realized she'd been making a faulty assumption: that people and cars respond the same way in a collision. She sighed. "All right, I get it. What can I do?"

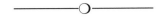

Keiko suffered what is commonly called a flexion-extension or whiplash injury to her neck. This shorthand barely begins to describe the tsunami of damage unleashed by the powerful forces that assaulted that region of her body. While a car accident was the mechanism of Keiko's injury, the same mechanism can be at work whenever the neck is rapidly accelerated or decelerated, such as in a fall or a football tackle.

How exactly did Keiko get injured? In the last twenty years, an explosion of research has given us some surprising answers. We used to think that a flexion-extension injury occurred because the head was pulled backward too far and then snapped forward too far, causing sprains and strains to the muscles and ligaments. But sprains and strains generally heal; this scenario couldn't account for the fact that so many people are in pain for two years or more after a low-speed collision.

We now know that this assumption is wrong. The latest research, which includes high-speed videography and dynamic X-rays of volunteers, demonstrates that the neck is subjected to tremendous compressive and shearing forces in rear-end collisions. These forces wreak havoc

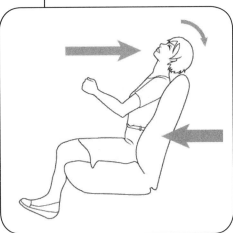

In a rear-end collision the neck is caught between shearing forces.

with the neck's architecture. They can strain or tear ligaments, muscles, and fascia, and create disc or facet injuries, vertebrae microfractures, brain injury, and injuries to the blood vessels, spinal cord, and spinal nerves. Let's look at what happened to Keiko in this relatively low-speed collision.

TYPES OF NECK DAMAGE

Shearing forces. Because the flexible neck lives between the seven- to ten-pound head above and the massive torso below, the neck is cracked like a whip in a rear-end collision. As Keiko's car was accelerated sharply forward, the seat pushed her torso and the lower part of the neck forward along with it. The upper part of the neck, held in place by the heavy head, stayed behind until the rotating head pulled it backward. In that instant, when the lower vertebrae were pulled forward by the torso and the upper vertebrae pulled backward, the vertebrae of her neck were sheared in opposite directions. The brunt of this shearing force typically impacts the fourth, fifth, and sixth cervical vertebrae. These are the most common

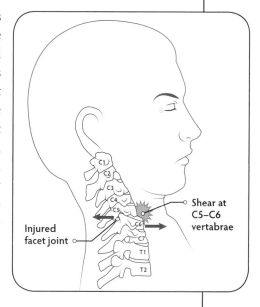

levels for cervical disc and vertebral injuries after a flexion-extension injury.

These forces injured Keiko's neck—from the fascia and muscles on the outside to the ligaments and facets joints trying to stabilize it and the nerve roots leaving the spinal canals. Even the spinal cord itself deep within the spinal canal may not have escaped unscathed.

Damage to muscles and fascia. The muscles of the neck work in a balanced fashion to keep the heavy head upright and level. In order to do that, many large muscles attach to the skull and then crisscross the neck and anchor into major structures of the torso, such as the shoulder blades, the collarbone, sternum, and upper ribs. (See image page 186.)

When the neck is flung rapidly backward and forward, the neck muscles and their connective tissue wrappings are strained. In Keiko's case, the strains were worsened because her head was turned at the time of impact, adding rotational or twisting forces to the mix. Muscle and fascial pain is typically aching, gnawing, burning, and/or searing.

181

Muscle and fascial strains accounted for some of the pain Keiko experienced immediately after the accident: the aching pain she felt when she tried to turn her head, the soreness of her jaw when she attempted to eat her bagel, and the burning pain in her neck and upper back.

Keiko was still experiencing burning and aching pain months after the accident. A significant part of this discomfort was actually fascial pain. Fascia has a much poorer blood supply than muscle tissue and takes significantly longer to heal. An injured muscle typically mends within weeks; it can take fascia months to recover. If fascia is left in a distorted position and not able to recover, it can solidify into a contorted shape.

Injury to ligaments. Flexion-extension injuries like Keiko's are notorious for injuring the small ligaments that tie the vertebrae together and help stabilize the neck. Like silly putty, they can snap. Ligaments are not designed to resist rapid, violent stretching. If a ligament is strained past 7 percent of its normal length, its capacity to fully heal is jeopardized. Ligaments are laced with a rich supply of pain nerves, so when they are injured they are good at screaming with pain. Ligamentous pain tends to be aching, sharp, or searing and is generally better with rest.

Ligaments also have sensory fibers that tell us where we are in space, called proprioceptors. When ligaments are injured, people tend to have balance problems. I used to get annoyed at my car accident patients because often, after they started to get better, they would trip and fall, reinjuring themselves. (Of course, I never show my annoyance.) Then I realized that they fell because of balance problems caused by ligamentous and facet injuries, as facet joints also have proprioceptive fibers.

Ligament damage is potentially quite serious, as a stretched or torn ligament cannot properly stabilize a joint. Treatment for strained ligaments includes proper nutritional support and rest and ensuring that no bony, muscular, or fascial distortions are still straining them. Rest is a difficult task for the ever-moving neck. The neck muscles sometimes go into temporary protective spasm in order to stabilize the neck while the ligaments are healing. Even though the ensuing muscle pain can be very uncomfortable, it is important not to release muscle spasm too soon with either massage or Botox injections. Either one can jeopardize the ligaments' chances to heal.

Poorly healed ligaments can result in wobbly, unstable vertebrae. If the neck remains chronically unstable, the bones will eventually try to do the ligaments' job and send out bony growths to stabilize the region, causing arthritis.

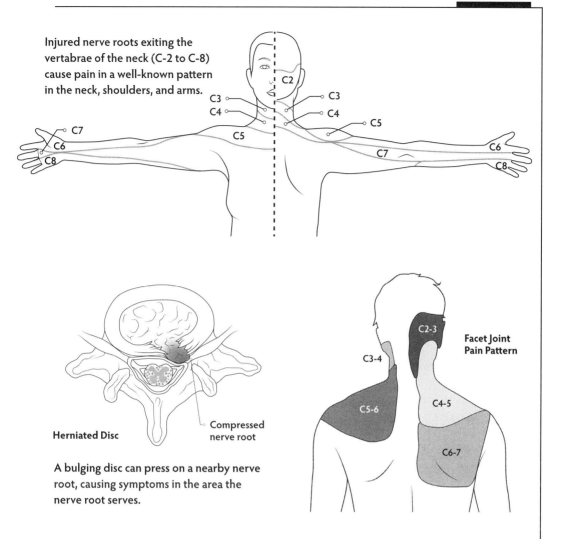

Injured nerve roots exiting the vertabrae of the neck (C-2 to C-8) cause pain in a well-known pattern in the neck, shoulders, and arms.

Herniated Disc

Compressed nerve root

A bulging disc can press on a nearby nerve root, causing symptoms in the area the nerve root serves.

Facet Joint Pain Pattern

Facet-joint injury. The shearing forces in flexion-extension injuries commonly damage the facet joints, compressing and grinding the facets against each other. I talked about these joints in the chapter on back pain. The facet joints control and limit the movement of the spinal vertebrae.

The tenderness Keiko experienced in her neck after the accident was in part the result of inflamed facet joints. Facet injury is usually accompanied by tenderness over the inflamed joint itself and muscle spasm as nearby muscles contract to protect the joint and limit motion while it heals.

Facet joints also have nerves that spread to the muscles and fascia of the head and upper back. Injured or inflamed facet joints create a fairly predictable pain pattern in these regions. Some of Keiko's head pain probably came from injury to the facet joints high in her neck. The deep, aching pain around her right shoulder blade probably came from damage to the facet joint low in her neck, specifically, the joint between the sixth and seventh cervical vertebrae. Like most people with cervical-facet problems, her pain was worse with backward bending.

While this pain probably came from damage to her facets, in other victims of car crashes, that pain can come from microfractures to the cervical vertebrae. Autopsy studies done on people who died from other causes (such as a heart attack) during a low-speed collision showed that a number had suffered from hairline fractures or microfractures in their vertebrae. Hairline fractures often cause a similar deep, aching pain that worsens when the person lies down. Such bone pain is usually resistant to all painkillers.

Nerve and disc injury. Eight pairs of nerves exit the bony canals in the cervical vertebrae and innervate the hand, arms, neck, and upper back. When the head and neck are whipped around in a car crash, the nerve roots are often banged against the neck's particularly treacherous bony canals. Given the knobby nature of these canals and the extreme mobility of the neck, this kind of "karate chop" is much more common in the neck than elsewhere in the spine. Irritation or compression of a nerve root can cause transient or prolonged pain, pins and needles, numbness or even weakness in the muscle group the nerve root serves. Karate chops to the nerve roots in the lower part of Keiko's right neck probably caused the pins and needles she experienced in her right hand. As long as nerve impingement doesn't persist, these symptoms should resolve in several weeks.

I was more concerned about the continued intermittent aching and weakness in her left arm. The neck, the nerve roots, and the discs tend to take the biggest beating on the side of the shoulder

Traumatized spinal cord

Traumatized nerve roots

The bony vertebrae can karate-chop the spinal cord or the nerve roots in the neck.

harness. (However, people need to wear seat belts to prevent far worse injuries.) Rear-end collisions typically propel the torso both forward and upward two inches or more into the shoulder restraint. The additional compression from the shoulder harness gives the nerve roots on the left side an especially brutal blow, which probably contributed to the weakness in Keiko's arm. Weakness indicates more serious damage to a nerve than does pain or numbness. Pain is actually the least serious consequence.

The weakness in Keiko's left arm may have also indicated that a disc had protruded or broken and was pressing on the nerve root. While discs can withstand extreme compressive forces, they are not equipped to deal with the shearing (tearing) forces generated by falls, car accidents, or football tackles. Shearing forces can cause discs to bulge, split, tear, or fragment to the side and press on a nerve root.

I don't think Keiko's disc actually herniated, or the leaking gel would have burned like acid on her nerve root. She could have had a bulging disc, however. I released the compressive forces pushing up from her chest and down from her skull, which gave her cervical discs more room to plump back up. Releasing the compression also allowed the vertebrae to move apart, releasing pressure on the facets and nerve roots. If the weakness had persisted after two or three treatments, I would have ordered an MRI to visualize the discs in her neck.

Headaches. Neck trauma has a wealth of ways to cause headaches. Injury to the upper cervical nerve roots that supply the back of the head can cause headaches and might have contributed to Keiko's. Smacking her head against the headrest may have traumatized the sensitive arteries trying to shimmy through the narrow passageway between the head and neck. Injury to the muscles and fascia strapping the skull to the neck and torso could have also precipitated headaches. To treat Keiko's headaches, I didn't have to know which injury caused her suffering. I planned to treat them all.

HEALING THE NECK

Over thirty years, I've developed an order for treating the neck that garners the best results. I first treat the injury shock, next the chest, and then the base of the skull before I pay attention to the neck itself.

Injury shock. Keiko's anxiety, fatigue, and difficulty breathing indicated that she was suffering from significant injury shock. I find this exceedingly common after car accidents, both because of the massive force even a "minor" car accident pounds into the body and because of the way car crashes traumatize the nervous system. Collisions typically whip around the slender stalk of the neck, shaking up the spinal cord, smacking nerve roots, and even slapping the brain. I have found that most neck injuries from car crashes, even low-speed ones, do the brain some damage, even if it's transient. I have not focused on that aspect of Keiko's injury here, as I leave discussion of brain injury to Section IV.

There is yet another way that neck trauma provokes injury shock: nerves from the upper and middle neck go to the diaphragm and orchestrate its motion. When these nerves get irritated, the diaphragm tends not to move as well or as fully. Poor breathing and weak diaphragmatic movement amplify injury shock.

My examination of Keiko's nervous system confirmed that it was shuddering with injury shock. To help Keiko heal, I addressed that first.

I discuss treatment of injury shock in the first section of the book. I start by releasing the diaphragmatic spasm. In her case the diaphragmatic restriction has been made even worse by the karate chop to the nerves feeding it. The nerve roots had mostly recovered, but the diaphragm remained seized up. The fear the car crash engendered compounded the diaphragmatic spasm as well. Once I gained partial release of the diaphragm, Keiko was breathing better and her nervous system began to calm. Full release required several more treatments. As it is rare to see a neck injury exist in isolation from chest problems, I further assisted her breathing and diminished her injury shock by freeing up her ribs and treating the rest of her chest.

Treating the chest. Trying to fix the neck without treating the chest is like ignoring the 800-pound gorilla in the room. The neck is dwarfed by the solidity and massive bulk of the torso to which it is anatomically tied. Large fascial planes and powerful muscles connect the neck to the breastbone, collarbones (clavicles), shoulder blades, upper ribs, and thoracic vertebrae. My next job was to release all the distortions in the muscles, fascia, bones, and ligaments caused by the compressing, twisting, and shearing. Keiko, like most

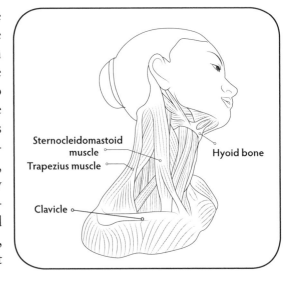

Sternocleidomastoid muscle

Trapezius muscle

Clavicle

Hyoid bone

drivers, had twisted around the restraining shoulder harness, compressing her left shoulder and her rib cage. As I released strains in her torso, her chest stopped pulling on her neck as much. A number of other improvements also occurred: her diaphragm released more and her rib cage expanded more, and both of those improved her breathing and further lessened her injury shock.

Next, I addressed the other master of the neck: the base of Keiko's skull.

Treating the base of the skull. Large muscles and dense fibrous bands stream down from the skull and attach to the neck and chest. Spasm in the muscles and fascia that bind the chest to the skull can compress the neck and squeeze the cervical discs. The meninges (the dural membrane) that is attached to the inside of the skull exits through a large opening in the base of the skull called the foramen magnum and fastens to the inside of the first two cervical vertebrae. This dural attachment helps keep these vertabrae stable, but it means that the position of the skull can alter the position of the neck.

Over several visits, I used cranial osteopathy to relax these muscular and fascial restrictions. Once those were attended to, her muscular and fascial tension relaxed and her neck pain diminished.

The first cervical vertebra is unique among all the bones of the spine. It is called the atlas because, like the Greek Titan who carried the world on his shoulders, the atlas bone bears the heavy weight of the head. The proper alignment of this small bone can dramatically influence the health not only of the neck but also of the head, brain, nervous system, and back. Fascia, ligaments, and dura provide stability to this critical area. However, trauma can distort it. When the atlas is twisted or misaligned, the weight of the head bears down unevenly, forcing the structures below to compensate. The result can be muscle spasm, twisted and painful facet joints, and pressure on the spinal discs anywhere from the neck to the low back. After an accident like Keiko's, I usually find there is compression between the atlas and the base of the skull.

The meeting point of the atlas

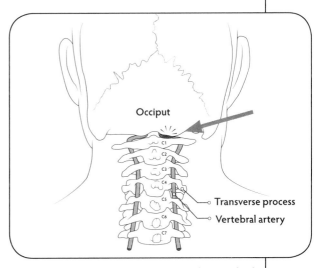

A misaligned atlas compresses the right vertebral artery as it weaves its way into the skull.

187

bone and the head, called the atlanto-occipital junction, is a treacherous place. Nerves and blood vessels to and from the brain must safely traverse this narrow space. When the atlas bone is even minutely rotated or out of alignment, it can cause symptoms as diverse as brain fog, headaches, and digestive problems. The anatomy of this crowded region explains why this happens.

The vertebral arteries that provide half the brain's blood supply must shimmy to the brain across the tight space separating the atlas and the base of the skull. When the space narrows, it can squeeze one or both arteries and decrease oxygen and glucose supply to the hungry brain. I suspect that Keiko's brain fog may have resulted from misalignment of the atlas, caused when her head smacked into the headrest.

Rotation of the atlas can also narrow the spigot through which cerebral spinal fluid (CSF) flows from the brain into the canal around the spine. Radiographic studies have confirmed that this occurs. When CSF flow diminishes, the brain is at risk for inflammatory damage from a backup of toxic debris that can't get out of the brain. As you can see, the health of the neck and brain are intimately related.

Since blood vessels are rife with pain nerves, irritation of the vertebral arteries can cause headaches. Keiko's throbbing neck pain could have been reflective of irritation to one or both of the vertebral arteries pinched by the distorted atlas and the base of the skull.

Digestive problems. One of the most frequent complaints I hear from my neck-injured patients is digestive upset such as nausea and queasiness. While their digestive problems can have a number of causes, the most common I have found is irritation of the vagus nerve, which also can be irritated by a distorted atlas bone. The vagus (vagabond) nerve is the master of the rest-and-digest parasympathetic nervous system, which we met in the section on injury shock. The vagus travels throughout the body to supply our organs with autonomic nervous system fibers. Compression here most likely accounted for the severe nausea Keiko initially suffered.

To help the atlas return to its home, I loosened the muscular and fascial tension that was holding the distortion in place. I sat in back of Keiko's head and curled my fingers so the tips were on the fascia and musculature between her atlas and the base of her skull. I let the weight of her head provide some pressure into my fingertips. As I felt the fascia and musculature begin to release, I applied gentle traction toward myself. Patients almost always sigh with relief when I do this because this technique feels so good. After this area released, I could more directly reposition the atlas. With the atlas in a better position, Keiko felt the fog in her brain begin to clear. Later, she reported that the occasional nausea that she'd been experiencing was also gone. I attributed that to the removal of pressure on the vagus nerve.

Once I restored motion to the chest, the base of the skull, and the atlas, I could successfully address the rest of Keiko's neck. I released the remaining fascial strains and muscle spasm. Then I paid attention to the facets and vertebrae. Studies show that restoring motion to the facet joints soon after neck trauma helps speed up and assist full recovery. Typically, I use very gentle traction and slight rotation of the injured neck to gradually open up one facet at a time. The whole time I treat, I carefully listen to the patient's cranial rhythmic impulse to make sure their body likes what I am doing. If my slow, small movements make the patient's central nervous system more irritated, I back off.

I never use sudden, jerky motions on the neck, also known as high velocity, low amplitude (HVLA). That technique is known in slang as "rack 'em and crack 'em." In my opinion, there are far better and safer methods for treating the neck than such fast, forceful techniques. Here, I differ from some in the osteopathic profession as well as some in the chiropractic profession. I believe that HVLA should never be used on an injured neck. I have found that very few practitioners are gentle and precise enough to use HVLA even in chronic

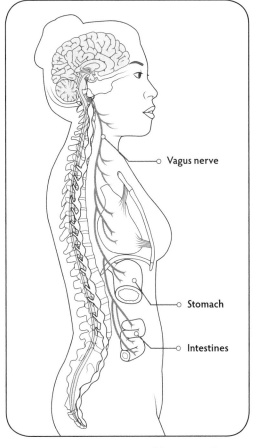

The vagus nerve, master of the rest-and-digest parasympathetic nervous system that controls digestive function, can get squeezed as it exits the skull.

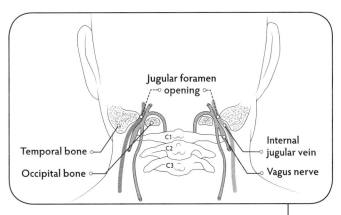

The Neck and Neurological Disease

Distortion of the atlas bone has emerged in recent years as a possible culprit in the plague of neurological diseases afflicting the brain. Because cerebral spinal fluid (CSF) drainage carrying debris from the brain must traverse this region, displacing the atlas is like crimping the drain. Daniel Harshfield, MD, has correlated decreased CSF drainage through this region with neurological disease like multiple sclerosis, Parkinson's disease, and Alzheimer's disease. He has also found that adjusting the atlas and returning it to its proper position restores CSF flow. While this hypothesis demands further research, it would be consistent with what osteopathic physicians and chiropractic doctors have long asserted: brain and neck health are intimately related.

conditions. If someone does have the skill level to perform proper HVLA cervical techniques, the correction should feel as gentle as putting an expensive teacup down onto its $1,000 saucer.

I also pay attention to a small bone at the front of the neck that is often ignored. I make sure to balance the tiny hyoid bone, which is attached to the tongue and the sternum and is slung by ligaments from the temporal bones (see picture page 186). Distortion of the hyoid bone can constrict the internal jugular vein, which passes below it, and block venous drainage from the head.

Treating all of this takes time. After a car crash, I prefer to see patients twice a week for two weeks, then once a week for one to three months, then twice a month for another four to eight months. Hopefully, they have been walking during this time. After about six weeks of treatment, I want my patient to begin gentle movement therapy, preferably under the guidance of an experienced and skilled physical therapist. Movement and activity are absolutely essential to heal a neck. Posture is often critical as well. More than anywhere else in the body, the neck is affected by posture. Posture and activity are best reframed by intelligent, thoughtful movements such as the practices suggested in chapter 18.

RICHARD. My cousin Richard is a hard-driving San Diego lawyer with little interest in chitchat. When he called out of the blue one day, I hadn't talked to him in twenty years, but he was desperate. He had terrible arm and neck pain from two bulging cervical discs. The surgeons wanted to schedule immediate surgery. He refused. I referred him to an excellent osteopathic physician in his region. He would have none of it. "Tell me something I can do myself."

"Swimming is the best way to rehabilitate most neck problems. You've got to wear a mask and a snorkel so you don't turn your neck."

"Consider it done."

He hung up before I could tell him to swim in warm water.

Three months later, my aunt called to thank me. Richard had no more pain. The day Richard and I spoke, he bought himself a mask and snorkel. The next day, he started swimming in the ocean. He gradually built up until he was swimming one mile every day, rain or shine. Fifteen years later, Richard is still pain-free. He swims a mile every day before work. He won't vacation unless the place he goes has somewhere to swim. You don't have to be nearly as compulsive as Richard to benefit from swimming, however.

I have found swimming helpful for many reasons. First, because you are no longer upright, the heavy head no longer presses down on the neck. The buoyancy of the water helps relax strained muscles and fascia. Moving through water provides a gentle traction between the smaller head and larger shoulders. However, an injured or painful neck should never be forced to move beyond a comfortable range of motion. I recommend swimming with a mask and snorkel so you don't have to turn your head excessively. To avoid increasing neck spasm from cold water, I recommend swimming in water with a temperature of eighty-two to eighty-five degrees.

Here are the stories of other patients who used water creatively to heal neck injuries:

Yvonne was four months out from her third flexion-extension injury. She had tried swimming with a mask and snorkel, but that worsened her neck pain and increased her arm weakness. Not willing to give up, she bought a plastic neck pillow designed for sleeping sitting up in an airplane. She got in the pool, put the pillow behind her neck, and attached it in front. Then she swam the backstroke. With the airplane pillow carefully supporting her neck, she swam pain free three times a week. She gained the benefits of swimming, rebuilt the muscle strength in her body, and completely recovered.

Lynette, another patient of mine, had an acute and unstable neck. Every form of exercise increased her pain, so she designed her own water therapy. Holding her breath, she let herself sink down to the bottom of the pool, creating gentle traction on her neck. Then she floated back up. Doing that exercise three times a week helped her. Soon, she could safely swim with a mask and snorkel. She then layered on other exercises, eventually graduating to yoga and tai chi. Now, she has only occasional minimal neck pain.

Unusual Causes of Neck Pain

I mention three causes of neck pain that I and other practitioners have occasionally missed.

- The eyes and the neck: The brain insists that the eyes stay level, so your neck bends and shifts to keep your eyes level to the horizon. Chronically unlevel eyes can strain even a healthy neck; imagine what they can do to an injured one. Unlevel eyes can often be treated cranially or addressed with special lenses.

- The legs and the neck: To heal a bad neck, you must wear good supportive shoes. If one leg is significantly shorter than the other, the neck twists to keep the eyes level. A lift in the short leg can help tremendously. A collapsed arch in one foot can shorten that side and may require orthotics. I vastly prefer soft orthotics made out of leather, cork, or rubber.

- Chronic twisting or torquing of the neck: Always turning to one side to watch TV or having a desk too high or low can strain the neck. Desks are often too high for women, too low for men.

WHAT YOU CAN DO

There are many things you can do to help yourself recover. I must emphasize, however, the importance of limiting the damage that tends to occur after the initial injury. All too often after injury, people power on with their lives and make the situation much worse. To prevent that, I offer some helpful suggestions.

Five Things to Avoid

Don't do work where you have to look up. This includes painting the ceiling, hanging new curtains, and sitting in the front of a movie theater.

Don't lift anything weighing more than ten pounds (five pounds with a serious injury or pain). Don't carry anything heavier than five pounds for very long. That means your child, most grocery bags, or even your briefcase.

Don't spend too much time on the computer. Computer work tends to turtle the head forward on the neck, creating a shear between the upper and lower vertebrae or worsening one already created by the injury. You must have armrests for your arms, or they will pull on your neck and strain it more.

Absolutely do not cradle your phone between your head and neck. No one should do this, even healthy folks, or soon they will have neck pain. The neck is not made to bend in this way.

Don't wear high heels. Heels change the angle of your low back so that your butt sticks out. That extra curve in your low back increases the curve in your neck, putting additional pressure and strain on your neck.

Ten Things That Help

Sleep in a comfortable position. When you sleep on your back (the best position after a neck injury), make sure you have a comfortable pillow to support your neck. (See photo page 321.) Also, consider putting a towel or small pillow under each elbow. Support under the arms takes strain off your neck. Put a pillow under your knees to take the strain off your low back.

Use a slant board to read or write. Bending your neck down for long periods overstretches already injured or inflamed ligaments and fascia. To give ligaments the best possible chance to heal, keep your neck in a neutral position as much as possible.

Consider a cervical collar. Wearing a cervical collar can be helpful after an injury. Cervical collars can help to maintain the neck in a neutral position and partially splint the healing ligaments, blood vessels, nerves, and muscles. Only wear a collar if it feels good, and do not wear it all the time—a maximum of four to five hours a day. If you wear it all the time, you can lose valuable muscle strength and end up worsening your condition. Some of my acute patients need to wear it when they sleep. Talk to your doctor or physical therapist about the proper use of a collar.

Make sure you have an ergonomic setup for the computer. This includes armrests, the keyboard at a level that keeps your forearms parallel to the ground, and the screen positioned so the neck sits on the torso in an easy position. Limit time to thirty minutes maximum, then rest.

Move every day. Gently moving the neck left to right and nodding up and down to whatever point is comfortable can accelerate healing. Find time for other pain-free, gentle, and slow forms of movement as well. Walk with good supportive shoes. Movement increases blood flow to the injured areas, removes toxins, and promotes health. You might have to wear a cervical collar when you walk or move. You might even have to walk in water wearing a collar. Start moving a little bit twice a day, if only for ten minutes, and try to build up to thirty to forty-five minutes a day.

Work out in water. As you learned in Richard's story, the single best movement I have found for healing an injured or painful neck is swimming with a mask and a snorkel. I am pleased that there are increasing numbers of physical therapists and Feldenkrais practitioners who are working with people in water to help them heal from all sorts of pain and injury. I often refer patients to them.

Posture is critical. A slouched or head-forward posture beats up the neck.

Yoga can be very curative. I have seen people with serious neck injuries dramatically improve with excellent yoga instruction. Proper yoga strengthens the core and lengthens the spine. Patricia Sullivan's suggested practices in chapter 18 for strengthening the neck and improving posture are simple and effective.

Certain poses like shoulder stands, headstands, and the plow can put necks in potentially dangerous positions. In a weak, injured, or arthritic neck, these postures can cause a disc to bulge or rupture. Even the bridge pose, done incorrectly, can injure a vulnerable neck. I am horrified by how often patients tell me they've been hurt after a teacher came up to them when they were doing a vulnerable pose and pushed on them to help make the pose look better.

Find out from your physician and other trained professionals who are the safe, effective yoga practitioners in your region. Then take personalized individual lessons first.

Try tai chi, qigong, and other healing modalities. These have remarkable healing abilities if done regularly and carefully. Tai chi and qigong use slow, precise movements to strengthen the body, lubricate the joints, and improve balance and blood flow. Meditation and visualization exercises help relax the neck and promote healing.

Breathe deeply. Full breathing helps increase oxygen to injured areas and promotes venous and lymphatic drainage of damaged tissue. Since the top of the lungs attach to the lower cervical vertebrae, neck health and lung health will often go hand in hand. The breathing practices in chapter 7 can be extremely helpful.

You don't have to do all that I suggest. Start with one suggestion and gradually build on it. You're in charge. With proper treatment, nutrition, and a movement program that helps encourage better posture, most of my patients who have suffered from neck pain start to feel significantly better in six to eight weeks. Full recovery can sometimes take as much as a year.

17

Hidden Structural Obstacles to Cure

Some people are in bone-crushing accidents and feel great six months later. Others stumble on a sidewalk and their health crumbles. What makes one person resilient while the other is devastated? In my more than thirty years of practice, I have asked myself this question with every patient I could not help. If you've undertaken many of the virtuous tasks I've suggested after an injury, yet you're not much better or you're getting worse, this chapter may have your answer.

Here are some of the factors I consider when evaluating a patient's progress:

- Genetics plays a role in how quickly a patient recovers from trauma, but so does the shape they were in before the trauma. Were they active? Did they consume healthy foods? Were they well rested? Or were they cramming for exams or taking care of a sick baby? Are they male, or female? Males tend to do better in accidents. Density of muscles and higher levels of testosterone seem to partly cushion men against the harmful effects of trauma.

- The patient may have unrealistic expectations about how quickly they will recover from trauma. Many patients (and many physicians) underestimate the amount of damage that trauma can do. Then both the patient and the physician, frustrated with what they consider the slow course of recovery, consider even successful treatments a failure.

  The success of antibiotics in treating bacterial infections has created a mythology of cure that makes everyone impatient about healing. Time and again, I've seen people try to reclaim their lives far too soon after an illness or injury. They demand too much of their bodies long before they have fully healed. This impatience with healing leads to many lingering health problems.

• I consider whether the patient has tried to strengthen injured areas too soon, before the damaging twists and compressions that trauma pounded into their bodies have been removed. If the patient did not first optimize their alignment and mobilize critical joints, they may inadvertently make the damaging distortions more permanent by strengthening the wrong muscles. Your body should be properly aligned and mobilized first, before you start a strengthening regimen.

I have also found that there are common—and commonly overlooked—structural conditions in the body that can profoundly affect recovery and make a person one of the few who does not get well even after their nervous system has returned to balance, inflammation has been addressed, and restrictions in motion resolved. I call these conditions hidden structural obstacles to cure.

1 Hypermobility

Symptoms:

- Extended healing times
- Lingering joint pain and muscle spasm
- Flat feet
- Unexplained anxiety

You've gotten many compliments in your yoga class for your wonderful flexibility, yet your joints and muscles continue to hurt no matter how much stretching you do. If joint and muscle pain lingers long after a trauma and nothing seems to improve it, consider whether your joints are unusually mobile. Has it always taken you longer than other people to heal from injuries? Even if you give your body a lot of time to heal, do you often end up with lingering pain? You may have lived your entire life with a generalized aching that you thought was normal. This aching coaxes you to keep stretching out the painful region, giving you temporary relief, but can ultimately make the situation worse.

Joint hypermobility syndrome is a condition in which a joint or joints move easily beyond the normal range of motion. It is often missed by practitioners, yet it seems to be increasingly common, so I put it front and center as a structural obstacle to cure.

Hypermobile people generally have a genetic condition that weakens the connective tissue. That means the ligaments stabilizing the joints aren't as strong as they should be, and the fascia linking bones, muscles, and organs are more easily overstretched. You've seen pictures of loose-limbed people who can twist themselves into a pretzel and fit themselves into a box. These people are extreme examples of hypermobility. Abraham Lincoln, with his tall, narrow frame, is thought to have had the Marfan's variety. In Marfan's syndrome, the connective tissue laxity can lead to weak blood vessels, especially aortic aneurysms—a potentially fatal condition. The twisting-themselves-into-a-box people usually have Ehlers-Danlos syndrome. They are usually quite athletic and start developing a lot of joint pain by the time they are in their twenties.

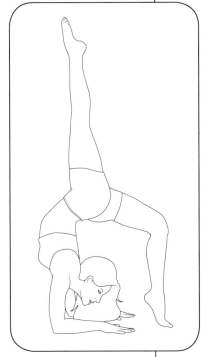

A mild form of hypermobility is fairly common. Some people have mild hypermobility throughout the body. Others may have hypermobility in just a few joints. Their shoulders might be extremely mobile, or their knees or elbows might bend too far backward. Hypermobility occurs nine times more frequently in females.

People with hypermobility syndrome generally have muscle spasm around the overly flexible joints. I believe that this spasm is the muscles' heroic attempt to help stabilize the otherwise too-flexible joints. Because of the increased muscle spasm, these loose-limbed people are constantly stretching to try to relieve the muscle pain. Unfortunately, in doing so they can easily overstretch their ligaments and tendons, which just makes matters worse. However, carefully strengthening these muscles can help stabilize the joints and decrease pain.

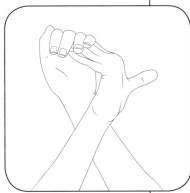

If your hand is this flexible, some of your joints may be hypermobile.

Most of the hypermobile adults I've treated are quite anxious. No doubt, some of this anxiety results from the chronic pain they endure. But I believe some of it comes from constant neurological stimulation. Joint ligaments are richly laced with nerves that inform us where we are in space (proprioception). In hypermobile joints, these nerves are constantly stimulated, flooding the brain with more input than the nervous system can handle. Also, the constantly strained fascia is laced with nerves that report pain and positioning.

All this excess neurological stimulation can lead to anxiety, which sometimes causes them to be branded as hypochondriacs. In fact, these often-athletic individuals are actually in a great deal of pain that they have learned to live with. Having their pain discounted by physicians becomes yet another burden for them. Instead, practitioners need to help them manage their pain, carefully strengthen key muscles, and encourage them to take additional time to recover from injury.

Kids can have excessive backward bending but improve as they grow older. When I diagnose hypermobility in a child, I strongly advise against activities such as gymnastics and ballet that can further overstretch and damage their joints. A person with hypermobility syndrome, whether an adult or child, is more easily and severely injured and their recovery takes longer, so I strongly advise against contact sports such as football and karate as well.

By gently evaluating the patient's range of motion in joints such as the knees, shoulders, elbows, and hands (commonly known as the Beighton score), a health professional can diagnose hypermobility fairly easily. This test does not reveal whether other joints are too flexible, but it's a good general guide. There are some costly genetic scans for some of the connective tissue disorders, but part of the problem with diagnosis stems from the absence of a definitive, reasonably affordable lab test.

If You Suspect You Are Hypermobile

- Obtain a proper diagnosis. Hypermobile people often suffer alone for years with friends and physicians alike discounting their pain. They usually feel a tremendous sense of relief at knowing the reason for their suffering.

- Get flat feet treated. Hypermobile people almost always have loose connective tissue at the bottom of their feet. Flat feet can cause them additional knee, hip, back, and/or neck pain and should be treated with soft orthotics. Once the flat feet are compensated for, hypermobile patients will usually feel better and recover more quickly and completely from injury.

- Allow additional time to recover from injury.

- Find practitioners with experience treating this condition. Any manual therapy must be exceedingly gentle. Postural corrections and muscle strengthening should be addressed by a practitioner (such as a physical therapist, Pilates teacher, or Feldenkrais, Alexander technique, or Egoscue practitioner) who is patient and precise and experienced with hypermobile individuals. Cortisone injections are almost always contraindicated, as they can weaken the already weak connective tissue structures.

- Surgeries that might be appropriate for other people may not be appropriate for people with hypermobility and may carry significant additional risks. The surgeon must be knowledgeable about the consequences and treatment of hypermoblilty.

- My hypermobile patients tell me Ligaplex II, a nutritional ligamentous support system from Standard Process, helps strengthen their ligaments.

- Proper nutrition is essential. Make sure you have a rich supply of minerals in your diet, because they are desperately needed to support the overworked connective tissues. Bone broths and mineral-rich foods such as nuts, yogurt, peppers, and green, leafy vegetables can provide abundant minerals. A good mineral supplement containing calcium, magnesium, zinc, selenium, and potassium is also critical.

- Address inflammation aggressively, as it can further weaken vulnerable ligaments.

- Smoking is an absolute no-no. Smoking increases inflammation and prevents the absorption of critical minerals necessary for ligamentous health.

2 Undiagnosed Foot Problems

Symptoms:

- Unexplained headaches
- Neck and shoulder pain
- Pelvic and back pain
- Knee and ankle pain
- Shoes that wear unevenly
- Stinky feet
- Shin splints

If you have headaches and/or constant pain in your neck, shoulders, upper or lower back, pelvis, knees, or ankles that is not relieved by exercise, stretching, or physical therapy, consider looking at the foundation of your structure: your feet.

Our feet were not designed to pound against pavement for decades. Nor were feet designed to be shoved into pointed shoes. The amazingly complex and delicate toe bones are not engineered to hold up the weight of the body in high heels or stand en pointe in ballet.

If you insist on wearing heels, whether they be cowboy boots or stilettos, you are putting strain on everything above your feet. High heels make your butt stick out by increasing the curve in your low back. That increased angle between your butt and low back may hurt not only your low back but also the shoulders and neck. I recommend all my patients forgo high heels. Luckily, Sarah Jessica Parker isn't my patient.

RANDI came to see me complaining of severe low-back pain. I treated her several times with manual medicine, but the treatments didn't help. Then I watched her play tennis. She looked like she was running over hot pebbles. I realized that her feet were causing her back problems. When I reevaluated her, I found that, indeed, her feet were very flat, and they stank, and the heels of her shoes had worn very unevenly. I sent her to get a decent pair of athletic shoes and soft orthotics.

After she wore soft, custom-made orthotics for two weeks, her back pain disappeared and her feet smelled much better. I've found that people with really smelly feet usually have structural foot problems. However, you may need support for your feet even if they smell delightful.

Time after time, I've found that uncompensated flat or distorted feet can cause back, knee, hip, and even neck pain and can even affect the person's general health. A few minutes of manual medicine to realign the foot bones and tissues can't rectify hours a day of people standing and walking in improper or unsupportive shoes.

People with high arches may also need proper orthotic support. I have quite high arches, but at fifty-five, I found I needed the support of soft orthotics. Once I put them in my shoes, my knee pain disappeared. Sometimes Dr. Scholl's, Superfeet, or other inserts found in good shoe stores can provide enough support. Other times, you need to go to a specialist who makes orthotics. I prefer people wear soft orthotics made with cork, rubber, or leather or a combination of those flexible materials.

How can you tell if you need orthotics? Look at how your shoes wear. If the heel wears unevenly, that can be an indication that you need orthotics. Or have a friend stand behind you while you stand barefoot with your feet about six inches apart. Your Achilles tendon should go straight down the middle of your heel. If the tendon curves in or out, you probably need orthotics.

Of course, you may also need manual therapy to help treat an old ankle or foot strain that is reflected in otherwise recalcitrant knee, hip, shoulder, or neck pain.

3 A Bite Imbalance

Symptoms:

- Unexplained headaches
- TMJ
- Sinus problems
- Tinnitus
- Vision problems
- Neck pain
- Teeth grinding
- Snoring

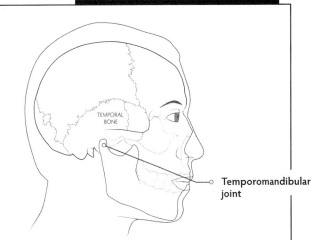

Problems with the bite can compromise the whole structure. Many powerful muscles attach the jaw to the skull and neck. The jaw is connected to the skull at a joint with the temporal bone, called the temporomandibular joint, or TMJ. Through its connection to the temporal bone, a distorted jaw can pull on the head, neck, and upper torso, distorting one or all of them. Bite problems can result in headaches, neck pain, TMJ disorder, sinus problems, tinnitus, and vision problems. Distortions of the bite can also create snoring problems.

Do you grind your teeth at night? Grinding often is your body's attempt to fix your distorted bite. If you grind your teeth, I recommend seeing a dentist who understands how bite affects the motion of the cranial bones. Both your upper and lower jaw have a suture in the middle that must be able to flex. I have seen fixed bridges placed across the top midline cause terrible headaches. While fixed bridges across the midline of the bottom teeth are not as bad as fixed bridges across the top midline, they, too, can cause headaches and neck problems. I always recommend that any dental bridge that spans the midline have a flexible component.

A knowledgeable dentist or orthodontist in some areas can be found through the Osteopathic Cranial Academy (www.cranialacademy.org).

I have seen disastrous health problems result after a dentist has aggressively filed down natural teeth to create a "perfect bite." These patients have lost the proper physiological relationship between the top and bottom jaw, resulting in terrible spasms and pain in the face and jaw as the various muscles frantically try to create the bite the patient was meant to have. The skilled orthodontists I refer to know that most change has to happen gradually. Instead of filing teeth, they move the teeth in a way that does not compromise cranial motion. Filing down fillings, crowns, and bridges is totally different and can be an important method of restoring a proper bite.

4 Problems from Scars

Scars significantly restrict the motion of joints, ligaments, muscles, and fluids. Several times, I've seen the restrictions created by Cesarean sections cause low-back or sacroiliac pain and dysfunction. I've found that by gently stretching the scar through its layers, I can resolve the pain and dysfunction. I now make it a point to ask each patient about scars and always release the restrictions the scars cause. The homeopathic ointment *Thiosinaminum* can also be helpful in releasing scars, and patients can use it themselves.

5 Improper Organ Alignment

Trauma has a knack for throwing organs around inside the body, often twisting them on their stalks. This can weaken the organ's function and create seemingly bizarre pain patterns. When I treat the usual suspects and yet the person still suffers, I evaluate the internal organs and figure out if they are in the wrong place.

Gastroesophageal reflux disease, or GERD, as it is sometimes called, is fairly common after trauma. The stomach is the Waring blender that mixes food and enzymes in a highly acidic environment so nutrients can be absorbed in the intestines. Two mechanisms at the top of the stomach keep this potent acid from flooding up into the esophagus and burning its delicate tissues. A valve directly between the stomach and the esophagus helps keep the acid contained. The diaphragm provides a second mechanism for containing corrosive stomach acid. The esophagus pierces the diaphragm on its way to the stomach where the diaphragmatic fibers weave a second valve around it. This forms a second critical mechanism for preventing acid from escaping the stomach and searing the esophagus. If the diaphragm is out of position, pulled to the side or up or down, this second protection often fails to function properly, allowing acid to stream upward and causing reflux. That's what happened to Giuliana.

GIULIANA had looked forward to a long-planned family trip to Italy to visit her relatives. The trip turned into a nightmare when she walked into her room at a small hotel in Florence. The air reeked of a common household pesticide spray. Apparently, the housekeeper had decided that Americans didn't like the springtime bugs and had doused the air with poisonous insecticide.

Giuliana felt ill instantly. By evening, her achiness and nausea had resolved, but she began to experience a terrible burning sensation in her stomach and throat. The next day, she was rushed to the hospital suffering from uncontrollable acid reflux as her highly corrosive stomach acid leaked into the esophagus and burned its delicate tissue.

When she returned to California, tests confirmed the diagnosis. The specialist was at a loss to explain how pesticide exposure could cause reflux. He put her on a prescription drug to reduce her stomach acid. For two years, Giuliana tried to stop the burning with special diets, herbal teas, and recommended supplements, all to no avail. When her prescription medication started to fail, in desperation she went to an osteopathic manual medicine practioner.

The injury shock created by the pesticide exposure had caused her diaphragm to go into spasm. To make matters worse, the toxic chemicals that flooded her liver caused it to become congested and swollen. The liver has a firm fascial attachment to the diaphragm, so the swollen liver further distorted the diaphragm, rendering the diaphragmatic valve between the stomach and the esophagus ineffective and letting stomach acid course upward and burn the esophagus.

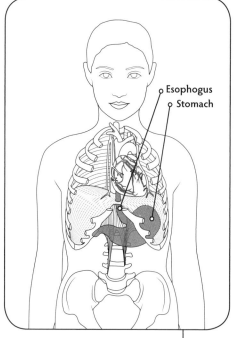

The diaphragm helps keep stomach acid contained, but when it is out of position, that protection can fail and acid reflux can result.

The osteopathic physician took the twists and spasm out of her diaphragm. He helped drain the liver of its toxic congestion. All the strain had dragged the stomach upward, partly into the chest (a mild form of hiatal hernia). He pulled the stomach down and stretched the restricted fascia that had helped maintain the pathology.

After six treatments, Giuliana was able to cut her prescription medicine by two-thirds. After four months, her reflux had totally vanished, and she never again needed medication for it. She goes to her osteopath three times a year to help her liver, diaphragm, and digestive system. But her two-year nightmare of pain had ended.

Any chest or abdominal trauma can twist one or both valves that keep stomach acid contained and allow acid to flood up into the esophagus. Then, like Giuliana, the person can end up with reflux or heartburn. Once the twists are removed and both the stomach and the diaphragm are restored to their proper position, reflux resolves much of the time. I've seen this happen dozens of times.

LYDIA. For months after her car accident, Lydia kept having back pain in the region of her left kidney. She also had two kidney infections. I treated and helped resolve her neck pain, but I couldn't fix her back pain or resolve her kidney infections with antibiotics, manual medicine, or homeopathy. I sent her to a colleague who specializes in osteopathic treatment of the internal organs. He repositioned her distorted kidneys with visceral manipulation, resolving her thoracic back pain. He told me that during car accidents, the fascia holding the kidneys is often pulled upward and twisted. In Lydia's case, the accident had pulled up the left kidney (the one that kept getting infected), partly closing off the urethra, producing pain and leading to repeated infections. After three treatments, the kidney infection was gone and her midback pain resolved.

With all these problems, an understanding of anatomy leads to the proper solutions. As Andrew Taylor Still, MD, said, you need to know three things to be successful as a physician: anatomy, anatomy, and anatomy. Understanding the body's structure and function shows us not only where to look when there is a problem but also how to fix it.

18

A Program for Restoring Motion

Movement is the heart and soul of healing. In chapter 7, I shared ways to release injury shock by restoring the breath and calming the nervous system. This chapter builds on that knowledge so we can further dissolve pain and help restore motion to the rest of our body.

Here, Patricia Sullivan and I focus on simple and effective movements and postures that address problems and pain in the low back, pelvis, chest, upper back, and neck. These practices will also help realign posture so that sitting, walking, and moving will no longer strain painful or injured areas.

Since the lower parts of the body generally have to be put right for the upper parts to follow, Patricia and I will focus on the low back and pelvis first.

A few things to keep in mind as you enjoy your practice:

- Exercises are most effective if done on a regular basis. Try for three or four times a week initially, and, if possible, build up to doing some every day.

- Listen to your body. Start out slowly and increase gradually.

- An exercise should not cause pain. If it does, stop. The next day, try a different one.

- Enjoy! The more you do these, the more your body will crave them.

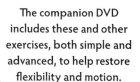

The companion DVD includes these and other exercises, both simple and advanced, to help restore flexibility and motion.

To help you navigate our recommendations, groups of exercises particularly beneficial to certain parts of the body are listed below. However, most of these movements and postures will help multiple areas of the body. This is especially true of the first set of poses, which help the low back but also help line up and heal the whole body. But do not continue a movement if it hurts. Even the simplest exercises can be wrong for certain people. Let comfort be your guide. See a movement specialist to make sure you are doing them correctly.

POSTURES FOR THE LOW BACK

PELVIC AND SACRAL EXERCISES

STRETCHES FOR THE UPPER BACK AND NECK

RELAXATION

Maud   Child's Pose, page 220

Rest Pose, page 220

GENERALLY SAFE TO DO AFTER A RECENT INJURY

Alternate Reaching, page 208

Standing Against the Wall, page 209

Legs on a Chair, page 65

A Pencil in Your Cheeks, page 212

Pelvic Tilt, page 213

Pelvic Clock, page 214

Sleep with a Pillow Between the Knees, page 214

Kegel Exercises, page 215

Child's Pose, page 220

Rest Pose, page 220

DO WHEN YOU HAVE IMPROVED

Cat/Cow, page 210

Downward Dog, page 211

Abdominal Strengtheners, page 212

Squatting, page 215

Shoulder Rolls, page 216

Thumb Circles, page 217

Hands Behind the Head, page 217

Arms Above the Head, page 218

Snow Angels on a Blanket, page 219

ESPECIALLY HELPFUL AFTER BRAIN INJURY

Pelvic Tilt, page 213

Snow Angels on a Blanket, page 219

Child's Pose, page 220

Rest Pose, page 220

when you are feeling better, add:

Cat/Cow, page 210

Downward Dog, page 211

POSTURES FOR THE LOW BACK

PATRICIA: Pain is often created by an asymmetrical load on the body from a forward-leaning posture. The back is strained as it tries to pull the body upright. The neck muscles are not designed to support an off-center head.

Aligning our posture is one of the most powerful ways of restoring liveliness to the pelvis, sacrum, low back, chest, neck, and head. Yoga poses that require equal demand of the body's many planes enable us to be at ease. When we are centered with respect to the forces of gravity and the dynamic tensions of left to right, forward, and back, we can carry ourselves easily and without strain.

Alternate Reaching

I often begin my classes on the floor with this reaching exercise. This helps wake up the lumbar spine and then lets that wakening travel up and down the whole spine. It helps to loosen the rib joints where they connect to the spine, a spot that tends to get locked up after trauma. By gently reaching and bowing the rib cage, these connections become softer and looser. This exercise also calms the fight-or-flight sympathetic nervous system that runs along that part of the spine and allows the calming parasympathetic nervous system to wake up.

▶ Lying on the floor, reach long through the left arm and left leg, release, and then gently lengthen through the right arm and right leg. As you reach to one side, the rib cage will bow on that side; this means the spine is also bowing. It's a small movement, but these small movements can be very powerful. Do about ten on each side.

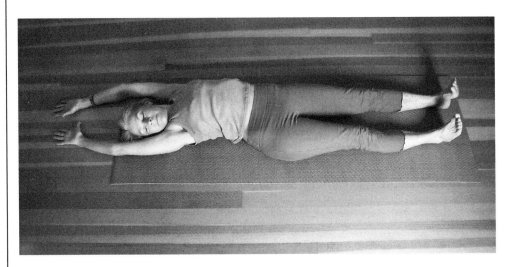

Standing Against the Wall

Working against the wall is a good way to begin reversing a forward-leaning posture. It wakes up the musculature that may have gotten lazy due to a hunched alignment. Notice that it takes a lot of work just to stand straight!

◑ Stand with your heels at the wall and bring the whole body straight back: the buttocks, the upper back and shoulder region, and, if possible, the head, without tilting the head back or deeply tucking it. Try to touch the wall equally at all points. Let your palms rest on your thighs. Let the breath flow as freely as you are able. Stand for a minute or two and feel the body realign itself with the feedback from the wall.

- As you step away, observe if your body can remain in the same position as against the wall. The more we stand against the wall with the head over the shoulders, the more normal that begins to feel to our nervous system.

- Don't let your arms fall forward out of habit. You should feel some portion of your arms touching the wall. This brings the shoulder blades into a better position with respect to the spine.

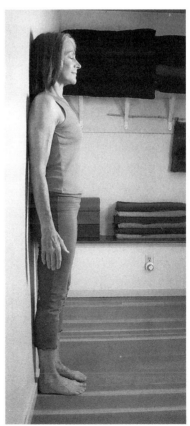

Cat/Cow

Cat/Cow is a classic yoga sequence used to stretch the chest, mobilize the upper back, release the neck, and move the low back in and out. This movement helps pump fluid into the discs of the spine. Any part of the spine that doesn't move freely means another part has to take up the load; it also can compress our nerves and our discs. By pumping up the discs, we help release pressure on the nerves leaving the spine. Moving smoothly and rhythmically through the range of motion in the spine allows all sections of the spine to become flexible. As we do this repeatedly, it helps release the diaphragm and relax the neck.

◐ Start on your hands and knees, with your hands directly underneath the shoulders and your knees directly under the hips as best as you can manage. Take an in-breath, and as you exhale, move your tailbone and your head toward each other, pressing the whole spine toward the ceiling. As you inhale, drop the chest toward the ground, allow the shoulder blades to sink and collapse toward each other, and then lift the head.

Cat

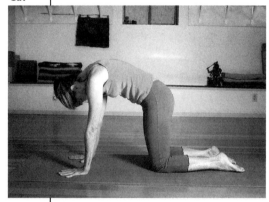

• As you move into the Cat position, keep the shoulder blades away from the ears and let the neck release down. It's much more relaxing to the neck.

• As you move into the Cow posture, wait toward the end of the movement, then slowly lift the head to about 70 percent of its full extension—even less if your neck is in pain. Lifting the head too vigorously can increase neck pain.

• Keep the elbows straight if you possibly can. You may not notice that you're bending your elbows, so every time you take your head down, watch the elbows.

Cow

210

Downward Dog

In Downward Dog, a tractionlike quality happens in the spine. This is especially good for the low back and the neck. The traction benefits the joints and the weight of gravity releases all the little connections in the neck that might be tight. The pose also helps stretch the chest. Downward Dog is an excellent pose to follow Cat/Cow.

▶ Put your weight on your hands and feet and lift your tail to the sky. It's more important to keep your spine straight than to keep your heels on the floor. Let your head rest between your arms. Hold for 15 to 20 seconds and then release. After a brief rest, repeat several times.

- The arms and legs should be lined up parallel to each other. Everything else should be symmetrical—hips at the same height, shoulders at the same height. This trains your joints to work with balanced effort.

- To do Downward Dog, you need to be able to take some weight on the arms. It's helpful if the back of your legs are a bit stretched out. If they aren't, don't straighten the legs as you come up.

- If the pose is too difficult on the shoulders, wrists, or hamstrings, do a modified pose with the arms resting on a chair or up the wall. It doesn't require as much leg stretch but still allows the shoulders and upper back to release.

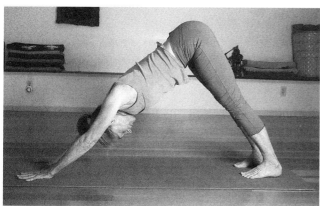

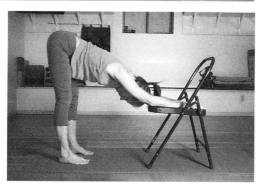

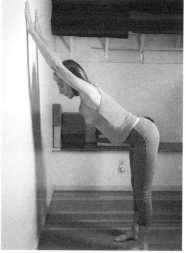

211

MAUD: My turn now. Along with the poses Patricia just covered, I've found that the Legs on a Chair pose on page 65 is one of the most important for people with low-back pain. I recommend that people with low-back pain take a break two or three times a day and do this pose for five to fifteen minutes each time. All poses where the head is down, I suspect, help cerebral spinal fluid flow into the brain and better flush debris out of it. My mentor, Stanley Schiowitz, DO, gave his patients these simple exercises to keep their backs healthy. I recommend them to my patients once the acute injury has calmed down. As always, start slowly, one at a time, and gradually increase the repetitions.

A Pencil in Your Cheeks

These movements help the sacrum reseat itself in the pelvis and strengthen weak muscles in the pelvis and abdomen.

◗ Stand in a relaxed fashion with your feet hip width apart. Pretend you are holding a pencil between your buttocks cheeks. At the same time, rotate your thighs inward. If this seems hard to do, put your hands on your inner thighs and gently encourage your thighs to turn in toward each other. Do this three times, holding for 15 seconds each. Try to build up to 30 seconds each.

Abdominal Strengtheners

These small movements strengthen stomach muscles and help improve posture, the first step toward building core strength.

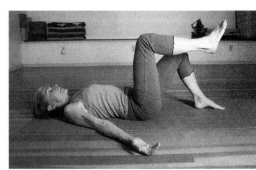

Lower Abdominals
◗ Lie on your back with your feet on the floor. Keeping your right leg at a constant angle, bring your right knee up toward the head just a little past your hip. Hold for 5 to 10 seconds, then place the foot back down.

Upper Abdominals
◗ With your feet on the floor and your arms relaxed at your sides, lift your chin slightly toward the ceiling. Lift your chest and head one inch off the floor, then place it back down.

  • On day one, do each of these five times slowly. Build up to twenty times.

PELVIC AND SACRAL PROBLEMS

PATRICIA: It's important to release the sacrum so that the lumbar spine doesn't have to do the sacrum's work. In car accidents and other kinds of trauma, the sacrum often gets jammed into one side of the pelvic bones. When that happens, the pelvic area becomes frozen and everything above is affected. The Cat/Cow and Downward Dog poses begin the process of releasing pelvic restrictions. The following sequence of postures can also help.

Pelvic Tilt

Tipping the pelvis forward and back starts releasing a jammed sacrum from where it nestles into the hipbones. It also helps awaken muscles that may have weakened. Once the pelvis has been repositioned into the proper alignment, performing pelvic tilts helps keep the pelvis in balance.

In this pose, the connection between the sacrum and the neck is very direct—more direct than almost anything else you can do. It allows release in both the pelvis and the neck.

◗ Lie on your back with your feet comfortably away from your hips and knees, the arms out at a 45-degree angle and the head and neck relaxed. Gently rock the pelvis head to tail, alternately having the lower back on the floor and off the floor. The head and neck should be gently rocking with the pelvis. If it isn't, you're actually tightening and holding something you want to let go. Do this ten to fifteen times.

- As simple and relaxing as this exercise seems, it's very potent. The neck and sacral areas are connected by the dural membrane that wraps the spinal cord. When one end is jammed or frozen, the other end is going to be pulled on as well. This exercise moves both ends in a very rhythmic and coordinated fashion, helping move fluid into the dural membrane and softening both the neck and pelvis.

- The parasympathetic nerves live in the neck and sacrum. Releasing the neck and pelvis stimulates the PNS, which makes us feel calmer.

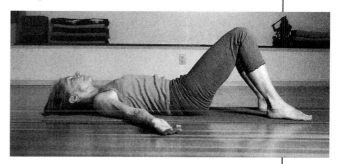

The Pelvic Clock

The way the pelvic bones connect to the sacrum is like a jigsaw puzzle. Unevenness of the connection can distort the pelvis. By accessing a third dimension of movement, the pelvic clock exercise starts to loosen up some of those connections and create more freedom in the pelvis. It's safe and really fun. Since the sacrum is tied into the nervous system, this movement also quiets the nervous system.

In my mind's eye, I draw a clock that starts near my navel and circles around to my pubic bone and back around again. The top, near my navel, is twelve on the clock, the pubic bone is six, and the hipbones are three and nine.

▶ Lie on your back with your knees bent and your feet flat on the floor. Go around in a circle, pressing your pelvis to the floor at each of the numbers on the clock in sequence. I start at twelve and then go to my right: eleven o'clock, ten o'clock, nine o'clock, back to twelve. Then I go back the other way: one o'clock, two o'clock, three o'clock, and so forth, back to twelve. Stay relaxed as you do this, and keep the breath flowing. I recommend doing this five or six times in each direction.

- Once you feel comfortable with this movement, you can go a little faster, in one direction a couple of times, and then the other way. You will feel like you're floating on water.

- You might find that you're moving your jaw at the same time you're moving your pelvis. That's okay.

- When you sit up, take time to notice how you feel. The tendency is for everything to feel a little sweeter.

MAUD: Everyone can benefit by paying attention to their sacred bone. Balancing the sacrum and pelvis are two of the most effective things you can do for low-back pain. If the imbalance in the sacrum and pelvis is not severe or long-standing, here are three things you can do to help reposition the sacrum.

Sleep with a Pillow Between the Knees

I advise people with a pelvic or hip problem to sleep on their side with a pillow between the knees. This position takes strain off the sacroiliac ligaments and puts the pelvis into a much more balanced position. A pillow under the upper arm can help, too (see photos page 321).

Kegel Exercises

Kegel exercises help strengthen and balance the pelvic diaphragm, which helps pump the fluids and organs in the pelvis. Many women and men have a weak pelvic diaphragm.

There are two sets of opposing muscles in the pelvic diaphragm. Initially, it is easiest to identify the relevant muscles during urination. When someone quickly stops urine flow, they're tightening one set of the muscles within the pelvic diaphragm and relaxing the other. If they actively push urine out, they are relaxing the first set of muscles and toning the second. Tightening and actively relaxing each of these muscles are the two parts of a Kegel exercise. People can do this any time, as it isn't visible to others.

◗ Tighten your pelvic floor muscles for 5 seconds, then actively push them out for 5 seconds. Try to do this five times in a row, building up to 10 seconds of contraction and pushing down five times in a row. Be careful not to tighten muscles in your abdomen or buttocks as you do the exercise.

Squatting

Squatting with both feet flat on the floor and some of the weight supported by the hands helps open up the wings of the pelvis, allowing the sacrum to reseat itself between them. Gently rocking forward and back can help coax more healthy motion into the pelvis.

◗ Come down on all fours and gently press your elbows into your knees. Stay in this position for 10 seconds and up to a minute, depending on comfort. Occasionally, rock back and forth gently.

- If this position is uncomfortable, come out of the pose. The sacroiliac joints may be too jammed or mis-aligned for the posture and you may need the assistance of a practitioner skilled in sacral realignment to help release them.

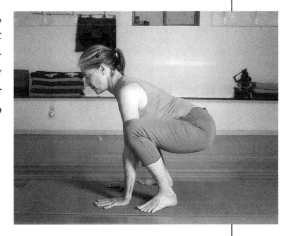

STRETCHES FOR THE UPPER BACK AND NECK

PATRICIA: In this series, we are working to both relax and strengthen the upper back. Since the torso dominates the neck, it is absolutely essential to restore motion to it first. When the upper back and the shoulders are relaxed and easily holding the body upright, the neck is much more readily released. Getting the back stronger can also help realign our forward-leaning posture and take pressure off the neck. I've already introduced Standing Against the Wall, Cat/Cow, and Downward Dog poses, which also address the upper back and the neck. Here are a few more suggestions:

Shoulder Rolls

The simple movement of rolling the shoulders forward and back recenters the shoulders where they should be and awakens the areas of the upper back that hold us upright.

▶ Start by rolling the shoulders back and down. As you roll your shoulders backward, feel the squeezing motion as the shoulder blades come together. Then release the shoulder blades and continue rolling the shoulders forward and up. Your hands should be gliding over the thighs so you don't do anything overly dramatic with the arms. Do about twenty or thirty of these. Then pause, relax for a moment, and do twenty to thirty in the reverse direction.

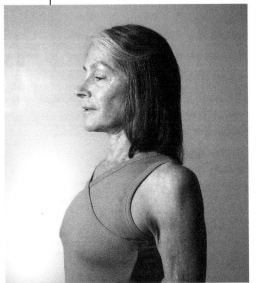

• If you overemphasize how much you lift the arms, you're actually tightening the neck. Just use the shoulders, gliding them around in a circle.

• Notice whether these movements tend to push your head forward. Keep standing upright as though you're standing right against the wall, breathing, squeezing, releasing, breathing, squeezing, releasing.

• If you feel fatigued after twenty or so rotations, stop. You can build up to thirty over a week or two.

Hands Behind the Head

This movement opens up the back and is very relaxing for the neck!

▶ Bring the hands up and interlace the fingers lightly behind the skull. Let the head rest back into the hands. As you begin to bring the elbows back, you will start to feel your shoulder blades pressing more firmly on your back. Your back has become more alive!

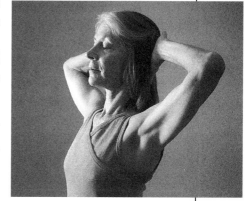

When the arms come down, pause to feel how wonderful that feels. Hold for 20 seconds if it feels good. Repeat two more times.

- Don't let the hands push the head forward.

- Try walking in this position. It helps open and strengthen the upper back.

Thumb Circles

This simple exercise is a great one for opening the upper chest and strengthening the mid-thoracic region. If one shoulder blade is stronger and works harder than the other one, this exercise helps equalize them.

▶ Stretch out your arms to the side, palms down. Curl your fingertips toward your palms in an open fist and point your thumbs to the front. As you gently squeeze the tips of your shoulder blades together, make small, six-inch circles with your outstretched arms, down, then up. After making fifteen circles, flip your palms up and move the arms, shoulders, and thumbs in a circle the other way, circling up, down, and around like a hitchhiker.

- This can be very tiring the first time you do it, so build up gradually. Usually, people can do fifteen at first. Progress gradually up to thirty.

- Be sure you're not jutting the head forward.

- Make small movements while the body remains steady and stable.

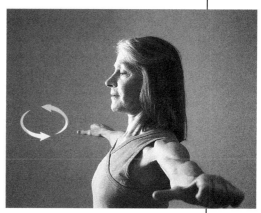

Arms Above the Head

This is a great opener for the upper ribs and the back, too. It not only calms the nervous system but also helps the diaphragm relax and the ribs expand.

▶ Interlace your fingers and start to bring them in front of your face. Squeeze your shoulder blades together. With palms down, push your hands toward the ceiling. As you pull your arms toward your ears, go only as far as you can without pain. Hold for 5 seconds.

Then, slowly flip your palms over so that the palms now point toward the ceiling. Keep your chest lifted and your shoulder blades together. Hold for 10 seconds. Repeat three or four times.

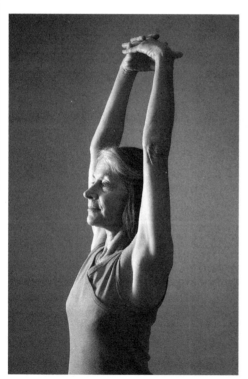 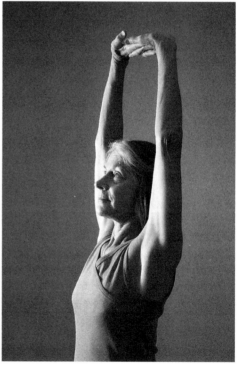

Snow Angels on a Blanket

This pose is a wonderful release for the chest and neck. Lying on a rolled-up blanket placed vertically along the spine will begin to loosen the muscles of the spine. It also helps loosen the connections between the rib cage and the spine, thus calming the sympathetic nervous system. This exercise is usually offered late in the yoga class, when the person has moved and stretched and loosened everything in the body.

▶ Fold the blanket three or four times lengthwise and lie down on it. Feet should be on the floor, arms out to the side, palms up. Starting slowly at first, move the hands up a bit higher than where they started, then back to the middle and up again as if you are making snow angels. If you have tight shoulders, make very small movements close to the body. Do this for about 30 seconds.

- If you have any kind of neck injury or neck stiffness, use a small towel under your head, or roll the blanket up under your head so that your chin is lower than your forehead. This elongates and stretches the neck so it's not arched backward.

- This posture bows the rib cage forward and opens the diaphragm, allowing it to move more freely.

NOTE: The exercise also can be done with a foam roller or a softer M.E.L.T. roller placed under the head, upper back, and pelvis and the feet flat on the floor. Use of the roller helps strengthen the abdominal muscles, as you must maintain your balance on the roller as you move your arms.

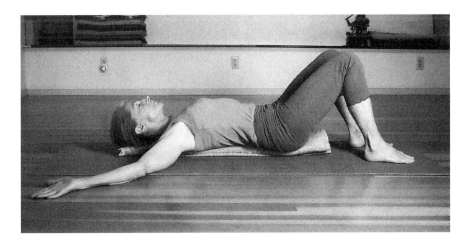

RELAXATION

MAUD: Here are two wonderful poses for the end of your practice.

Child's Pose

My mentor, Ann Wales, DO, who lived to be 101, told me that doing the Child's Pose every day makes for a long life. It certainly feels good, and now I will remember to do it more often. It is a good pose to put toward the end of your movement time.

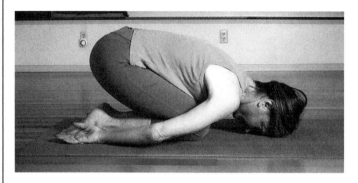

Rest Pose

Yogis say that resting your body in a comfortable position at the end of the session is the most important part of the practice. Let your body ease into relaxation. If you are cold, be sure to cover yourself with a blanket. You may need a little height or softness under your head, a cloth or eye pillow to cover and relax your eyes, or pillows or blocks to relax your legs. As you rest and let your body soak in your experience, the nervous system can absorb the changes that your practice has orchestrated for it.

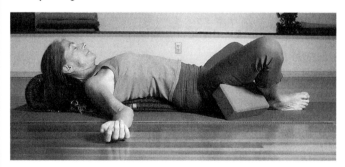

IV.

Healing Head and Brain Injury

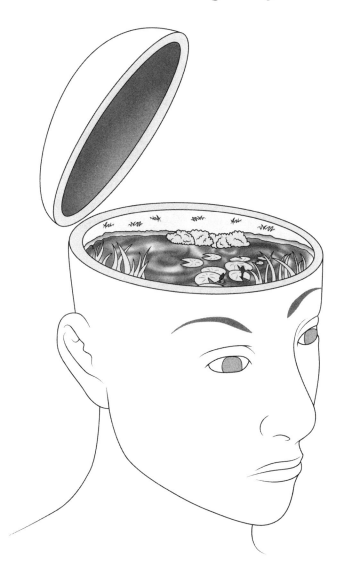

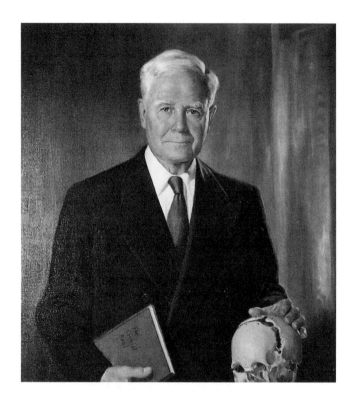

William G. Sutherland, DO
1873–1954

William G. Sutherland was an early student of Andrew Taylor Still, MD, the founder of osteopathic medicine. A reporter turned physician, Will Sutherland remained endlessly curious and inventive. Upon discovering the movement of the cranial bones and the pulsations of the brain, he created cranial osteopathic medicine.

19

The Skull:
The Brain's Formidable Protector

Life is motion. Therefore, it should not be strange to us that the master of life—the brain—is constantly moving as it orchestrates life. It's a novel concept to most people because they can't see, feel, or hear the beating of the brain. It took two brave physicians to buck the common wisdom a hundred years ago. Not only did they claim that the brain pulsates, but they also found ways to feel those pulsations and designed treatments to help the brain heal following injury.

Throughout this book, I have focused on many critical aspects of the nervous system. We have seen the wonders of the autonomic nervous system as it regulates our breathing and heartbeat and provides the richness of our sexual experience. We have learned how nervous system dysfunction not only contributes to injury shock, PTSD, breathing and cardiac problems, and digestive distress but also stokes the fires of inflammation. I have shown you many ways to address these problems.

Now I turn my attention to the master of the nervous system: the brain itself. In this section, I explore how the brain lives and thrives, how it gets hurt, how it responds to trauma, and its role in pain. I discuss some straightforward methods practitioners can use to help the injured brain.¹ I also discuss some critical things people can do for themselves to help restore health to the brain.

The brain does not live alone. Extensive layers of protection embrace it. First, it is surrounded and penetrated by flowing cerebral spinal fluid (CSF). The CSF cushions the brain from insults and nourishes it. Second, a system of dural membranes surrounds the fluid and the brain. These membranes attach to the inside of the skull, then form several sickle-shaped dividers that separate parts of the brain and help diffuse forces that pound the head. The membranes also send delicate fibers deep into the custardlike brain to feed it and anchor it within the protective skull.

The skull is not a rock. It is made up of 108 joints that glide over one another or function like gears. The skull expands and contracts in coordination with the motion of the membranes and the brain. For optimal health, all three—bone, brain, and membranes—must move synchronously together.

Though osteopathic physicians have been exploring the brain's pulsations for decades, we don't know what propels them. Perhaps it is an electromagnetic or hydraulic force. We do know, however, that this motion helps propel nutrients into the brain and pump waste products out of the brain. When this motion slows, the brain's sea becomes soiled and the brain struggles. When the motion is optimized, the sea regains its pristine nature and the brain thrives.

Free movement of the skull is essential for optimal brain health. The skull provides essential channels that allow oxygen, glucose, and other nutrients to reach the hungry brain. The skull also provides gateways for toxic debris to leave. So I begin this section with the skull. I also begin here because the skull gives us critical access to the brain. We can put our hands directly on it to open the channels. Furthermore, lots of times, people smack their head without injuring their brain. Compression of the skull by itself can create problems like headaches, dizziness, sinus problems, or the myriad of symptoms listed above. Often these problems can be resolved by treating the skull.

As I talk about treating the skull, remember: the dural membranes attach to the inside of the skull. They send their fibers deep into the brain. So the skull, the dura, and the brain all move together. By freeing up the skull, we can help the three components of the head regain their synchronized movement. When that happens, seemingly miraculous healing of brain and body occurs.

THE MYSTERY OF THE DISARTICULATED SKULL

At the beginning of the twentieth century, two young osteopathic physicians realized that the skull is not a solid ball of bone. Independent of one another, each realized that the joints of the skull, just like joints in the rest of the body, were designed to move. From that profound realization, William G. Sutherland and Charlotte Weaver made remarkable discoveries about both the normal and abnormal motions of the skull and the medical—especially neurological—problems that can result from abnormal motion.

My cranial training has followed in the tradition of Dr. Sutherland. So let's go back to the beginning of the twentieth century, when a curious medical student saw a disarticulated (split-apart) skull positioned on a metal stand—a skull very similar to the one in the picture that begins this chapter. Seeing all the bones separated from each other, Sutherland noticed a curious fact. The edges of the joint (suture) between the temporal bone on the side of the skull and the sphenoid bone in front were beveled like the gills of a fish. He suspected that these gill-like joints were designed to allow for motion. Looking more closely, he realized that all the bones of the skull were designed to move. Some looked like gears, and some had the same beveled edges designed to slide over each other. "Why?" he asked himself.

Taking his exploration further, Sutherland examined the heads of his colleagues. With his perceptive touch, he discovered that the skull pulsates at a different rate than the beating of the heart or the rhythm of the breath. What could cause such pulsations? After searching through the body for an explanation, he found an answer. Inside the skull, the brain expands and contracts. A healthy brain has a strong, even amplitude (strength of pulsation) throughout the skull. Optimally, this pulsation occurs six to fourteen times a minute. If the head is traumatized, however, and the expansion of the skull's joints is diminished or distorted, the strength and fullness of the brain's pulsation is also diminished.

As years went on, this insightful physician examined countless patients and found that when certain cranial sutures got jammed, patients experienced symptoms such as headaches, dizziness, or hearing and vision problems. These symptoms corresponded to the specific areas of the skull that had been compromised. When the restricted region was released, the symptoms usually resolved. Since the head is lined inside by a dense web of dural membrane, Sutherland also realized that a blow or restriction in any part of the skull could have ramifications in other parts of the skull. Because the membrane links the expanding and contracting skull with the pulsating brain, a blow to the head not only reverberates throughout the skull but also affects the brain and its intricate membrane system.

Sutherland and his students found that by using these new cranial techniques, they could also cure previously untreatable problems such as migraines, trigeminal neuralgia, tinnitus, colic in newborns, and some hormonal and nervous system problems. He and his followers also claimed that the brain could heal and regenerate, something that the rest of medicine has only recently acknowledged. In the 1980s, medical science began catching up with Sutherland's discoveries. Movies taken during neurosurgery showed the brain pulsating in the way Sutherland had described. Other scientific studies confirmed that the skull minutely expands and contracts to accommodate this motion of the brain. Now, cranial osteopathy is a prominent specialty commanding respect from the osteopathic and allopathic medical communities.

FOUR TROUBLE SPOTS

I have been using cranial osteopathy for more than three decades, and its ability to cure countless problems never ceases to amaze me. Besides its powerful ability to treat headaches, immune problems, and balance, digestive, vision, hearing, and hormonal disorders, I have found that proper alignment and free movement of the skull's many bones is essential for the health of the brain.

In this chapter, as I introduce the brain's bony home, it's not my purpose to go into detail about the techniques I use to diagnose a jammed suture or separate and realign the bones of the head. Working with these bones is an exacting

A Healing Moment

At my first cranial course, within a few hours, every other physician in the room could feel the elusive cranial rhythmic impulse; I couldn't. Then, on day three, eighty-year-old Rebecca Lippincott, DO, joined us. She had spent decades working with the founder of cranial osteopathy, William Sutherland, DO. Seeing my struggle, she put her hands on the patient's head and had me sit down next to her, telling me, "Put your hands on my hands and listen." I gently placed my hands on her wise hands and felt them move ever so slightly. After I'd gained a sense of the head's rhythm, Dr. Lippincott moved away. I put my hands directly on the patient's head and suddenly felt that slight expansion and contraction of the skull that reflects the brain's pulsation. That moment was one of the most magical of my life, transforming my sense of the human body. Feeling the nervous system's pulsation filled me with amazing awe for the life force within us. Having been given this gift by Dr. Lippincott, I now teach it to others.

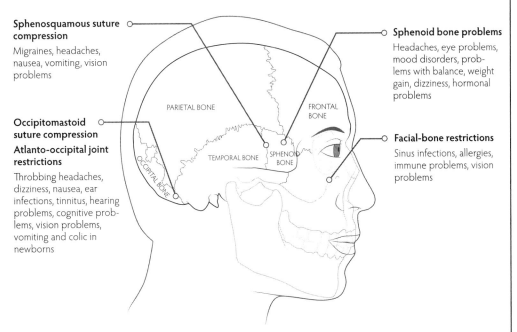

Sphenosquamous suture compression

Migraines, headaches, nausea, vomiting, vision problems

Occipitomastoid suture compression

Atlanto-occipital joint restrictions

Throbbing headaches, dizziness, nausea, ear infections, tinnitus, hearing problems, cognitive problems, vision problems, vomiting and colic in newborns

Sphenoid bone problems

Headaches, eye problems, mood disorders, problems with balance, weight gain, dizziness, hormonal problems

Facial-bone restrictions

Sinus infections, allergies, immune problems, vision problems

PARIETAL BONE

FRONTAL BONE

TEMPORAL BONE

SPHENOID BONE

OCCIPITAL BONE

Four major trouble spots in the skull's web of bones can cause a whole host of problems.

and precise undertaking, demanding intimate knowledge of anatomy and years of medical training and experience. What I do want people to know is that if they suffer from seemingly intractable problems caused by restrictions in the skull's bones or sutures, those problems can, with proper diagnosis and treatment, go away.

The skull's remarkable flexibility is a two-edged sword. Because the skull's twenty-nine bones can minutely expand, slide, flex, and twist at the jagged joints called sutures, the head can expand and contract to accommodate the pulsations of the healthy brain. In turn, the beating brain helps keep the skull's joints freely moving. The skull's flexibility allows it to absorb a blow more easily than could a rigid structure.

The skull's flexibility has a downside. If a person hits their head too hard or in the wrong place, the sutures can jam together and compress the nerves and arteries that pass through or over the area. The sutures also can lose mobility due to an infection, allergies, or pulls from the rest of the body. Think of the skull like a big, three-dimensional Swiss watch with bigger gears in back and smaller gears in front. If you smack the watch, the gears jam. Just as a person needs a watchmaker to fix a bent watch, to fix a jammed skull, they usually need a practitioner trained in cranial treatment.

Although blows to the skull can reverberate anywhere in the head's intricate web of bones, I find five areas to be the most vulnerable and troublesome, including the head's connection to the neck. I always evaluate these regions and take special care not to compress them when I treat a patient.

THE BACK OF THE HEAD
The Occipitomastoid Suture
The Atlanto-Occipital Joint

Symptoms:

- Colic
- Deafness and hearing problems
- Digestive problems
- Dizziness, vertigo, and nausea
- Headaches
- Tinnitus

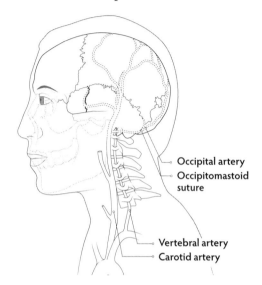

JULIE. Nine-year-old Julie had just joined a children's choir. Her luminous voice thrilled her teacher. But one day, as she stepped off a curb into the street, a speeding car forced her to jump back. She tripped and fell backward, hitting the back of her head on the curb.

A few days later, she developed headaches. Over the next year, she started having one ear infection after another. No one connected her headaches or chronic ear infections to her fall. She was completely deaf in her right ear by the time the doctors removed the mastoid portion of her right temporal bone to deal with the chronic infections.

By the time she was fourteen, Julie was crippled by severe, unrelenting headaches. Attempting to control the pain, her physician gave her large amounts of pain medication, which caused dangerously irregular heartbeats. Her mother took her to a cardiologist who, being an osteopathic physician herself, was familiar with osteopathic manual medicine. She referred Julie to me.

Julie and her mom drove three hours to my office. When Julie walked in, a hatch line of pain marked her forehead. I asked about head injuries, but neither Julie nor her mother could recall one. Her mother handed me a ten-page spreadsheet on which she had meticulously logged all of the drugs her daughter had been taking to try to control her pain.

While this was a seemingly complex case, the answer was relatively simple once I looked at the patient's anatomy. Julie had injured an area that is rich in blood vessels and nerves. When injury compromises this area, the results can be disastrous for health, but the solution is relatively straightforward.

To explain what caused Julie's constant headaches and her hearing loss—and how she got better—I need to introduce you to the first trouble spot: the place where the back of the head meets the side of the head. The large bone that forms the base and the back of the skull is called the occiput. The occiput shares an inch-long joint with a bone on the side of the head called the temporal bone. (There is one temporal bone on each side). The place where the occiput and temporal bone come together is called the occipitomastoid, or OM, suture.

The temporal bones are fan-shaped bones that sit on either side of the head, like snug little hats circling your ears. If you put your thumb gently in your ear and fan your fingers above it, you have a general idea of where the temporal bones are. These are the very bones Dr. Sutherland so famously realized looked like the gills of a fish. Because unhappy temporal bones can cause many health problems, cranial osteopaths call them "the troublemakers of the head."

When I touched the back of Julie's skull, I could feel the occipital bone was pushed forward on the right side into the temporal bone; the suture between them felt like it had been soldered shut. This was the side on which Julie had lost her hearing. The left side didn't feel much better. These findings made me quite sure that a powerful blow to the back of her head had locked up these bones. When I asked again about head trauma, Julie remembered falling backward and hitting the curb, and said, "It's true I haven't felt right since then."

Julie's suffering makes sense to me. Trauma that locks up the temporal bones—such as a blow to the back of the head—is notorious for causing ear infections. I often see ear infections in children when head trauma of some kind (including a difficult birth) has locked up their temporal bones. It's simple anatomy. The inner ear runs through the temporal bones. The movement of the temporal bones pumps the ear canals and keeps them free of fluid so the ears don't brew infection. Julie's fall had shoved the temporal bone and the occipital bone together and restricted the temporal bone's motion. Its pumping action became very unenthusiastic, and fluid in her ear canals stagnated. When that happens, bacteria grows. The result was Julie's repeated ear infections.

Why did this blow cause Julie such severe headaches? Again, the anatomy of this crowded region gives the answer. The head has efficiently created passageways for the hundreds of nerves and blood vessels that crisscross this

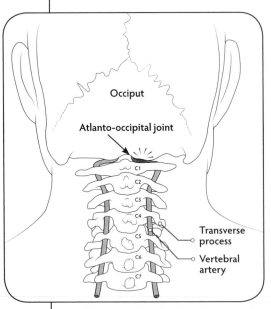

Occiput

Atlanto-occipital joint

C1
C2
C3
C4
C5
C6
C7

Transverse process

Vertebral artery

region in their journey between the brain and the rest of the body. Two important—and pain-causing—structures run right over the OM suture. The occipital nerve and the occipital artery that supply the scalp run behind the ear and over the channel of the OM suture. This artery and nerve are covered by a sleeve of connective tissue (fascia) that weaves through the suture. When the suture is jammed together, it pulls the connective tissue, pinching the vulnerable artery and/or nerve and causing severe headaches.

My job was to restore motion to the occipital and temporal bones so the temporal bones could pump the stagnant ear canals and the vulnerable artery and nerve could move freely. Freeing up that area was only part of the battle, however. I knew I had another job to do to completely eliminate Julie's headaches.

Given the force of Julie's backward fall, the back of her head also had been shoved downward into her first cervical (neck) vertebra. I often find that blows to the back of the head jam this atlanto-occipital joint. When it is jammed or misaligned, all kinds of health problems can result.

As we learned in the neck chapter, the neck's first vertebra is unique among all the bones of the spine. Because the first cervical vertabra balances the heavy head on its shoulders, it is called the atlas, after the Greek Titan, Atlas, who held up the world. For the head to stay balanced on top of the spine, the skull and the atlas must be properly aligned and moving freely together.

The two vertebral arteries—which provide half of the blood supply to the brain—must cross the space between the atlas and the base of the skull. If trauma narrows that space, as it did with Julie, one or both arteries get squeezed. Arteries have many pain fibers. These compressed arteries probably contributed to Julie's headaches.

I had my job set out for me. Using the precise techniques of cranial osteopathy, I pulled the temporal bone away from the occipital bone in order to free the occipital nerve and artery and get the temporal bone pumping again. Using a technique William Sutherland named the "cookie jar" to separate these two bones, I held the base of the skull steady with one hand while I gently rotated the temporal bone until it came free. I repeated this technique on the other side.

To free up the vertebral artery, I separated the occipital bone from its weld to the top of the neck. Using one of Dr. Ann Wales's favorite techniques that she learned from Sutherland, I held the back of Julie's head with one hand—always careful to not compress either OM joint. I had Julie hold her breath. At the same time, with my other hand I gently balanced the back of the first cervical vertebra on the tip of my middle finger. As Julie struggled for breath, that effort released the compression. When she finally inhaled, the bones separated and were back where they belonged. I also gave Julie homeopathic *Naja tripudians* to address the initial trauma and her subsequent symptoms.

By her third visit, Julie had almost no headaches and the ones she had were mild. She had stopped taking all pain medication. As her cardiologist had hoped, once off the medication, her heartbeat returned to normal. After two more visits, her headaches were gone. If Julie had not been treated, I suspect, she would have also gone deaf in her other ear.

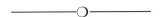

I started with Julie's story because injuries to the back of the head are so common, and the devastating problems they cause can be relatively easy to fix when the practitioner understands the anatomy and has the skills to make the precise corrections.

RELIEVING COLIC IN NEWBORNS

The healing power of cranial work can be especially dramatic in treating a newborn suffering from colic. Years ago, a friend of mine who had lived in England told me, "There's no colic in England."

"Why is that?" I asked.

"Because physicians immediately send symptomatic babies to osteopathic physicians."

I'm sure there's still colic in England, but since osteopathic physicians are part of Britain's National Health Service, more of the babies there receive cranial care.

The main nerve to the baby's tummy, the vagus nerve, runs through a passageway between the temporal bone and the occipital bone called the jugular foramen. Pressure in this region can compress the vagus nerve running through the canal. Vagal compression can irritate the parasympathetic nervous system and cause the gut spasm called colic. The two nerves to the baby's tongue also go through openings on each side of this area called the hypoglossal foramen (canals). Pressure here can pinch one or both hypoglossal nerves and make it hard for the baby to suck properly. When a baby's suck becomes weak and ineffective, they pull in excessive air, which also causes abdominal pain and bloating. Since a baby's skull is so flexible, the birth process can compress the vagus and/or the hypoglossal nerve(s).

When I treat a colicky baby, I gently reposition the temporal bones on the side of the baby's head. I pry them apart from the four pieces of the occipital bone, which, in infants, have yet to fuse into one bone. I also take the pressure off the poor nerves to the baby's abdomen and tongue so the belly will quiet down and the baby can suckle contentedly.

LYDIA. Six-week-old Lydia was so tiny and weak, she looked one week old. She constantly arched her body backward in pain. She slept only twenty minutes at a stretch and then woke up whimpering. Her suck was so ineffective, her devastated mother had trouble nursing her.

Lydia's parents showed up at my office frantic with worry and exhausted from lack of sleep. I examined Lydia and found distortions in sections of the occipital bone, as well as in the occipital bone's relationship to the neighboring temporal bone. The compression of the baby's head during labor had probably pounded the temporal and occipital bones together. The compressed bones were squeezing and compromising both the vagus and hypoglossal nerves. The irritated vagus nerve gave Lydia terrible intestinal cramping and further compromised her ability to absorb nutrients. No wonder she had not grown enough. All the neurological irritation also kept Lydia from sleeping well.

Like many colicky babies, Lydia desperately tried to suck; the pressure of sucking her mother's breast slightly expanded her compressed head and temporarily relieved some of her pain. All sucking of objects (pacifiers, fingers, bottles) can be helpful, but the mother's nipple and breast provide the best resistance. When an older child sucks their thumb, they may be trying to provide themselves emotional comfort, but I almost always find the child is mechanically trying to expand their compressed head themselves. (Try sucking hard on your thumb and feel how you can open up your palate and release some pressure in your face.) Proper cranial treatment will usually remove their need for thumb sucking.

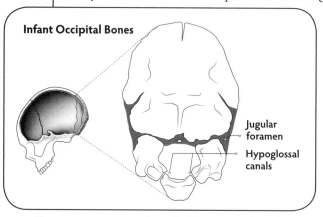

Infant Occipital Bones

Jugular foramen

Hypoglossal canals

The vagus nerves pass through the openings (jugular foramen) between the occipital and temporal bones. In an infant, the occipital bone is in four parts.

As with treating many serious problems, I started far from the most tender area. With Lydia, I started at her feet. As I worked my way up, I paid special attention to the sacrum because the sacrum mirrors much of what happens in the skull. When I touched her bloated, painful abdomen, I was well aware of her suffering. Sometimes my touch soothed her, and sometimes she frantically tried to curl away from my gentle hands. When I reached the base of her skull, I was ever so careful. Just as a little movement of my fingers could give her relief, done incorrectly it could increase her suffering.

Lydia hated to have me touch the back of her skull; it probably felt sore to her. With my two little fingers, I coaxed the base of her skull to minutely move away from the first vertebra of the neck. Then I gently worked to free the four parts of the occipital bone from each other. Later, using my thumb and index finger, I carefully lifted her frontal bone. Soon, I felt her head expand and push me away. This quiet but powerful expansion was her body's way of saying "Enough." The treatment took twelve minutes. More treatment would have been too much and could have made the situation worse.

After Lydia's first visit, she slept longer and cried less. After four treatments at weekly intervals, she could suck vigorously, her bloated belly was gone, she'd gained weight, and she had a full, lusty cry, not a whimper. With the pressure taken off her vagus and hypoglossal nerves, she recovered and remained healthy.

PEGGY's head struck the headrest in a low-speed rear-end collision. Other than having a sore neck for a few days, she felt fine and thought nothing of her accident. Then winter flooding occurred in her neighborhood. Gamely, she helped her neighbors pile sandbags in front of their homes. As she lifted one of the sandbags, she heard a pop. Then everything went quiet. She had completely lost hearing in her left ear.

Days later, an audiologist confirmed the total loss of hearing in that ear. The doctors were at a loss to explain her problem. The structures of her ear looked fine on a scan. No one could relate lifting a sandbag to sudden, profound deafness. "A mere coincidence," said one physician. "One for the medical textbooks," said another. She was treated with cortisone and other powerful drugs, all to no avail. She came to see me on a wish and a prayer after she had tried everything else.

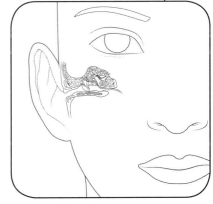

The bones of hearing run through the temporal bone. If the temporal bone is stuck, hearing can be affected.

233

Any trauma that damages the eardrum or other inner-ear components can damage hearing. However, Peggy had been tested for all of these things, and none of them appeared to be present.

I looked for structural causes of her problem. In particular, I was looking for a history of blows to the head that might have twisted her temporal bone, thereby affecting her hearing. The minute bones of the inner ear run through the temporal bone and link together in a very particular fashion. If their connections aren't precisely positioned, hearing suffers.

My physical exam revealed a severe compression between the left occipital bone and the left temporal bone. I suspected that hitting the headrest partly jammed this suture, but not enough to affect her hearing. Lifting the sandbag, however, pulled the sternocleidomastoid muscle, which attaches the upper chest to the temporal bone, ratcheting the bone into an even worse position. As a result, the small bones of the ear that transmit sound to the brain were pushed out of alignment, disrupting her hearing in that ear.

I gently separated the temporal and occipital bones and rebalanced the temporal bone with its twin on the other side of her head. I also gave her homeopathic *Crocus sativus* to address her deafness.

After her second treatment, her hearing was restored. She was thrilled. Her other physicians were shocked. Not having considered the functional anatomy, they decided it was a spontaneous, unexplained cure.

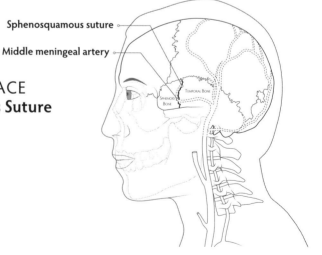

Sphenosquamous suture

Middle meningeal artery

THE SIDE OF THE FACE
The Sphenosquamous Suture

Symptoms:

- Headaches
- Migraines
- Nausea and vomiting
- Vision problems

GERHARDT developed his first migraine two months after a touch football game where he slammed the right side of his forehead into his opponent as they both reached for a pass. He didn't feel dazed and no bruise appeared, so he thought nothing of the event. He and his opponent went out for beers after the game was over.

A year later, to appease his nagging wife, he came to see me. "I don't expect you to do anything for my headaches. They're pretty recent, and I can't think of any reason I have them. Probably age. But maybe you can help my knee. I twisted it playing tennis."

I took Gerhardt's history and learned that twice a month, Gerhardt got classical migraines that started with twenty-five minutes of flashing lights and ended in eight hours of excruciating pain. The medications he took were only somewhat helpful. I asked him about injuries. He denied any except a knee injury from skiing as a teenager.

Why Problems May Start Long After an Accident

It is not uncommon for a headache or other problem to begin suddenly, months or years after an acute injury. Even though the body is pushed out of alignment by the injury, often it can compensate until a simple activity of daily living or another strain or injury breaks the camel's back and pushes the structure over the edge. The resulting conditions—such as headaches, ear infection, and dizziness—appear to flare up out of nowhere. A sudden, severe new headache, however, must always be evaluated immediately to rule out one of the rare but serious medical problems that can cause them.

In Gerhardt's case, the blow to his forehead shoved the frontal bone—the one that forms the forehead—backward. Starting a chain reaction, this force jammed the frontal bone into the nearby sphenoid bone surrounding the eye, which was then shoved into the dastardly troublemaker: the temporal bone. Running under the suture that joins the sphenoid and the temporal bone (the sphenosquamous suture) is an important artery supplying the brain called the middle meningeal artery, which is surrounded by a connective tissue sleeve that feeds through the suture. When the suture gets jammed together, the connective tissue gets tightened and squeezes the artery. Besides being ripe with pain fibers, this artery has a specialized talent. When it constricts, it sends out a kaleidoscope of flashing lights to warn of the headache to come. After I pointed out what I suspected to be the cause of his migraines, Gerhardt remembered the blow to his forehead during touch football. Though Julie and Gerhardt could later correlate their problems to trauma, many people can't pinpoint a specific injury.

To treat Gerhardt, first I gently lifted the frontal bone off its weld to the sphenoid bone. The sphenoid bone now had more room. Then I minutely distracted the sphenoid bone from its neighbor, the temporal bone, to release the tissue wrapping the middle meningeal artery. After several visits, Gerhardt had no more headaches. I also used the visits to resolve the twist in his knee.

235

Recently, allopathic medicine has linked many migraines to problems with another nerve in the skull, the trigeminal nerve. The ganglion (root) of the trigeminal nerve lives in a cave provided by the temporal bone. Temporal bone distortions that squeeze this large root can also cause the terrible pain of migraines. So can pressure on any of this nerve's numerous branches as they make their way to the face and jaw. Given the osteopathic profession's meticulous attention to the temporal and sphenoid bones, cranially-trained osteopaths find most migraines relatively easy to cure.

THE ORBITS OF THE EYES
The Sphenoid Bone

Symptoms:
- Headaches
- Strabismus
- Sinusitis
- Dizziness
- Hormonal problems
- Weight gain
- Mood disorders
- General malaise

The position of the eyes is dictated by the bony caves in which they live, known as the orbits. The sphenoid is the main bone forming the orbits. The sphenoid bone is a batlike mask of bone that spans the front of the head from one side to the other, with a ledge running deep into the skull. Eleven other small bones contribute to the orbits, and each of them is vulnerable to trauma. When healthy, the eyes' delicate cone-like caves expand and contract several times a minute. This motion bathes the eyes in fluid and then draws it away.

Distortions of the sphenoid bone can distort the orbits and lead to congestion around the eye, causing visual distortions and/or headaches. Distortions can also change the relative position of the eyes in their sockets so that the eyes are no longer level. The winged sides of the sphenoid share a long suture with the head's troublemaker, the temporal bone. Anything that distorts the temporal bones can also distort the eyes' orbits and affect vision. Blows to the back of the head, for example, can push the temporal bone forward into the sphenoid bone and distort the orbit. Since the jawbone (mandible) snuggles tightly into the temporal bone, any trauma to the jaw, such as a difficult tooth extraction or a punch, can also affect vision. Repeated ear infections can inhibit the rocking motion of the temporal bone and inhibit the motion of the orbits as well.

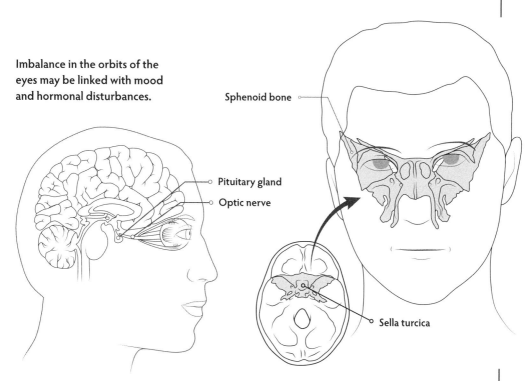

Imbalance in the orbits of the eyes may be linked with mood and hormonal disturbances.

Sphenoid bone

Pituitary gland

Optic nerve

Sella turcica

Cranial osteopathic physicians can often correct traumatically induced orbital, temporal, and occipital bone imbalance linked to visual problems. Some cranial osteopaths are so concerned about the effect of vision on the body's function and structure that these practitioners test their patient's vision even more precisely than most optometrists. These osteopathic physicians then prescribe very finely tuned lenses, which they have found can improve a person's general health.

In my clinical experience, there appears to be a connection between orbital imbalance and hormonal and mood problems. This may be partly explained by the fact that the sphenoid bone that creates the orbits is also the home of the body's master hormonal gland, the pituitary. The pituitary, which lives within the four-pronged bony platform called the Sella turcica within the sphenoid bone, regulates the behavior of virtually every hormone in the body, including those regulating mood. A trauma anywhere in the head can distort the sphenoid bone and compromise both the orbits and the hormonal output of the pituitary gland.

The eyes and the pituitary are also linked by connective tissue. The optic nerves in back of the eyes are covered with a thick layer of dural membrane that attaches to sister membranes near the pituitary. Distortions of the orbits can pull on the optic nerve and transmit distortions to the pituitary.

I have a number of methods to address distortions affecting the pituitary, and rebalancing the orbits is one of them. I have found that gentle and precise realigning of distorted orbits and rebalancing the eyes in their sockets can improve mood and hormonal balance.

THE FACE

Symptoms:

- Allergies
- Immune problems
- Sinus infections
- Vision problems

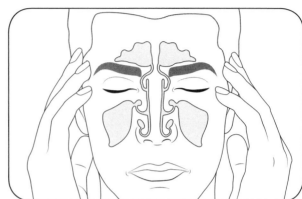

CHERISE. Two months after catapulting over the handlebars of her bike and landing on her face, forty-eight-year-old Cherise got her first sinus infection. Twelve months and four more sinus infections later, she wound up at my office.

The face is made up of many delicate bones working together in a gear-like fashion to pump the sinuses free of fluid and provide lymphatic drainage to the face and eyes. Jam up this complex movement with a blow to the face, and the bones can't do their job. This stagnant, sticky pool of mucus provides a lush breeding ground for bacteria. The face burns and aches. The growing pus can cause a fever.

Once that cascade of symptoms develops, a person may need antibiotics to cure the infection. But the mechanical cause of the sinusitis must be addressed as well or the compressed facial bones will soon brew another infection. Precise treatment of the traumatized area can restore each delicate gear's function, open up the sinus caves, and take the twist out of the surrounding connective tissue. That's what I did with Cherise. I released the compressions between the bones in her face so her sinuses could drain—and drain, they did. Big clumps of mucus dislodged, and suddenly she could breathe again.

Most injuries to the face and head also cause injuries to the neck. Nerves coming from the neck supply the sinuses and tell them how to function. To help Cherise's sinuses, I also had to treat her neck and make sure the vertebrae were aligned so the nerves were not being compressed. Rear-end collisions can compromise the neck enough to affect the sinuses, something we saw earlier with Sam. The relationship between the neck and the sinuses

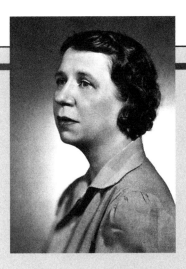

The Story of Dr. Charlotte Weaver

Until recently, most of osteopathy's understanding of cranial maladies came from the groundbreaking work of William Sutherland, DO, and the physicians who followed in his tradition. But there was a brilliant woman physician in the early 1900s who also had profound insights about how the bones of the head move and the pathology that could result from cranial distortion. Her pioneering work had been lost to history until recently. Thanks to Margaret Sorrel, DO, Doctor Charlotte Weaver's insights are once more seeing the light of day.

Doctor Weaver believed that the two bones at the base of the skull (the sphenoid and occipital bones) are modified cervical vertebrae, and that, like cervical vertebrae, those bones can move and function well or become misaligned. With her background as a neurologist and psychiatrist, Weaver correlated disruptions at the base of the skull with psychiatric and medical pathology. Like Sutherland, she used her hands to correct the lesions and address some serious neurological problems, such as failure of children to thrive and hormonal problems stemming from pituitary dysfunction.

explains why so many people have colds, sinusitis, and allergies after car accidents. The good news is that once cranial treatment restores motion to the skull, face, and neck, the chronic cold or sinusitis caused by trauma frequently disappears.

I often recommend to my patients a variation of a treatment I learned from my mentor, Ann Wales, DO, that helps them pump their own sinuses. I tell patients to put one thumb in the middle of their palate—that's the top of the mouth, where it still feels hard. I tell them to put the tip of the second finger of the other hand on the forehead just above the bridge of the nose. With a few ounces of pressure, I have them push up on their palate until they catch the feeling of the exerted pressure with their index finger on the forehead. Then they press back down on the forehead until they catch the pressure on their thumb. This is kind of like playing Ping-Pong on their head.

When a person first starts, they may not feel the Ping-Pong sensation on their fingertips, but the pumping pressure in their mouth and forehead should feel good. They should do this about twelve times a minute for about two to three minutes. Then they should feel some mucus drain down the back of their throat. I recommend drinking a glass of water afterward.

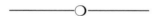

These are but brief sketches of some of the problems that can result from trauma to the skull. I've seen hundreds of patients thrilled to regain their health—even decades later—once full motion is restored to the bones of the skull.

THE SKULL/BRAIN CONNECTION

Treating the skull profoundly helps the brain. The skull, the brain's formidable protector, controls the gateways in and out of the brain. The brain can perform magnificently only when all the sutures are open and all the gears in the three-dimensional watch of the skull are running smoothly.

I recently received a letter from Sumi, a patient of mine in the late 1990s. She came to me a year after a serious car accident. In addition to her neck pain and other trauma, she was having trouble thinking. Previously, she had been an excellent student; after the accident, she had difficulty focusing and was failing her college classes.

I found numerous anatomical distortions in her body typical of victims of car accidents. Here I want to focus on what I found in her skull. As with Julie, her occipital bone was jammed into her right temporal bone and into her first cervical vertebra. The pulsations of her brain, instead of being six to fourteen times a minute, occurred two and a half times a minute—markedly decreased from normal.

Over several visits, I worked to release the base of the skull. By the third and fourth visits, the jammed sutures in her skull were regaining some of their normal motion. But during the fifth visit, something dramatic occurred.

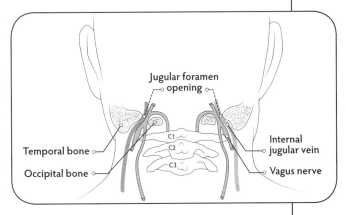

Two crucial passageways—the jugular foramen—open between the occipital bone and the temporal bones. We met them before with baby Lydia who suffered from colic, and we will meet them again in upcoming chapters on brain injury. Not only do the vagus nerves snake through these passageways, but the internal jugular veins do as well. These veins carry deoxygenated blood full of debris out of the brain. These openings are therefore major exit routes for an important trash removal system in the brain.

The brain cannot fully heal from trauma until the toxic debris of injury is flushed out of its tissues. When trauma jams together the bones that form the jugular foramen, as they did with Sumi, these openings can narrow and debris-laden fluid can back up behind the obstruction, affecting the brain's ability to function. Studies have shown that, even years after a brain injury, venous blood flow through this exit route is sluggish, causing increased backpressure in the brain and poorer fluid flow out of the brain. In all my head trauma and brain-injured patients, I make sure that these canals are wide open.

In her letter, Sumi stated that on her fifth office visit, "I was lying on my back on your table and experienced a very distinct pop in my head, much like one's ears pop at changes in elevation. Instantly, I felt my brain to be clearer, and had not realized I had been in a mental fog for over a year. I have told this story many times to others who have experienced head injuries to illustrate how deep the damage can be and how miraculous the healing possibilities."

The pop Sumi experienced was the right temporal bone finally pulling away from its compression against the occipital bone. Once these bones sat in their appropriate homes, the jugular canal was more open and the fluid buildup in the brain—with its toxic debris and deoxygenated blood—flowed out in a rush. I suspect that the twist in her temporal bone had also kinked a major artery that snakes along the inside of the bone, called the internal carotid artery. Untwisting the bone removed the kink, and fuller blood flow surged into the brain. With blood flowing freely in and out again, her brain started to clear.

When I reviewed her chart notes for that fifth visit, I found that her cranial rhythmic impulse practically doubled to four and half times a minute after the temporal bone release. She soon made a complete recovery.

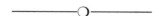

I tell Sumi's story to illustrate how enthusiastically the brain responds to the revival of its fluid flow and how important the dynamism of the skull is to the health of the brain. The brain can perform magnificently only when all the gateways of the skull are open, the fluids are flowing freely, and the sutures and gears in the skull are moving, humming, and singing like opera stars.

20

Mild Traumatic Brain Injury

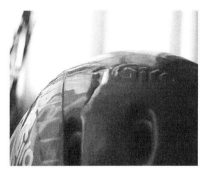

Almost home, twelve-year-old Phillip dutifully dismounted from his bike and walked it across the street in the crosswalk. Pity he didn't break the law and ride across. He might have made it to the other side before the truck plowed into him. The collision slammed the bike into his right hip, spun him into the air, and threw him headfirst into the curb. The truck driver was apologetic to the neighbor who, upon hearing the crash, rushed to help Phillip lying sprawled on the sidewalk. "The sun was in my eyes—I didn't see him," he said. "I was going about twenty-five miles per hour," he said to the police who arrived shortly thereafter.

Phillip stood up, remembering none of it. His hip hurt. His bicycle helmet was cracked. When his mother arrived ten minutes later, Phillip proudly displayed the helmet. "See the big dent? He hit me pretty hard. But I don't remember it."

In a panic, his mother called me. "Take him to the emergency room," I said. "As soon as they clear him, bring him in."

Three hours later in my office, Phillip seemed his normal, articulate, funny self. "I'm not hurt badly," he said. "Look, nothing's bleeding." His only complaints were a mild headache, some scrapes and bruises, and some hip pain. I repeated the neurological exam done in the ER and found no apparent abnormalities. When I told his mother that the initial findings did not yet indicate more serious damage, she said, "I want to kiss his helmet."

This was just the beginning of Phillip's journey with mild traumatic brain injury. As Phillip and his family would soon learn, nothing is mild about a traumatic brain injury.

What is mild traumatic brain injury? What are its symptoms? How does trauma damage the brain, and how does a person heal from it? I explore these questions in the next three chapters.

Complex and mysterious as brain injury is, helping the brain heal is actually quite straightforward once you understand some basic facts about its anatomy and physiology. Brain injury seems to cause intense injury shock, a kind of hyperexcitability of brain tissue that interferes with the brain's ability to function. The brain is a water creature, utterly dependent on its fluid flows to function and survive. More than any other cells in the body, the cells of the brain are attuned to the motion of the fluids that bring them oxygen and nutrients and take out the trash. The magnificent brain is the most voracious user of energy and oxygen in the body, and it must be brought these things in great abundance by the blood circulation, or it will falter. Great ponds of fluid, called ventricles, live inside the brain. These ponds feed the rivers of cerebral

The Sobering Evidence on Brain Injury

Research about the long-term effects of brain injury is disquieting.

- Even a single mild traumatic brain injury can leave measurable scars in the brain and cause lasting cognitive and emotional problems.
- Ten to twenty percent of MTBI patients continue to experience neurological and psychological symptoms more than one year after their injury.
- A single MTBI can cause structural changes in the brain; regions that control mood, executive function, and learning take the worst punishment.
- Athletes show a measurable drop in cognitive function after a single concussion. Most recover, but if they sustain additional injuries, their cognitive decline becomes more pronounced, even permanent.
- Some victims suffer continuing, widespread damage from inflammation in the brain decades after their injury.
- Brain injury is associated with seizures, sleep disorders, neurodegenerative disease, sexual dysfunction, depression, endocrine disorders, and systemic metabolic dysregulation, any of which can persist for years.

spinal fluid that course through the brain. If the brain's fluid rivers are stagnant and its cells assaulted by a swill of toxic debris, the brain will slowly perish.

Once the brain can frolic again in its liquid home, surrounded by healing nutrients, lots of oxygen, and cleansing torrents of fluid, the brain has a remarkable ability to heal. Removing injury shock and restoring fluid flow can create amazing changes in brain health. But before I can talk in more detail about healing the brain, I must first describe how we diagnose brain injury.

MILD TRAUMATIC BRAIN INJURY: Invisible and Devastating

Diagnosing a mild traumatic brain injury (MTBI) can be very difficult. The symptoms are often subtle and overlap with other medical conditions like stress, hormonal imbalance, or mood disorders. The symptoms can take weeks or even months to develop, long after the injury that caused them has been forgotten.

MTBI is often an invisible injury. If there are no wounds, bleeding, or other obvious physical trauma and the person can walk about and talk fairly coherently, then they seem to be no worse for wear. The victim's friends and family can miss brain injury's subtle signs, thinking the person needs more sleep or should just stop being so irritable. The victims themselves are often the most blind to what is happening. When the brain isn't working very well, people can't tell that there is anything wrong with them. Just as vampires can't perceive themselves in a mirror, people with brain injuries often can't see themselves in the mirror of life.

Then, out of nowhere, weeks or months after the trauma, problems start appearing—difficulty in focusing or with completing tasks, outbursts of anger, forgetfulness, sexual problems, extreme fatigue. Due to coordination problems, people feel clumsy and off-balance and may take a fall. Performance suffers at work or school. Perhaps the person's partner notices that their mate is not themselves, but since no one ever mentioned that collision on the sports field or the minor motor vehicle accident, the fact that it might be brain injury never occurs to anyone. The brain injury remains invisible.

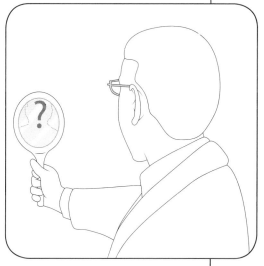

The signs of traumatic brain injury are often invisible even to the person suffering from the injury.

One reason that brain injury is constantly missed is that patients often think, mistakenly, that injuring the brain is like bruising a bone: it hurts for a while, and then it heals. Brain injuries are different. A brain injury, even a mild one, can behave more like a chronic disease—causing injury and dysfunction long after the precipitating incident. While some people recover with no long-term consequences, many others enter a long night of endless, debilitating suffering.

It is also easy to miss brain injury because people often can do familiar tasks for a while afterward, a phenomenon known as the training effect. Their habits carry them through life for a time. They can give a lecture they've given before, or finish up architectural plans they have been working on. As the training effect wears off and the brain is asked to perform new or unfamiliar functions, however, cognitive difficulties become apparent. But because so much time has passed since the injury, no one links the mental deterioration to a brain injury.

One of my patients, a brilliant lawyer, was in a serious accident in which he briefly lost consciousness. He returned to work fairly quickly, apparently in good health. Then, over the next six months, the quality of his work deteriorated. He found it difficult to concentrate. He had increasing trouble following a legal argument. Finally, one night, he found himself staring at a law book for ten minutes and having no idea what he had read. For months, the training effect had masked the silent damage ravaging his brain. When it wore off, he could no longer function at his high-powered job. His formerly crystal-clear mind felt like a murky pond.

As the brain-injured person's life unravels, their family, boss, or friends may tell them they aren't working hard enough or focusing enough. They might accuse the person of malingering from what seemed like a minor trauma. But nothing is minor when the brain is involved.

How to Find Out If You've Suffered a Brain Injury

Why can't a doctor slide the patient into an MRI machine that takes illuminating pictures of the brain and tell them what's wrong? The doctors on *Grey's Anatomy* and *House* are endlessly putting their thinly garbed patients into large white machines and later uttering incomprehensible diagnoses. While brain-imaging technology is constantly improving, for the most part the damage caused by an MTBI will not show up on an MRI or CT scan. Those scans are generally used to visualize extensive damage, where the bleeding, bruise, or swelling is so substantial that a neurosurgeon might need to cauterize the broken blood vessel, remove a pool of blood, or open up the skull so the swelling brain has room to expand.

Just as no machine can diagnose an MTBI, it's easy for practitioners to miss them because there is no one symptom or group of symptoms unique to MTBI. Diagnosing an MTBI requires good detective work. When I suspect a brain injury, I take a thorough history of the accident and then cast a wide net to catch brain injury's subtle symptoms. Are there changes in the person's vision, hearing, smell, or taste? Do odors seem stronger; are loud noises more bothersome? Does bright sunlight hurt their eyes? Those are considered changes in the sensory systems. I inquire about mental changes and cognitive and memory function. Are they having trouble focusing or multitasking? Are they now keeping an endless supply of sunglasses and keys around because they keep losing them

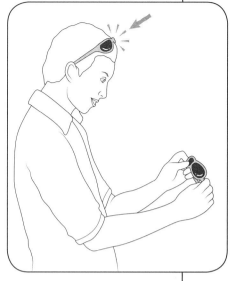

or forget that their glasses are on their head? Do they forget where they are going or what they were doing? I ask about physical symptoms that correlate with injury to the nervous system: Are they nauseated, dizzy, or constantly exhausted, yet have trouble sleeping? Do they have unexplained headaches?

Finally, I ask about state of mind as it reflects behavioral changes. MTBI is almost always accompanied by changes in mood. I find out if they are unusually quick to anger or cry easily. Are they overwhelmed and upset by seemingly minor problems? Do the ordinary tasks of life suddenly seem unbearable? Have they become extremely irritable for no reason? Are they uncharacteristically depressed or anxious? Have they lost interest in sex?

Rarely does anyone have all these symptoms. Some people have symptoms only in one category, others in multiple categories. The symptoms depend on which part of the brain was injured and the seriousness of the injuries. The more categories involved and the more severe the symptoms, generally the more extensive the damage. The categories roughly correspond to the areas of the brain that are injured.

Stephanie, the woman in the horrendous car crash in chapter 5, had problems with smell, taste, and concentration, along with extreme fatigue, revealing that she had problems in the sensory, mental, and physical clusters. As we will see, Phillip had visual problems, trouble concentrating and staying organized, headaches, and problems with anger. So he had problems in the mental, physical, sensory, and behavioral clusters. I've included a chart of the most common symptoms in each of these groups.

Symptoms of Brain Injury

MENTAL SYMPTOMS	PHYSICAL SYMPTOMS	BEHAVIORAL CHANGES	SENSORY SYMPTOMS
Short-term memory problems	Headaches	Depression	Increased sensitivity to light
Forgetfulness	Dizziness or vertigo	Anxiety	Increased sensitivity to noise
Attention difficulties	Fatigue	Irritability	Increased sensitivity to smell
Inability to focus or concentrate	Immune problems	Emotional fragility	Decreased sensitivity to smell
Inability to multitask	Vision problems	Impulse control	Changes in hearing
Difficulty making decisions	Insomnia	Anger or rage	Decreased sensitivity to taste
Problems comprehending language	Tinnitus (ringing in the ears)	Loss of interest in sex	Difficulty with visual focus
Unable to find words or using the wrong ones	Sexual performance problems	Sleep problems, including nightmares	
	Menstrual irregularity Weight gain Constant thirst Infertility Temperature instability Hormonal problems	Problems relating to other people	

THE PARTS OF THE BRAIN

Although the brain works as a unit to coordinate all its different parts, it can be useful to understand the functions of each part of the brain to get a sense of what problems occur after injury to each part of the head. The three areas most prone to injury—the front, back, and side—account for the vast majority of symptoms.

The Cerebral Cortex

Think of the brain as a sphere with multiple layers. The custardlike outside layer of the brain is best known as the cerebral cortex (sometimes called the cerebrum). It contains about a hundred billion neurons, and trillions of loyal companion cells called glia that protect the neurons and help them function. The large size of the cortex differentiates our human brain from that of other creatures.

The uniquely human cortex is divided into four regions: the frontal lobe, in front; the temporal lobes, on the side; the parietal lobes, on top; and the occipital lobe, in back. The cortex is also split down the middle into two halves, or hemispheres, by a sickle-shaped membrane called the dural falx, which means the two sides can't talk directly to each other. If the halves want to communicate, they have to travel down deeper in the brain to the central highway, the corpus callosum.

Each hemisphere of the brain tends to have different functions. The right side tends to be creative and imaginative. The left tends toward the more orderly. Injuries to the right hemisphere can cause problems with memory, problem solving, attention, spatial orientation, and social interaction. Injuries to the left hemisphere can cause problems with memory, organization, speech, writing, cognitive processing, and mood.

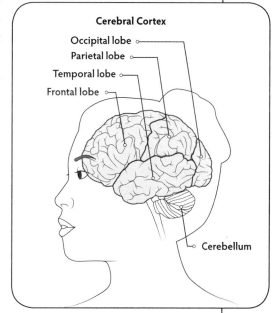

The Frontal Lobe

The area behind the forehead, which will turn out to be the region of Phillip's most serious injury, is called the frontal lobe. The frontal lobe maintains attention and is in charge of executive function. The frontal

Warning Signs of Serious Brain Injury

If you have any of the following symptoms after an injury to the head or a violent blow to the body, go to an emergency room:

- Problems with balance, vision, or hearing
- One pupil larger than the other
- Slurred speech
- Nausea or vomiting (if vomiting, call an ambulance, as it can mean life-threatening pressure on the brain)
- Severe headache that continuously gets worse
- Serious bleeding from the head or face
- Bruising behind the ear (Battle's sign)
- Clear fluid drainage from the nose or ear
- Confusion, drowsiness, and lethargy
- Weakness on one side of the body
- Loss of consciousness or memory

This is by no means a complete list. You must take any potential brain injury seriously and err on the side of caution. Remain alert for any signs of discomfort and get evaluated by a physician if anything unusual develops, particularly a headache. Brain injury may take hours, weeks, or longer to manifest itself. When in doubt, **go!**

Know that your brain can be hurt even if you don't lose consciousness. This is a main source of confusion about brain injury among physicians and patients alike. I cannot tell you how often my patients tell me that a health care practitioner dismissed the possibility of a brain injury because the patient did not lose consciousness. Loss of consciousness is only one of many possible symptoms of brain injury. It is no longer even used as a key sign of concussion. More significant than a loss of consciousness is whether there has been any change in mental status—no matter how temporary—after an injury.

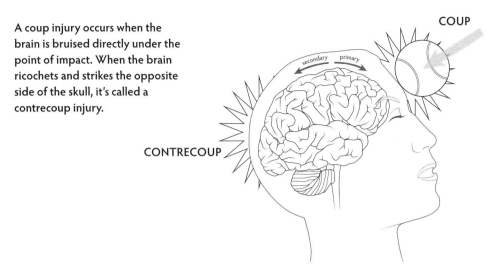

A coup injury occurs when the brain is bruised directly under the point of impact. When the brain ricochets and strikes the opposite side of the skull, it's called a contrecoup injury.

lobe orchestrates complex thoughts such as goal planning and multitasking and governs parts of memory, language, and awareness. As if the frontal lobe didn't have enough responsibility, it also governs emotional response and impulse control.

Because of its position, the frontal lobe is commonly injured. Injury to this area can occur when someone trips and strikes their face, or when the forehead bangs into something. These forces can slam the brain's frontal lobe against the frontal bone of the skull, which has sharp, protruding ridges right below it. When the brain is bruised directly at the point of impact, it's called a coup injury.

The frontal lobe also can be damaged when the head is struck from the back, such as when the head slams into a car's headrest, or the person falls backward and hits the back of the skull. That's because the impact can fling the brain forward against the frontal bone. When the brain ricochets and hits the opposite side of the skull, the second blow is called a contrecoup impact. The frontal lobe is one of the most common victims of a contrecoup injury.

The frontal lobe can be injured even if nothing hits the head. A powerful blow to the body that causes the head to snap violently backward or forward can sling the frontal lobe against the frontal bone. A football tackle to the torso is a common culprit causing such an injury.

Like Phillip, any person with a frontal lobe injury can have trouble paying attention. The victim of a car crash often can't focus on what the police officer asks them. Later, when they go home or to work, they can have difficulty understanding or doing tasks. A person can forget where they put their checkbook, or when they were supposed to pick up their children. Patients with frontal lobe injury often forget how to get to my office even if they've been seeing me for years. Feeling overwhelmed by the activities of daily living, people often become irritable, angry, depressed, and weepy. Calm people can become violent. Symptoms might arise immediately, but they can also take weeks or months to develop.

The Occipital Lobe

The occipital lobe, at the back of the head, is the second region of the brain commonly injured. The occipital lobe orchestrates vision and partly functions like a movie screen as images are projected onto it from the eyes. If the back of the head is struck, the occipital lobe can get injured. Then it is as if the movie screen becomes wrinkled, making objects appear out of focus. The distortions can be almost imperceptible. A person's eyes may become more tired when they read. They often go back to their eye doctor to ask for new glasses, but changing their lenses will not help them. To take the wrinkles out of the movie screen and fix their vision, motion must be restored to restricted bones in back of the skull, and any compression by the occipital bone on the brain's occipital lobe must be released.

The occipital lobe can also be damaged from a blow to the front of the head. If the force is strong enough, the brain ricochets and strikes the back of the skull, causing a contrecoup injury there. As you will see later, when Phillip's forehead struck the sidewalk, the blow was so powerful that his brain struck the back of his skull, affecting his vision.

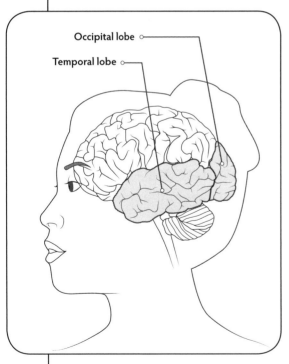

Occipital lobe

Temporal lobe

The Temporal Lobe

The temporal lobe is the third area extremely prone to injury. The temporal lobe sits inward from the ear and that troublemaker of the skull, the temporal bone. If a person's head is twisted or turned at the moment of impact, the rotational force of the collision can slam the temporal lobe into a rugged shelf of bone that protrudes into the brain called the petrous ridge. Falls, car accidents, and sports injuries often have a rotational component. A blow to the side of the head also can damage this area.

The temporal lobes are involved in long-term memory formation and organization of sensory input, shapes, sounds, language, and emotional responses. The hippocampus, the area responsible for consolidating information from short-term into long-term memory, is located in the temporal lobe. The amygdala, which processes emotional stimuli including fear, is located toward the tips of the temporal lobes.

Injuries to the temporal lobe can cause long-term memory problems and personality changes, and damage can alter desire and sexual behavior. Damage to the left temporal lobe can cause problems with language: people talk more slowly, and are unable to formulate sentences, or understand other people's words. They can have trouble understanding directions as well as other subtle language cues. Damage to the right temporal lobe can result in decreased recognition of visual content. Injuries to either temporal lobe can cause problems with hearing, tinnitus, and balance, and difficulty recognizing faces and shapes. The front of the temporal lobe lives near the middle meningeal artery. Injury to this artery can cause everything from migraines to epidural hematomas, a form of bleeding in the brain that is extremely serious.

The Corpus Callosum

Underneath the cortex, connecting the two halves of the brain, is the corpus callosum. This is a neurological superhighway that passes information back and forth between the two sides of the brain. It's actually more like a super telephone exchange, with messages flying back and forth among the different parts of the brain. The corpus callosum, sometimes called white matter, is made almost entirely of axons—the long wire-like extensions on brain cells that transmit electrical signals to other cells. As we will see later, injury to the corpus callosum and its axons is frequently involved in ongoing brain injury.

The corpus callosum is made of

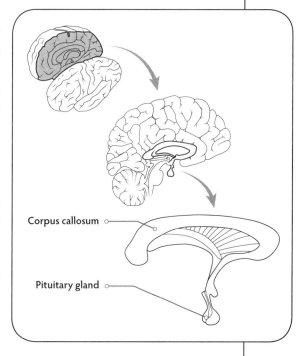

Corpus callosum

Pituitary gland

denser tissue than the cerebral cortex that surrounds it, with a consistency more like Silly Putty than Jell-O. When force is applied to objects of different densities, physics dictates that the objects then accelerate or move at different speeds. When the brain is rapidly flung about, particularly when the body is subjected to rotational forces, the fluffy cerebral cortex on the outside moves more slowly than the denser corpus callosum beneath it. Consequently, the nerves that bridge the two areas are easily sheared, stretched, and torn. This type of injury is called diffuse axonal injury, because it's spread throughout the brain and involves damage to the long arms of the neurons, called axons.

If the connection between the corpus callosum and the frontal lobe is damaged, people tend to have executive-function problems, as we will see happened to Phillip. For others, when their boss says, "I need you to add a window to the architectural plans for the bathroom," the person understands the words as they go into the temporal lobe and into the corpus callosum. But due to damage between the corpus callosum and the frontal lobe, the information does not get to the executive-function area that carries out the order. The brain-injured architect may leave out the window or put it in the kitchen.

If the connection between the visual interpretation center of the brain (the occipital lobe) and the corpus callosum is damaged, a fielder might see the baseball coming, but since that information doesn't make it to the corpus callosum, the corpus callosum can't transfer the data to the movement centers of the brain to tell the person to catch the ball. The ball hits the fielder in the face.

Shears between the corpus callosum and parts of the cerebral cortex explain a common phenomenon I've often found after a brain injury: people are much more likely to be uncoordinated, and trip, fall, and get in other accidents. Their lack of proper brain processing make them much less aware of their surroundings and more prone to accidents and falls.

The Cerebellum

In the back of the head, below the occipital lobe, is the cerebellum, or little brain. It looks like a walnut shell. The cerebellum controls movement as well as balance and orientation in space. Patients who have a cerebellar injury describe feeling off-kilter or dizzy.

The cerebellum has another critical job that is worth mentioning here: it must remain proudly lifted up and away from the funnel-like opening to the spine directly beneath it, the foramen magnum. When the cerebellum is even minimally displaced downward by trauma, it can block an important exit route for drainage of cerebral spinal fluid (CSF) out of the brain and into the spinal cord. The spinal cord needs the CSF to stay moist. The brain needs the CSF to flow freely out of the brain, removing toxic debris and keeping excess fluid from building up in the brain and squeezing it. Some researchers suspect that blockage of the route below the cerebellum may play a role in ongoing brain jury and even in some neurological diseases such as multiple sclerosis and Parkinson's disease.

Compromise of any escape route for toxic debris, I believe, can not only affect neurological diseases but also significantly aggravate brain injury and keep it going.

The Pituitary Gland

A tiny gland in the middle of the brain orchestrates almost all of the body's hormonal functions. The pituitary gland, uniquely part gland and part brain, swings from a thin stalk of tissue connected to the brain region called the hypothalamus. The hypothalamus is constantly talking to the pituitary, telling it, for example, that the body needs more energy, more sex hormones, or more insulin. The pituitary gland then sends chemical messengers to the appropriate organ, thereby directing almost all of the body's hormonal functions.

Nestled in a bony nook of the sphenoid bone called the sella turcica, or Turk's saddle (which I called a four-poster bed in the chapter on sexual healing), the pituitary lives under a canopy of dural tissue. It affects sexual arousal and performance by telling the sex organs how much testosterone, estrogen, and progesterone to produce. By its regulation of the thyroid hormones, it can determine if we are fat or thin, or whether we feel hot or cold, energetic or fatigued, or whether our skin is vibrant or dry. It stimulates the adrenal glands to produce cortisol, the powerful hormone that plays such an important role in regulating the fight-or-flight response, blood sugar levels, immune system function, blood pressure, and inflammation. The pituitary regulates the function of the kidneys and orchestrates or influences growth, mood, memory, and fluid and mineral retention, as well as a whole host of other functions critical to life.

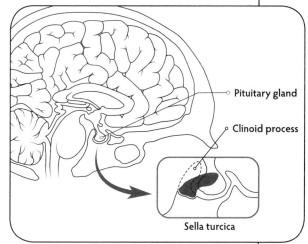

Pituitary gland

Clinoid process

Sella turcica

A distorted posterior clinoid process puts pressure on the pituitary gland.

Suspended as it is above its bony perch, the pituitary is very vulnerable to trauma. Injury can bang the tiny pituitary against the bony bedposts (called clinoid processes), injuring its delicate tissue and impairing its function. Trauma can also distort the bedposts. Once a post becomes bent, I find its distortion can compromise the rhythmic pendulum swing of the pituitary that corresponds with the brain's pulsations, even causing the pituitary to repeatedly smack the post. Trauma can also damage the thin stalk of tissue that connects the pituitary to the hypothalamus.

Because the pituitary orchestrates the function of every gland in the body, I suspect that injury in this region accounts for some of the more unusual problems I've seen after brain injury. These include menstrual irregularity, excessive thirst, sexual difficulties, weight gain, depression, fatigue, and temperature imbalance. Because injury to the pituitary can cause dysfunction in any of the hormone systems it regulates—including adrenal, thyroid, and reproductive—I always consider the possibility of injury to the pituitary and accompanying hormone disruption after a head trauma. The symptoms can be very subtle and can overlap with other common symptoms of head injury, such as memory problems, fatigue, and mood disorders.

———○———

LASHAWNA. A distraught mother brought her three-year-old daughter, Lashawna, to see me after Lashawna developed uncontrolled bleeding from her kidneys. Standard medicine, despite massive amounts of cortisone, could not stop it. Her doctors were considering a kidney transplant.

I put my hands on little Lashawna's head. After careful evaluation of the bones of her skull, I found that her forehead (the frontal bone) was pushed back significantly, compressing the sphenoid bone which holds the pituitary gland. Furthermore, since the dural membranes connect to the clinoid processes, I could feel from the dural tugs that the front clinoid processes were pressing against and compromising the pituitary.

I told her mother that I felt that her daughter's forehead was compressed backward, compressing the pituitary's home and thereby affecting the hormone regulating her kidney. She replied, "Lashawna has looked different since her fall nine months ago. Her forehead is pushed back more. I told other doctors that the bleeding started after Lashawna fell on her face, but no one took that seriously, so I stopped saying anything."

"Well, it makes sense to me," I replied.

I lifted Lashawna's frontal bone, pulling it away from its compression into the sphenoid bone behind it, releasing some of the pressure on the pituitary. Then, using the dural membranes as pulleys, I helped straighten out the bedposts so the pituitary was no longer being compromised. Since the optic nerves to the eyes are covered with a sheath of dural tissue that links up to the dura covering the pituitary, I very gently used the eyes to help balance the bedposts.

After two treatments, her mother remarked that Lashawna's forehead had come back out and she looked like the old Lashawna. I agreed her forehead was now better shaped. After three treatments, Lashawna's kidneys stopped bleeding.

This successful result was not just coincidence. Six months later, Lashawna again fell on her face. The kidneys started bleeding, but this time it took me only one treatment to stop her from urinating blood.

Of course, most children who fall on their face don't damage the pituitary or the brain, but when someone does, it's good to know what might help.

USING THE BRAIN'S PULSATIONS TO GAUGE BRAIN HEALTH

My training in cranial osteopathy has given me an essential tool for evaluating the health of a patient's brain: using touch to discern the quality and frequency of the brain's pulsations.

Like the dancers in an exquisite ballet, different parts of the healthy brain have unique talents yet move in miraculous harmony. The nerve cells that make up the brain—the neurons—talk to each other and sway in unison. The neurons are assisted by nurturing cells called glial cells. Glial cells engulf and protect neurons and guide the blood vessels to snuggle up to the neurons so they receive proper nourishment, kind of like the music that orchestrates the dance. Glial cells also give the brain structure, in essence also providing the stage that the neurons perform on. As the neurons and glial cells dance together, perhaps it is their motion that causes the brain to pulsate. Since life is motion, it only makes sense that the prime mover of love, compassion, and wisdom moves like all the other vital organs in the body.

Because the brain is tethered to the skull by a series of membranes, the brain's subtle motions can be felt throughout the skull. As I mentioned earlier, cranial osteopathic physicians call this pulsation the cranial rhythmic impulse (CRI). When the brain, the skull, and its marvelous membrane system are all functioning optimally, these pulsations exhibit a good power (amplitude) that expands evenly throughout the skull six to fourteen times a minute. This coordinated dance of the skull, membranes, and brain helps pump the brain's fluid flows.

Trauma to the skull, the membranes, or the brain itself can slow down the brain's pulsations, making them weaker and more erratic. If a particular area of the skull and/or brain has been injured, the injury is reflected in sluggish and uneven motion in that part of the brain, the membranes, and the skull. I use my ability to palpate these restricted or weakened areas to design appropriate cranial treatments that will assist the fluid flow and help the brain regain its mobility and health. I can use improvements in the CRI to measure the success of my treatments as well as the success of other therapies.

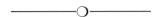

Soon after the terrible blow to his head, Phillip started to suffer from debilitating headaches. He had trouble concentrating in school. Before the accident, Phillip kept a notebook of all the books that he had read. After the accident, he stopped reading because he couldn't follow what he read. Phillip had also been a math whiz, but after the accident his math grades grew steadily worse. He often felt so frustrated, he started slamming doors.

In order to understand how the accident caused Phillip's problems and what I did to help him heal, I need to take you on a tour of the smallest parts of the brain and its critical fluid channels, for both are so different from what we can imagine. Inside the skull, like the deepest part of the ocean, is mysterious, powerful, and full of amazing currents that provide life itself. And like the depths of the sea, the brain seems inaccessible. So imagine you are on an even tinier submarine than the one James Cameron used to explore the *Titanic*. From this vantage point, you are about to enter a magical world.

—— | 21 | ——

The Long Night of Brain Injury

*"Essentially, all neurodegenerative diseases are associated
with the accumulation of cellular waste products."*
—Maiken Nedergaard, MD, DMSc
Professor, Department of Neurosurgery, University of Rochester

Brain injury happens first at the level of the brain cell. It is the destruction of
neurons, glial cells, and their networks that we experience as loss of memory,
changes in mood, and difficulty thinking. To understand how brain injury
affects these and other functions, we need to understand how the cells of the
brain work together and how injury destroys and disrupts them. With our
minuscule submarine, we enter the microscopic world of the brain cells.

MEET THE CELLS OF THE BRAIN

Opening before us is an endless spider web of cells, some star shaped, others
with long arms and octopus tentacles, still others like links of sausage. If the
different kinds of cells flashed in different colors as they talked to each other,
the signals would blink down long networks of cells into the distance, and all
the colors would perform in synchronicity.

For a hundred years, science regarded a cell called the neuron as the superstar
of the brain. These magnificent cells were thought to be the source of the brain's
power, with a hundred billion neurons linked across millions of miles of connecting structures. This fantastical world has only started to reveal its other secrets
within the last two decades. Neurons certainly are important, and I'll talk about
them first, but they've been joined in recent years by a new cast of characters.

Most of us imagine cells as little boxes with lots of important stuff inside.

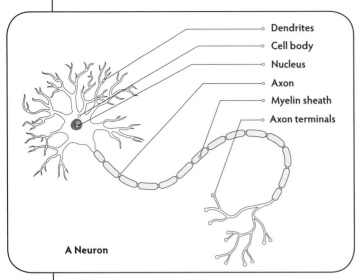

- Dendrites
- Cell body
- Nucleus
- Axon
- Myelin sheath
- Axon terminals

A Neuron

The neurons in the brain look quite different. They have tentacles on their heads called dendrites that receive information from other neurons and spidery appendages on their feet that send information. Their long, wire-like arms, called axons, speed information coded in electrical impulses from one end of the neuron to the other.

Neurons communicate using chemical messengers called neurotransmitters. These chemicals escort the neurons' messages across gaps, called synapses, between the neurons. Messages constantly flash back and forth among the untold billions of neurons, like the action of a supercharged pinball machine. There are trillions of synapses in a single human brain, perhaps more than there are stars in the universe. Neurons are also unique because they transmit and receive information in intricate circuits—a single neuron can be connected to ten thousand others. These networks link many different parts of the brain and travel from one side of the brain to the other. Complex cognitive and executive functions depend heavily on these immense brainwide networks. Their vast interconnectedness means that damage to an axon or the death of a neuron can cause far-reaching damage around the brain, as widespread waves of destruction ripple through the dying neuron's networks.

Much of this information exchange passes through the corpus callosum, the dense white-matter structure that sits underneath the fluffy cerebral cortex. The corpus callosum is basically made up of the long axonal arms of neurons. In the average person's brain, there are thousands of miles of axons. Axons that cross the junction between the lighter and denser parts of the brain are at particular risk during head injury.

Brain injury cuts neurons off from the two things they most need to function: oxygen and fuel (glucose). The voracious brain, which consumes 20 percent of the body's energy when it's healthy, needs even more when it's injured. Even in the best of times, neurons can barely survive five minutes without oxygen. However, trauma frequently causes swelling, which squeezes and closes off the pipes that bring these supplies to the brain's cells. With their food and oxygen supply cut off, the starving and suffocating neurons grow weak and eventually die.

Neurons will also die in a dirty brain. Neurons are so exquisitely sensitive to the cleanliness of their surroundings that they can be poisoned by their own neurotransmitters if these chemicals are not constantly swept away. The brain has two fluid systems to take out the trash: one that connects to the venous blood circulation system and one that pushes cerebral spinal fluid rapidly through the brain's tissues. Trauma quickly pollutes the pristine environment neurons depend on to function at their best; unfortunately, the cleansing systems can also falter when the brain is injured. I am convinced that the impairment of the brain's fluid systems—the venous system and the system of cerebral spinal fluid—can cause a backup of toxic debris and prolong brain damage, stoke the fires of inflammation, and set in motion a vicious cycle of increasing damage and decline. Restoring fluid flow to bring in necessary nutrients and clean out the trash is a matter of the greatest urgency for the health of the brain following trauma.

The shape of the neuron makes it extremely vulnerable to injury. With such long and delicate axonal arms, the neuron's axonal fibers easily get overstretched or ruptured, especially when subjected to rotational forces. Because axons are thin, swelling or bleeding can smother them. Traumatic injury to axons may trigger a cascade of destruction in the brain that can go on for decades following even a single insult.

HIDING IN PLAIN SIGHT: The Glial Cells

The prima donna neurons have garnered much of medicine's attention, yet by some accounts they represent as little as 15 percent of brain cells. The leftover 85 percent are a family of cells called glia. Glial cells don't send electrical signals, like the flashy neurons do. Their very name gives a hint of how they were regarded: *glia* comes from the Greek word for "glue"—not a very enticing name. Long dismissed as mere packing material that held the neurons in place, glial cells were known to provide some mundane housekeeping services like feeding the neurons and mopping up after them. They were described as housewives or handmaidens and mostly ignored.

But like scorned Cinderella, the glial cells are the ultimate beauties. It turns out the neurons are utterly dependent on them for every kind of function. Without the glial cells' dutiful attention, neurons would starve to death, suffocate, be unable to fire their electrical impulses, or send their messages to other neurons, and they would swim in a backwash of toxic trash. Only

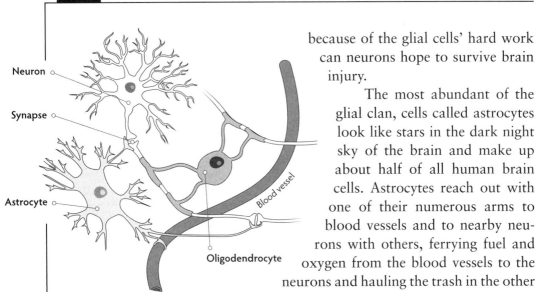

Neuron

Synapse

Astrocyte

Blood vessel

Oligodendrocyte

because of the glial cells' hard work can neurons hope to survive brain injury.

The most abundant of the glial clan, cells called astrocytes look like stars in the dark night sky of the brain and make up about half of all human brain cells. Astrocytes reach out with one of their numerous arms to blood vessels and to nearby neurons with others, ferrying fuel and oxygen from the blood vessels to the neurons and hauling the trash in the other direction. With their feet, astrocytes create the channels through which life-giving cerebral spinal fluid brings nutrients to the cells and flushes away debris. Astrocytes are masters of the blood vessels, modulating their fluid flow. They boost the strength of the electrical impulses in neurons and ferry signals across the synapses between them. At the same time, all of these structures are in motion.

Like housekeepers throughout history who know their masters' secrets, astrocytes listen in on the conversations of the regal neurons. Then they transmit information through their own networks by waves of calcium that speed information rapidly across great distances.

Because science has only recently realized that a cell involved in housekeeping could be important, we are just beginning to really appreciate the astrocytes. We know that Einstein's brain had a normal number of neurons but a far higher-than-normal number of astrocytes. We know that the number of astrocytes is abnormally low in the cortex of people suffering from chronic depression and schizophrenia. On the other hand, they are high in number in people with seizures. Perhaps astrocytes develop in people with seizures as an attempt to regulate the electrical activity of hyperexcited neurons as they spin out of control. Scientists think that is possible, since causing a seizure with shock treatment stimulates astrocyte production at the same time that it helps some people with depression or schizophrenia.

When injury attacks, astrocytes keep neurons alive by providing them with growth factors and nutrients, working to keep the cellular environment free of toxins, protecting neurons from further damage, and producing antioxidants to protect them from the ravages of inflammation. The explosion of toxins that contaminates the brain after injury, unfortunately, can overwhelm and damage the astrocytes. When astrocytes die or become dysfunctional, the neurons shortly follow. One astrocyte can be connected to 160,000 synapses, so when astrocytes falter anywhere, the effects can be felt everywhere.

Another flavor of glial cells, with the tongue-tying name of oligodendrocytes, or ODs, make up the omega-3-rich myelin covering of the axons. Each tentacle of an OD grips a segment of an axon and wraps up to 150 layers of insulation around it, like an electrician wrapping tape around a wire. The sausage-shaped myelin wrapper boosts the speed of an axon's electrical impulses by up to fifty times. When we learn a new skill, structural changes happen in regions of the brain that are rich in OD cells.

ODs protect the fragile axon from injury but are themselves injured by the toxins that collect in stagnant brain tissues after brain injury. When the OD cells are irretrievably damaged, it starts a process called demyelization, in which the myelin wrapper around the axon disintegrates and the neuron eventually dies.

Some glial cells, called microglia, function like macrophages, cleaning up debris and beginning the repair process. I suspect that, like the macrophages which manage inflammation in the rest of the body, microglia can lose their healing focus and become aggressively destructive when debris contaminates the brain for too long.

THE BRAIN'S HEALING WAR

To understand the cataclysm of damage to the cells of the brain that extends over weeks, months, and even years, let's look at what happened to Arturo.

ARTURO was driving through an intersection when a speeding car ran a red light and smashed into the right side of his small sedan. Arturo's car spun out of control. As he was tossed around his shoulder harness, his head twisted helplessly to the left, striking the window, and then to the right. I am going to talk not about how Arturo recovered afterward, but about what happened to his brain as a result of this accident.

Arturo was taken by ambulance to an emergency room, where the scans miraculously showed no patent brain damage. If we had taken our submarine into Arturo's frantic brain, however, we would have seen a scene of tremendous devastation.

Arturo's brain received its first insult when his head struck the window,

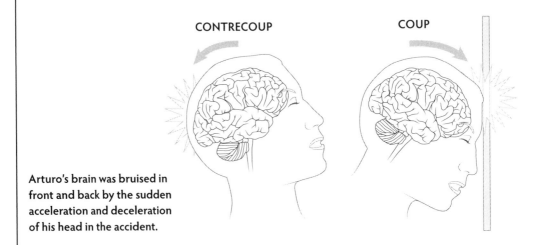

CONTRECOUP **COUP**

Arturo's brain was bruised in front and back by the sudden acceleration and deceleration of his head in the accident.

bruising the brain underneath it. As the car spun through the intersection, Arturo's brain sustained a second impact when his head snapped backward and his brain was catapulted into the back of his skull. Microscopic blood vessels burst in the front and back of his head and leaked acidic blood into Arturo's brain. The blood burned nearby neurons, damaging them. Since the brain, encased by the skull, has little room for extra fluid of any kind, the bleeding pressed against nearby brain tissue and uninjured blood vessels, squeezing the tissue and cutting off oxygen and nutrients to the damaged cells. The bleeding was too small to be detected by the scans, but it set up a cascade of destruction that went on for some time.

Far more serious than the bleeding was the devastation caused when the force of the spinning car found its way into the cells of Arturo's brain. Lighter and denser parts of Arturo's brain slid over each other and then pulled apart, creating damaging shearing forces. Some axons were torn apart, causing the death of neurons and spilling toxins and debris into the surrounding environment.

Most of the axons, however, were strained and stretched by the spinning forces. The stretching damaged their membranes, which developed holes, like in a leaky boat. Vital minerals that keep the neurons working poured out of the holes and harmful substances leaked in. Microscopic pumps inside the neurons sprang into action and tried to pump out the damaging substances. The stretching also damaged the girders that form the neurons' internal skeleton. While they struggled mightily to right themselves and keep from collapsing, the neurons became increasingly agitated by all of the debris pooling in their environment and they became ill.

————————O————————

Injured neurons are already under tremendous stress. In addition to being stretched by rotational forces, their membranes are deformed by the moving pressure waves that injury pounds through the skull. Their metabolism starts to falter. Under all this strain, the neurons panic and excrete a massive amount of neurotransmitters into their environment, as if they are trying to send distress signals in every direction. The neurotransmitters add to the building pollution in the neurons' environment. The loyal astrocytes try to sweep up as much debris as they can and keep dead cells away from the sensitive neurons, but the explosion of neurotransmitters cripples the astrocytes as well.

Diffuse axonal injury

As the neurons and their loyal companions struggle to deal with their damaged membranes, poisoned environment, and collapsing structures, inflammation brings them another round of misery. As we learned in the chapter on inflammation, the body does not negotiate with injury. When injury attacks, it goes to war. Within minutes of a traumatic brain injury, the body's ancient protective system—inflammation—leaps into action. Glial cells, blood vessels, and even the neurons themselves send out chemical distress signals called cytokines to inform the brain that it is under attack.

In answer to the cells' S.O.S., immune cells rush to the scene of injury. Highly destructive neutrophils release their powerful array of chemical weapons to burn away the blood and the dying cells, but these substances are highly toxic to the struggling neurons and astrocytes. Cells called microglia, which live in the brain, transform from calm little spiders to creatures out of a horror movie, raging beasts that release damaging chemicals of their own. The chemical weapons released by these cells are necessary to clear a space for the surviving neurons, but they cause significant damage to other brain cells and can contribute to their death.

Soon the site of injury is swarming with destructive immune cells, powerful cytokines, and cellular debris. Specialized astrocytes and microglial cells rush in to stop the bleeding and wall off the injury site. Nearby blood vessels become temporarily porous so that healing nutrients and fluids can rush in. The excess fluid is designed to jump-start the healing process. But, as we have seen, the brain, encased in the relatively inflexible shell of the skull, has little room for extra fluid. The fluid causes swelling and the swelling increases pressure inside the skull. The pressure pushes against the blood vessels, constricting them and cutting the neurons off from precious oxygen and nutrients. The swelling of nearby astrocytes further shuts off the flow of oxygen and fuel from the traumatized blood vessels.

Even if oxygen and fluid can make their way to the injured cells through undamaged blood vessels, the battle for healing has just begun. As the neurotransmitters accumulate in the stagnant fluid, the neurons become overstimulated by their own garbage, a highly dangerous state called excitotoxicity. The dangerous overstimulation triggers a self-destruct switch in the neurons, which begin to fall apart. Toxic protein debris, such as amyloid precursor protein, begins to accumulate around the damaged cells.

The pumps inside the neurons desperately try to set things right, but pumps run on energy. Just when the neurons' need for oxygen and fuel is greatest and most desperate, the neurons face an energy crisis. Oxygen and glucose are in short supply in the injured brain because swelling has restricted blood flow, the vasculature is in shock, and the pathways to the cells are backed up so that fuel and oxygen can't get in. Even if they could, the injured brain's needs are so great that they outstrip the available supply. The neurons can survive for a certain amount of time before they starve and suffocate, but eventually they fall apart.

Meanwhile, the long axons of the neurons are having their own problems. The valiant ODs that tried to protect the axons start to disintegrate under the assault of the destructive immune cells and cytokines. Their myelin wrappings slowly fall apart, a process called demyelination. Newer myelin is thinner and far more susceptible to damage from inflammation, which may explain in part why a second brain injury is far worse for the brain.

The naked axons can no longer protect the neurons, and destructive calcium ions flood into the dying cell. The cell's internal skeleton collapses, the balance of chemicals that spark the neuron's electrical signals is lost, and the cell dies. The cell's polluted environment triggers self-destruct mechanisms that cause other neurons to die, and the neuronal networks start to fail.

Despite this orgy of destruction caused by injury and inflammation, inflammation still is primarily a healing process. The same microglial cells that are such adept killers of neurons and their glial helpers also produce neuroprotective cytokines and growth factors and, like the macrophages in the rest of the body, should eventually move the process of inflammation toward healing. The problem is not that injury to the brain causes inflammation; it's that the brain has a far smaller capacity to accommodate inflammation's damage.

To shepherd inflammation toward healing is a far more complex task in the brain than in the rest of the body. Fluid flow is more easily disrupted, and the cells are far more desperate for oxygen and nutrients and far more sensitive to the backup of debris. Unless inflammation can be turned toward healing, however, the destruction will continue.

I am convinced that the basic principles of moving inflammation toward healing are the same in the brain as elsewhere in the body. Restoring fluid flow in particular is of the greatest urgency, as fluid flow reduces swelling and improves blood circulation. Then the anti-inflammatory chemicals that modulate inflammation's power can be reinforced with omega-3s, vitamins, and antioxidants. Then the cells' power plants—the mitochondria—can be repaired with protein and all of their membranes rebuilt with healthy fat.

ONGOING INFLAMMATION AND BRAIN INJURY

A traumatic brain injury can initiate a cataclysm of destruction that ravages the brain for years. Chronic inflammation takes hold, and axons are slowly destroyed along tracks far from the original injury. One group of researchers discovered that seventeen years after a single brain injury, activated microglial cells, a bellwether of inflammation, were found throughout the brain.

Chronic inflammation is not a healing process. It is a highly destructive, self-perpetuating disease that damages healthy tissue. In chronic inflammation, destruction and repair take place at the same time, but destruction is winning. Why does inflammation in the brain so readily get off track and become chronic? I believe that part of the answer can be found in the disruption inflicted on the brain's fluid flow by trauma. When toxic debris accumulates because fluid flow is stagnant, it sets off the vicious cycle of destruction that I just described. The immune system treats the debris pile as an invader and sends inflammatory chemicals and cells to destroy it, which cause more damage and produce more debris. Because the fluid is stagnant, the debris is never cleared. Thus begins an endless cycle of accumulated trash, destructive cells, and chemicals that cause more damage and more trash.

The brain cells whose job it is to shepherd inflammation toward healing—the microglial cells—lose their way. Microglia, like their macrophage cousins in the rest of the body, have great power both to harm and to heal. When the brain is injured, they leap into action. Their job is to clear away the debris of injury in the beginning of inflammation—a necessary but highly destructive process—and then, mission accomplished, release healing and growth factors necessary for repair and restoration. But when the brain is

The Risks of Bleeding in the Brain

Bleeding in or around the brain is always potentially serious. The brain has little room for excess fluid, and blood is toxic to brain tissue.

Head injuries can cause bleeding between any of the skull's membranes. Bleeding between the outermost layer of the dura and the skull is called an epidural hematoma, the injury that tragically killed the great actress Natasha Richardson. The most common place for this injury is on the side of the head, where the bony covering over the middle meningeal artery is relatively thin and weak. The patient may seem fine at first, but as the arterial bleeding continues, damaging and sometimes fatal pressure is placed on the brain. The person starts complaining of a headache and can lapse into unconsciousness. This is a true medical emergency and must be treated quickly.

Bleeding between the dura and the middle layer (the arachnoid mater) is called a subdural hematoma. This can occur when the brain is rapidly accelerated forward or backward, as in a fall or a sports collision. Tiny blood vessels between the two membranes shear apart, causing bleeding in the space between them. This injury can occur after even a minor head injury but is more common among those whose blood vessels are easily injured, such as the elderly or people on blood thinners. Symptoms can develop quickly or over a period of days to weeks, depending on the rate of bleeding. As blood accumulates, it puts pressure on the brain, causing headache, increasing confusion, dizziness, vomiting, drowsiness, and changes in behavior. If left untreated, this, too, can be fatal.

Bleeding between the spidery arachnoid mater and the tender pia mater is called a subarachnoid hemorrhage and can result from head injury or from a spontaneous rupture called an aneurysm. This is an extremely serious condition marked by sudden, severe headache—often described as the worst headache of someone's life—and is also a medical emergency.

Seek immediate medical attention when any of these symptoms occur after a head injury or a violent collision—even if the symptoms occur weeks later. It could save your life.

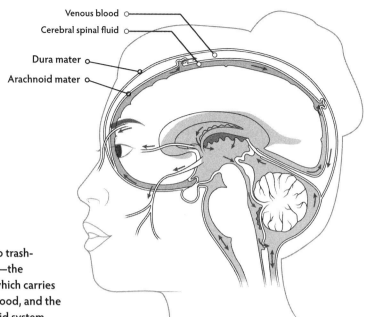

Venous blood
Cerebral spinal fluid
Dura mater
Arachnoid mater

The brain has two trash-removal systems—the venous system, which carries deoxygenated blood, and the cerebrospinal fluid system.

continually injured by toxic debris and the inflammatory entourage it attracts, the ongoing damage confuses the microglia. The microglia never get to rest and move the injured brain away from inflammation because the brain keeps getting injured and the microglia keep responding to the ongoing injury. Like a broken record, the healing process gets stuck. Eventually, the microglia end up destroying and healing the brain at the same time, and inflammation never turns off. In the rest of the body, chronic inflammation can be painful and disabling. In the brain, it is catastrophic.

To halt continuing brain injury and give the brain breathing room to heal, it is critical to restore full fluid flow. The shock must be taken out of the traumatized blood vessels so that they can move oxygen and glucose to the starving cells. The pipes through which the waste is flushed away must be cleared of kinks and twists. The drains out of the brain, which are often clogged or impeded by injury, must be opened. The pumps that push the fluid through must be working properly. As you will see in the next chapter, there are ways to do all of that.

The lymphatics are the heroes of health that help turn inflammation off in the rest of the body by removing the toxic debris of injury. The glymphatics and the brain's membrane mothers are the heroines that help turn inflammation off in the brain and allow the brain to heal.

HOW THE MOTHERS' HARD WORK HELPS THE BRAIN

The brain is a three-pound weakling, and its outer layer has the consistency of custard. It is always at risk of injury. In fact, you may wonder how the brain can survive any movement at all without fragmenting itself on the bony skull or impaling itself on the skull's protruding spikes and ledges.

The answer is that the brain has a unique protection system. That system surrounds the brain with a cushioning moat of fluid. It anchors the brain within the skull to stabilize it. It absorbs and disperses the forces that assault it. It creates channels for the fluids that nourish and cleanse the brain—and then helps pump the fluid. What could possibly do all this work—protecting, cleaning, nourishing, absorbing the blows of life, defending—and still be smiling at the end of the day? Mothers, of course. The brain has three of them. When the mothers are moving freely and seated evenly in the skull, the brain is healthy and happy. When they are twisted or lethargic, debris piles up, inflammation takes hold, axons are perpetually stretched and injured, and the brain can falter.

The mothers are a series of membranes called the meninges. I call them the mothers of the brain because each of the three layers is named after a mother and because, like good mothers, the meninges are tough and tender, protective and attentive, and geniuses at multitasking.

The dura mater. The tough, outermost layer of the meninges is called the dura mater, or tough mother, and it is one tough mother. The dura lines the skull and surrounds the brain, linking the two of them together. The dura has two layers. Its outermost layer adheres to the inside of the skull and sends fibers through the skull's sutures, which fuse with the outer layer of bone. By tying the brain and the skull together, the dura secures the brain so it doesn't move around too much. The dural coupling of brain and skull also explains why the brain and the skull move together like dance partners, harmonized by common dural tethers.

The dura also folds into the brain to create four interconnected, pulsating "sails" that divide the brain into different compartments. Like shock absorbers, these

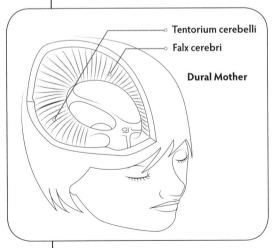

Tentorium cerebelli
Falx cerebri

Dural Mother

The brain's outer mother—the dura—divides, protects, and anchors the brain inside the skull.

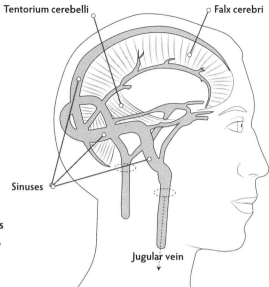

Tentorium cerebelli

Falx cerebri

Sinuses

Jugular vein

The dura not only pumps the fluids but also creates the large channels, called sinuses, that carry debris-laden fluids out of the brain.

dural sails absorb some of the force the brain is subjected to and help it resist rotational forces. A sickle-shaped sail called the falx separates the brain into its two hemispheres—the right brain and the left brain. Two dural "tents" (the tentorium cerebelli) rise over each side of the cerebellum, the nugget of brain in back that controls movement, and a fourth divides the cerebellum in half. The sails pulsate and move. The tentorium flaps up and down like the powerful wings of a bird, forming a diaphragm within the brain to help pump fluids.

The dura also creates the large channels (sinuses) that carry the fluids—in particular, used-up and debris-laden venous blood—out of the brain. In a brilliant feat of biological multitasking, many of the fluid-carrying sinuses are located directly on, under, or around the dural sails that pump them.

The sinuses carrying venous blood turn into the internal jugular veins that exit through openings in the back of the skull called the jugular foramen. We met the jugular foramen before. It's a set of openings between the occipital and temporal bones that can be obstructed by trauma. Sumi, whose story I told in chapter 19, came out of her mental fog when the jugular foramen opened up and the debris-laden venous blood from the sinuses was able to drain out of her brain.

The dura—in fact, the entire membrane system—is particularly vulnerable to distortion in trauma. Because the dura adheres to the skull, trauma that distorts the skull will distort the dura. The membranes move together, so distortions will be translated into the entire system and, I believe, into the brain itself. When the dural sails become distorted, so do the sinuses draining toxins from the brain. Much of my work in treating brain injury involves straightening out the meninges so that the venous channels are opened, strains are taken out of brain tissue, and the vigorous movement of the membranes is restored so that fluid flow is optimized.

The spider and tender mothers. Two more mothers protect and nourish the brain: the weblike membrane called the arachnoid mater (the spider mother) and the delicate pia mater (the tender mother). These two membranes form a moat around the brain, called the subarachnoid space, that is filled with cerebral spinal fluid (CSF). By being suspended in fluid, the three-pound brain effectively weighs about two ounces, enabling it to float harmlessly away from many of the forces that ordinary life pounds through the skull.

Besides creating the subarachnoid moat, these membranes help direct nourishment into the brain. Hundreds of miles of blood vessels penetrate the brain from the subarachnoid space, ferrying oxygen and nutrients to the hungry brain. Cerebral spinal fluid rushes in through pipes that surround the blood vessels, bringing vitamins, hormones, and growth factors and flushing out debris and toxins.

THE GLYMPHATIC SYSTEM

Osteopathic medicine has spent close to a hundred years refining techniques to assist the brain's two fluid systems. Both of the fluid systems that nourish the brain and clear away its trash can be compromised by brain injury, and both must be restored to full function for the damage to be halted.

Arteries and veins make up the first system. As we just learned, hundreds of miles of blood vessels penetrate the brain from the moat of the subarachnoid space. Tiny arteries bring in oxygen and fuel, and small veins carry away some of the debris. This system is slow and steady.

The second system is vigorous and powerful: it is a cleansing torrent of cerebral spinal fluid. CSF surrounds the brain in the subarachnoid moat and floods into the brain's interior from that moat through channels that follow the same pathways that the arteries use to carry blood. The pia mater folds in to start the channels. Then astrocytes wrap their feet around the arteries to create the channels, making a dual pipe system in which blood is carried through the inner pipe and CSF is carried through the outer one. Great jets of CSF flow under pressure deep into the brain through these channels. CSF then flushes out debris and trash at high speeds along channels that follow the exiting

Hope for Victims of Brain Injury

The destruction of axons in the suffering brain that goes on for years after trauma and has baffled researchers may not be solely the result of a self-perpetuating inflammatory process. Perhaps the continuing damage to the axons also comes from a second source. Is it possible that the brain's membranes have ensnared the weakened axons and subjected them to continuing stretch damage?

As I mentioned earlier, trauma can twist and distort the brain's membrane system (the dura). Because the dura orchestrate the brain's position inside the skull, dural twists can drag the brain into a somewhat contorted position. Perhaps these traumatic distortions of the dura hold the brain in an abnormal position that continues to stretch its already weakened axons, resulting in ongoing axonal damage. This may eventually cause them either to disintegrate or to be more vulnerable to future insults.

If dural distortions are actively injuring the axons, one would expect this continuing damage to be accompanied by continuing inflammation. One would also expect to find the damage—and inflammation—along the length of the stretched and disintegrating axons. Recent research has provided some evidence that this may, in fact, be happening. In 2011, researchers found deteriorating axons accompanied by a chronic inflammatory process in some subjects years after the brain injury. The researchers also found that the destruction was not confined to a single place, but frequently extended laterally throughout the brain's axons. The researchers speculated that this pattern of destruction may reflect the regions under the greatest biomechanical strain during the original insult. Since distorted membranes can be corrected by cranial osteopathic techniques, this provides a significant avenue for future exploration that might help redress the years of suffering endured by victims of traumatic brain injury.

veins. The CSF flows back into the moat, joins the venous system exiting the brain, or leaves the skull through pathways around the cranial nerves or down into the spinal cord.

In the rest of the body, the lymphatic system has the job of removing debris and cleansing the tissues. The brain has no lymphatic vessels, leaving that job primarily to the astrocyte-created drainage system. Since the system is formed by glial cells and acts like a lymphatic system, researchers have dubbed it the glymphatic system. The torrents of CSF pulsing along the glymphatic channels sweep the brain clear of potentially harmful substances, including used-up neurotransmitters and the amyloid proteins that are characteristic of Alzheimer's disease.

The discovery of the glymphatic system has created tremendous excitement in the research community. Increasingly, researchers are identifying static CSF flow as a primary contributor to the neurodegenerative diseases of aging—Alzheimer's disease, Parkinson's disease, ALS (amyotrophic lateral sclerosis), and multiple sclerosis. We know that the flow of CSF slows down as we age, as does the brain's ability to clear harmful substances. The brain's environment begins to deteriorate, and the buildup of toxins causes neurons and glial cells to malfunction. I believe a similar mechanism is at work in traumatic brain injury. After traumatic brain injury, just as in the neurodegenerative diseases of aging, the flow of CSF and venous blood is impaired, and vulnerable neurons and glial cells are sickened by the pools of waste the injured brain cannot clear. This explains why brain injury increases the risk of neurodegenerative diseases and why degenerative changes in the brains of some mild traumatic brain injury patients closely resemble those found in early Alzheimer's dementia.

Improving the brain's fluid flows is at the heart of the work that I and other cranial osteopaths do: we are mechanics of the brain's fluid flow. We restore motion to the mechanisms that pump it, the channels that carry it, and the drains that let it out of the skull. What I do and what you can do to heal the brain is the subject of the next chapter.

22

Healing the Brain

The brain longs to heal. After an injury, it frantically tries to regain its steady motion. That's what I find when I listen to the brain's conversations after trauma. Like a heart damaged by a heart attack, after significant trauma the brain wriggles erratically and pulsates in a much less effective manner. Even a small trauma can disrupt the brain's normal pulsations. The sooner the brain can find its way home to a regular rhythm and a powerful amplitude (strength), the quicker it—and the rest of the body—heals.

When the brain remains untreated and the injury is allowed to persist, the brain weakens to the point where it is crawling to exhaustion like a weary traveler struggling to find water in the desert. The brain remains feeble and erratic until injury shock is removed, inflammation tamed, and motion restored to the brain and its supporting structures. Then health will return.

The brain is the most complicated organ on the planet, and brain injury is incredibly complex. No one treatment modality, medication, hormone, or supplement can miraculously cure it. But helping restore the brain's motion and its fluid flow can galvanize the brain's remarkable healing powers.

As a cranial osteopathic physician, I'm lucky. I can feel how the brain is doing. I can feel which parts of the skull are restricting which parts of the brain's motion. I can feel how one or more of the dural sails have lost their flexibility or have become twisted, compromising the brain's expansion and contraction and restricting the brain's fluid pathways. Through my hands, I can feel how powerfully and completely the brain is pulsating.

I use my cranial skills not only to evaluate the brain's health but also to design effective treatments and monitor the success of those treatments. Years

275

of practice have shown me that with some essential help, regardless of whether the brain injury occurred yesterday or twenty years earlier, the brain has a remarkable ability to heal. But like the rest of the body, in order to heal, the brain must move. The brain, the brain's life-giving fluids, the brain's enveloping membranes, and its bony container must all move fully and freely to stop the damage and begin the healing.

Healing brain injury, as elsewhere in the body, requires a series of steps. First, the destructive parts of the injury process must be halted. Bleeding and destruction of neurons and glial cells must cease. That means that the inflammatory fires accompanying injury must be modulated. Proper fluid flow of both the cerebral spinal fluid and the venous system must be optimized to flush out the toxic debris that stokes up the inflammatory fires. All the exits for fluid removal must be wide open to channel toxins out of the brain and stop the swelling, which will otherwise cause more damage to the brain.

To manage all this, the hungry brain needs lots and lots of energy (primarily derived from glucose) and oxygen. However, trauma has created a number of impediments to the brain's energy supply system. The twists in the dura create detours or even roadblocks for venous blood and CSF to escape. If the exit pipes are constricted, that causes back pressure and swelling in the brain, making it harder for blood vessels to bring in enough glucose and oxygen. Normally, the brain uses 20 percent of our energy. Injury dramatically escalates that need.

There are solutions to all of these problems. Whether, as with Phillip, the person comes to me right after a trauma, or arrives months or years later, addressing these components of brain injury can reap tremendous rewards. The sooner treatment can be initiated, however, the better. I have repeatedly found that if a patient receives cranial treatment within forty-eight hours of the injury, as Phillip did, the symptoms of injury are markedly diminished and the patient recovers much more quickly.

HEALING PHILLIP'S BRAIN INJURY

I saw Phillip four hours after the truck hit him. The first thing I do to treat any bleeding and swelling in the brain is to give my patients homeopathic *Arnica montana* in a high potency (dose)—a minimum of 1M. Since Phillip's injury was fairly severe, I gave him the higher dose of 10M. This dose also helped his diffuse bodily trauma. Studies show that *Arnica* dramatically decreases bleeding and bruising and is especially effective in treating brain injury.

Then I very gently examined him. I had treated Phillip for many years for the mild bangs and bumps of an athletic kid. He had always been healthy.

Phillip's helmet had protected him from a skull fracture and a much more serious brain injury. Even with the helmet, however, as happens with many blows to the head or torso, the front and the back of the gel-like brain had slammed against the inside of his hard skull, causing bruising and bleeding of the brain.

That trauma was reflected in what I felt under my hands. Phillip's nervous system felt chaotic, as though he'd been spun around in a dryer. His brain, which should have been gradually expanding and contracting like a balloon gaining and then losing some air, wriggled around erratically. The bones in the front (frontal) and back (occipital) of his head were locked solid against their joints.

Treatment Methods

Some ways to help the brain heal have existed for a hundred years or more, and some are new. I generally prefer tried-and-true methods that have a long track record, like osteopathic medicine, Oriental medicine, and homeopathy. But I am also grateful for recent technological and pharmaceutical advances. The gruesome damage created by the latest weapons of war has led to wonderful medical breakthroughs. I do not pretend to know many of these latest advances that can make a tremendous difference right after a serious brain injury. I defer to my colleagues on the front lines of emergency medicine—physicians in the ER or the neurosurgery suite.

As I discussed in chapter 20, I had to start by addressing Phillip's injury shock, calming his nervous system, and helping restore his breath. To assist in this, I also gave him a high dose (10M) of homeopathic *Aconitum napellus*, a remedy specifically for terror and panic from a life-threatening event. Then I began the slow, gentle, and precise task of calming his deeply agitated nervous system with my hands. As it is almost always best to start treating trauma far from the worst damage, I began at Phillip's sacrum.

As I talked about earlier, the sacrum has profound links to the brain and nervous system. The membranes that surround the brain fall like a curtain around the spinal cord and then attach inside the sacrum. The nervous system ends its central core inside that bone. With such an intimate connection to the brain, the spinal cord and sacrum pulsate in rhythm with the brain's movement, the cranial rhythmic impulse (CRI). Like a puppeteer, I used my hand on the sacrum to influence that sheath of membrane to help diminish the brain's chaotic movements. I monitored my success by listening with my hands to the developing improvement in Phillip's CRI. Under the gentle treatment of my hands and the orchestration of the dural pulley, Phillip's brain calmed somewhat.

Concerned about possible abdominal-organ injury, I used only gentle pressure to help release the diaphragm to improve his breathing. I also applied gentle inhibitory pressure where the ribs meet the spinal vertebrae to help relax the sympathetic nervous system.

Then I examined and treated Phillip's head. All of my techniques were exceedingly gentle: I did not want to further tear the now exceedingly fragile blood vessels and nerves and increase the severity of his brain injury. His compressed skull was bearing down on his brain, which I worried was beginning to swell. To give the brain as much room as possible, I tractioned the frontal bone slightly away from its traumatically induced weld to the sphenoid bones on either side. I pried the frontal bone away from the ethmoid bone of the nose that forms the shelf below it. Both of these techniques increased the size of the skull and took the pressure off the brain, but they also did something else very important: they helped cerebral spinal fluid (CSF) drain out of the skull.

Cerebral spinal fluid is the life-sustaining fluid in the brain that streams into all the nooks and crannies of the brain. As it flows, it brings nutrients and healing factors to the brain's cells and cleanses away toxins and debris. If the CSF cannot clear the brain's waste products, brain tissue in the stagnant region can suffocate in a pool of toxins and inflammation can spin out of control. The downward spiral this provokes ends up causing far more damage to the brain than the original injury.

The CSF flushes out of the brain through all twelve cranial nerves (CN), but the olfactory nerves to the nose provide especially important escape valves. Small holes in the bone at the top of the nose, called the cribiform plate, allow CSF to drain through the olfactory nerves and then into the lymphatic channels of the face and neck. These holes also allow small substances to pass into the brain from the nose, which explains why sniffing cocaine has such a powerful and immediate effect on the brain. By releasing the bony compression above the nose, I opened up one

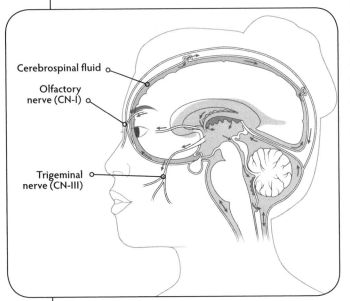

Cerebrospinal fluid

Olfactory
nerve (CN-I)

Trigeminal
nerve (CN-III)

of the main drainage pathways. This not only released some of the pressure building up in Phillip's head but also, most critically, helped remove some of the toxic waste products. Since a lot of CSF fluid drains into the venous system, I had to address that system as well. I did that when I moved to treat the back of Phillip's head.

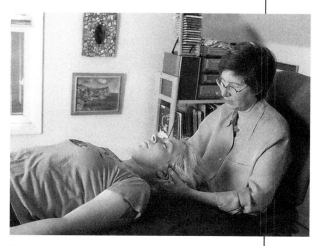

By opening up the bony channels in the back of the head through which the jugular veins pass, I help toxic debris drain more easily out of the brain.

Working at the back of Phillip's head, I ever so slightly pulled the welded occipital bone away from its grip on the temporal bones on each side. This accomplished two things. First, it gave his brain a little more room to expand and contract. Second, it opened up critical exit points for debris-laden venous blood to leave the brain. Much of this venous blood courses through the large internal jugular veins that must navigate the bony passageways between these bones. Trauma that pushes the bones together can narrow these openings (the jugular foramen). By gently pulling the bones apart, I widened Phillip's two jugular foramen. Pressure in his brain eased, and venous blood flowed more easily out of his skull and shunted away toxic waste.

Next, I worked on the pipes that carry the venous blood to the exit points. As we saw in the previous chapter, the dural membrane surrounding the brain separates in places to create sinuses (pipes) for the deoxygenated and debris-laden venous blood to travel out of the skull. In Phillip's case, as in so many victims of brain injury, trauma twisted the membranes and these channels had developed kinks. My next job was to iron out the wrinkles, large and small, from the membranes.

Because the dura orchestrates the brain's position inside the skull, dural twists can drag the brain into a somewhat contorted position. After Phillip's fierce rotational trauma, the contorted dura no longer kept his brain centered. I sensed under my hands that the pulsations of the brain, skull, and dura were causing the displaced brain to hit against ridges inside the skull, which can cause more injury. By working with the dura's attachment to the outside of the skull, I manipulated the membrane and the bones, using them like guy wires to straighten out the brain. One of my most essential jobs after brain injury—and one I do repeatedly—is to make sure the dural membranes are straightened out.

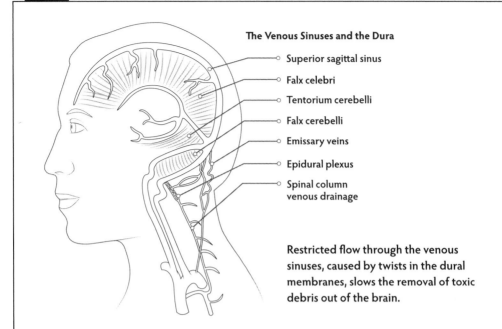

The Venous Sinuses and the Dura

○ Superior sagittal sinus

○ Falx celebri

○ Tentorium cerebelli

○ Falx cerebelli

○ Emissary veins

○ Epidural plexus

○ Spinal column venous drainage

Restricted flow through the venous sinuses, caused by twists in the dural membranes, slows the removal of toxic debris out of the brain.

Then the brain can sit balanced inside the skull and venous blood can stream more freely toward the exit routes once again.

All this gentle treatment helped calm the brain's panicked shuddering. That in itself prepared Phillip's brain to better begin its rebuilding process. Just as it's impossible to repair a damaged bridge in the middle of an earthquake, the trembling brain makes reconstruction difficult. The brain's chaotic wriggling also made it harder for the brain's housekeeping cells, the astrocytes, to hold onto the metaphoric brooms and dustpans necessary for waste removal.

As Phillip's brain began to pulsate more evenly and fully, I sensed that the skull, the dura, and the brain had regained some of their normal healing motion. The calmer brain indicated to me I had partially managed to dampen the damaging chemical cascade that was keeping brain injury going.

When Phillip rose from the treatment table, he said, "My head feels much better. But I'm really tired."

"Tired is good. Rest, and rest some more."

Before sending Phillip on his way, I reiterated to his mother the advice she'd been given in the emergency room to check him every two hours for twenty-four hours. During the night she was to wake him and shine a flashlight in his eyes to make sure his pupils dilated in response to the light. If the pupils didn't dilate, his head pain increased, or she had trouble waking him, she was to take him back to the emergency room immediately. I told her to take him to a neurologist in the morning. I also gave him a high dose of *Arnica* to repeat once a day to help prevent more bleeding and bruising, especially in the brain.

Phillip made it safely through the next day. He saw a neurologist, who sent him back to me. Two days later, I treated him again. As often happens after a brain injury, the body seems to forget much of the positive effects of any treatment and has to be frequently reminded how to heal. I have also found that homeopathic remedies have to be repeated much more often as well. By then, Phillip's head hurt a lot more, as did his neck, torso, pelvis, and especially his hip. After such a drastic insult to the nervous system, people generally have less initial pain. That's because the nervous system is too injured to appropriately communicate how much has been damaged. Then, as the nervous system heals, people start feeling what's really going on and the pain can explode.

I repeated much of what I had done in the previous treatment—opening the skull's sutures, straightening out the membranes, unblocking the drains and fluid channels, and settling the nervous system.

Phillip's Healing Journey

The road to healing can be long and have quite a few bumps. However, the path someone takes at the beginning of the journey can dramatically improve the final outcome. I forbade Phillip from playing basketball until I cleared him, because a second injury can be catastrophic if it occurs while the brain is still healing. The extensive guidelines now in place on the treatment of head trauma were not in effect then, but my experience had taught me the dangers of a second injury before the first had healed. The current guidelines prohibit athletes from returning to sports until they are cleared though a gradual, step-by-step evaluation process that takes a minimum of four days after the athlete is symptom-free.

I referred Phillip to an orthopedist for his hip injury, and the neurologist continued to monitor his brain injury. I continued to treat him osteopathically once a week. For several days after the treatments, his headache would lessen.

After being benched for a month, Phillip returned to his beloved basketball. Learning new, patterned movement is one of the best healers for brain injury. Basketball—with its complex movements—was a perfect vehicle for helping retrain his injured brain.

Not yet having a more comprehensive view of mild traumatic brain injury (MTBI), I did not warn his parents that Phillip should have his cognitive skills evaluated. The frontal lobe of the brain, where Phillip had his focal injury, is in charge of executive function. He also suffered diffuse injury elsewhere as a contrecoup trauma to the opposite side of his brain, the occipital lobe. These multiple injuries showed up later in many ways.

Before his injury, Phillip did mathematical problems for fun and was a voracious reader. After his injury, reading gave him a headache and he lost all interest in it, and he started flunking math. The problems didn't make sense to him. His math difficulty had probably resulted from frontal lobe damage. His reading problems could have resulted from the contrecoup trauma to the occipital lobe in back, the part of the brain that interprets visual images. It could have been caused by damage to the axons coming from the eye as they attempted to bring the visual images to the occipital lobe. Or the injury could have been anywhere in between. The ophthalmologist found nothing wrong with his eyes. I did work to resolve imbalance between his two orbits. That process decreased his headaches when reading, but did not re-spark his interest in books. For many years, Phillip also had trouble with anger. Frontal lobe injuries can cause that as well.

Luckily, Phillip was so bright and talented that, once his mother bought a video camera, he found he could write, direct, and edit captivating movies. That's how he makes his living, eighteen years later, as a talented film director and editor.

Phillip is doing well. His cranial sutures and dura still run on the tight side. He needs an osteopathic treatment approximately every two months and an occasional homeopathic remedy to help keep him headache-free. He has resumed his love of reading, and his math skills have to some extent returned. He can focus for fourteen hours a day doing the work he loves, but he's scattered about the boring details of daily living, paying bills, and staying on track with the annoyances of life. His parents, he, and I all attribute a part of his disorganization to his brain injury.

Even quick osteopathic and homeopathic care cannot completely stop all of the damage of brain injury. But the positive effects of osteopathy and homeopathy can be profound. Phillip, his family, and I are all convinced that without immediate and consistent osteopathic and homeopathic care, Phillip would have suffered from much more pain and could have been left with much more serious and debilitating cognitive problems.

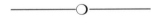

My experience with Phillip, as well as with hundreds of other patients, has repeatedly reaffirmed my conviction that the brain has a remarkable ability to heal, even years after a brain injury. I also know that when a person injures their brain, other parts of the body that were also injured tend to take a lot longer to heal. Now it's time for me to describe ways people can help repair a compromised brain.

WHAT YOU CAN DO

When you have suffered a brain injury, it's common to feel overwhelmed and unable to cope. So here are some of the simple things I recommend that my patients do—and avoid—within the first weeks after a brain injury:

Get evaluated immediately by a physician to rule out serious or life-threatening injury. I cannot emphasize enough that brain injury always must be taken seriously. When in doubt, err on the side of caution.

Get treated by a competent cranial practitioner. Once any serious pathology has been ruled out, I recommend seeing a cranial osteopathic physician as soon as possible after a brain injury. From over thirty years of experience and thousands of patient visits, I am convinced that cranial treatment decreases inflammation and its continuing cascade of damage, helps the brain mop up toxins, diminishes dangerous swelling, helps restore fluid flow, and assists the repair process.

If a cranial osteopathic physician or a medical doctor trained in cranial osteopathy is not available in your area, I recommend finding a trained health care professional who has taken several craniosacral courses. Craniosacral therapy is not osteopathic care. However, in the hands of an experienced and careful health care professional well versed in anatomy and physiology, it can be the next best thing.

Take homeopathic Arnica. I recommend that as soon as possible my patients take a couple of pellets of homeopathic *Arnica montana*. I recommend keeping *Arnica* in the car and in the backpack or purse. I do.

Arnica has a well-studied ability to diminish bleeding, bruising, swelling, and inflammation posttrauma. If someone is on the way to the emergency room, I tell them to take whatever strength they've got with them. I prefer my patients take a dose of 200C once a day for three days. Homeopathic *Arnica* is readily accessible in many health food stores and pharmacies. As always with homeopathy, if symptoms worsen, *stop* taking the remedy. I discuss homeopathy in more detail in chapter 27.

Rest. A person with a brain injury must rest their brain. Forcing the brain to concentrate or focus after being injured is like trying to race on a fractured ankle. Instead of soothing the damaged neurons and calming the cascade of trauma exploding in their brain, a person is whipping their limping, bleeding brain onward and pouring gasoline on the fiery cascade of injury.

"But I feel okay," my patient may say. "My head doesn't hurt. Doesn't that mean my brain's okay?"

"No." I tell them. "Some people have headaches; others don't." Anyone who's

Brain Injury in Children

For twenty years, I have been insisting that victims of traumatic brain injury, especially children, rest their brains even though lots of other physicians have told these patients to just get back to work or school. I am relieved that at the annual meeting of the Pediatric Academic Society in 2012, Dr. Kristy Arbogast, director of the Pediatric Injury Prevention Program at Children's Hospital of Philadelphia, unequivocally stated that after a concussion, children must give their brains a break. That means limiting "cognitive activities to a level that does not elicit symptoms." Which can mean forgoing homework, or reading for school, or avoiding noisy or busy environments, computer work, or other stressful activities.

read *Hannibal* knows that the brain has no pain fibers. Sometimes the brain can only let someone know it's hurt by increasing their anxiety, making them exhausted, not allowing them to think clearly, or making them forget or lose things.

I have repeatedly found that the people who truly rested their brains after a brain injury regained a more even and fuller cranial rate and healed much more quickly as well. On the other hand, a demanding school or work schedule resulted in a much slower return of a healthy cranial rate—instead of getting better, brain pulsations became weaker and more erratic and other symptoms kept getting worse.

Sleep. Sleep is one of the best things you can do to heal your brain. The brain makes healing growth factors and anti-inflammatory chemicals during sleep. Sleep improves cognitive function and headache severity. You must get enough sleep after brain injury!

Unfortunately, brain injury often interferes with sleep. The breathing exercises in chapter 7 and the suggestions in chapter 26 on sleep can help with this problem. Acupuncture has proved as effective as medication in treating insomnia, without the side effects. Sleep is not the same as resting. Rest your brain during the day and make sure you get eight-plus hours of sleep at night.

Stay hydrated. Hydration is absolutely essential after a brain injury. The cerebral spinal fluid needs lots of water to flush away debris. I suspect that the soothing and protective effects of sufficient water are not lost on the wise brain. Drink at least eight cups of water a day.

Supply your ravaged brain with clean fuel. The most powerful medicine for healing your injured brain resides on the end of your fork. Every day, researchers are rediscovering the power of a healing diet to halt and even reverse some of the devastation of brain injury. Your injured brain is starving and on fire with inflammation. Its membranes and metabolism are faltering, and its need for energy, vitamins, minerals, and antioxidants is gargantuan. Feed it inflammation-fighting foods that help it heal, not ones that fuel the inflammation and make it worse. The healing-from-injury diet in chapter 10 is a good place to start.

Feeding your injured brain a rainbow of antioxidant-rich foods—dark, leafy vegetables, as well as oranges, carrots, and berries—is one of the best things you can do for it. Antioxidants are the body's natural inflammation-fighting chemicals. Inflammation produces free radicals, the damaging molecules that are so toxic to neurons, glial cells, and blood vessels. Astrocytes are reservoirs of antioxidants, but brain injury can overwhelm them, and they need to be extensively replenished.

The humble blueberry is the superstar of antioxidants, containing the highest level of all the foods studied. If you don't feel like cooking, make a smoothie with frozen berries and a nutritious "green" powder such as Green Vibrance that concentrates nutrients from vegetables. However you do it, get those antioxidant-rich foods into your diet.

Your injured brain needs high quality protein, particularly during the first two weeks after a brain injury, to build neurotransmitters and reduce inflammation. Wild salmon and other cold-water fish are high in protein and inflammation-fighting vitamins and fats. Even though they're expensive, think of them as part of your medication. For those who eat meat, grass-fed meats are also a good source.

Healthy fats are essential to heal the brain. Fat makes up the membranes of brain cells and the myelin covering of their axons; a person with a brain injury has an extra need for healthy fats such as fish oils, coconut oil, and butter. There is growing evidence that pure, nonhydrogenated coconut oil may be protective against Alzheimer's disease and other degenerative neurological diseases. Though I have had no known brain injury, I usually use at least a tablespoon of organic coconut oil a day either on my vegetables or in a smoothie. I recommend it to everyone who has had a brain injury.

Feed your brain healing supplements. While I am generally quite cautious about supplements, there are some that have proven their worth in helping the brain heal. Vitamin D is known to have profound anti-inflammatory effects and, in combination with the steroid hormone progesterone, has been shown to dramatically improve the brain's repair mechanisms. We all should protect ourselves with sufficient levels of vitamin D. I recommend at least 1000 IU a day. Find a good supplement that contains vitamin D in combination with vitamin A and vitamin K2. Omega-3 fish-oil supplements are a good source of vitamins A and D.

Omega-3s are the superstars of brain health. Omega-3 fats form the structure of cell membranes, and the brain cannot survive without them. There is anecdotal evidence that megadoses of omega-3 oils can help the brain heal from what seems to be catastrophic, irreversible damage.

A 100 mg B vitamin with folate and a tablet of sublingual B12 once a day can also help. I have found B12 and folate injections to be even more helpful when used twice a week for approximately one month after an acute brain injury.

Brain injury decreases magnesium. Magnesium is needed for glucose utilization and proper nerve-protein synthesis. I recommend a minimum of 400 mg of magnesium a day.

Consider curcumin. I strongly recommend curcumin (turmeric) supplements, another emerging superstar of brain healing. I give it to many of my patients dealing with inflammation and brain injury. Patients report fewer headaches and better mental clarity when taking this supplement. Curcumin has been shown to protect the brain against inflammation's damage, enhance production of the brain's natural antioxidants, and counteract cognitive impairment caused by brain injury.

Tap into healing powders. I use two products that my patients report have helped them. Brain Vibrance Supreme Powder has proved helpful in improving the rate of recovery in my patients with MTBI. It contains three products that seem to support brain health: acetyl-L-carnitine, glycerophosphocholine (GPC), and phosphatidylserine (PS).

I have also found that the herbal extract of *Rhodiola rosea* helpful in diminishing fatigue and helping memory and cognition problems. This is a fairly well-studied herb with strong anti-inflammatory properties. I recently gave some of my brain-injured patients a product called E-Z Energy by Ameriden, which contains *Rhodiola rosea* as well as other herbal supports. When my MTBI patients take E-Z Energy, they report that it helps both their thinking and energy.

FIVE THINGS TO AVOID

There are some things you should be careful to avoid, or they could turn your injury into a much more serious disaster.

Avoid activities that could cause a second brain injury. A second brain injury is ***much more serious*** if it occurs before the first one heals completely. This is called the second-impact syndrome, and it can cause serious, even life-threatening brain damage. That means you cannot return to mountain biking, soccer, or any activity that has a danger of head injury until the first brain injury has thoroughly healed.

Avoid inflammation-promoting foods. The injured brain is on fire with inflammation. Your diet has to be front-loaded with the nutrient-dense foods I mention above. Brain injury is not a time for vacillation. Make a commitment to nutritious food, and help your brain heal.

I strongly recommend avoiding foods known to fire up inflammation, such as corn syrup, sugar, soda, and deep-fried foods. The nutritional suggestions I've made in the chapters on inflammation and food apply doubly to brain injury. Absolutely avoid trans fats—they love to fill up cell membranes and turn them hard and impenetrable. They are known to make nerve membranes more brittle. People who consume them are thought to sustain more brain injury than someone who does not indulge. That's the last thing someone wants when they are trying to heal an injured brain. Alcohol is very hard on the injured brain as well.

Avoid flying. I advise my patients to avoid flying and traveling to high altitudes. Significant changes in pressure can affect hydrostatic pressure in the closed space of the brain. A patient of mine, three weeks postconcussion, noted that her headache increased dramatically when she drove up a mountainside and reached 5,000 feet. She immediately turned around and went back down. Good for her!

Several patients have acknowledged that flying caused their brain-injury headaches to get much worse. Each of them felt that flying too soon after a brain injury markedly slowed down their progress. I have not had patients scuba dive soon after a brain injury, but that extreme change of pressure would be an even worse idea.

Avoid toxic chemicals. After brain injury, people should avoid exposure to toxic chemicals (of course, this is always a good idea). Since head injury can create small tears in the blood vessels and/or the dural membrane, creating damage to the brain's blood-brain barrier, there is a greater potential for toxins and bacteria to enter the brain. Many people experience an increased sensitivity to toxins after a brain injury. I recommend avoiding chemical and pesticide exposures until the blood-brain barrier has a chance to heal, which can be weeks or months.

To avoid such life-altering consequences, please avoid these common toxins:

- Pesticides in all forms, even household sprays for bugs.

- Percochlorohydrate dry cleaning, as that is hard on the liver and brain. Use nontoxic dry cleaners.

- New paint, and sealants and stains for wood, tile, and other chemical sealants.

- New carpet in the home or office.

- Perfumes and perfumed cleaning and personal-care products.

If you go shopping and find yourself suddenly feeling sick or sensitive, *leave!* You may find you are very sensitive to odors after brain injury: respect what your body is telling you.

HEALING FROM CHRONIC BRAIN INJURY

JOSEPH. Twenty years earlier, Joseph had been a defensive back for a Pac-10 college. He looked the part. Standing six-foot-four with a thick neck, large hands, and a solid frame, he commanded any room he walked into. For several years, he had had excruciating headaches seven days a week. He'd been to a number of neurologists. They could offer nothing but lots of painkillers. He tried acupuncture, which can often help headaches, but acupuncture didn't touch his pain, so his acupuncturist sent this wonderful gentleman to me.

I'm not much of a football fan: I'm too aware of the kind of damage it does. Baseball is more my sport. But I knew enough to suspect Joseph's head and brain had taken a beating. I asked him about concussions.

"I've never had a brain injury," he insisted. "But I did use my helmet to stop people." (Helmet spearing has since been outlawed because the risk of catastrophic brain and spinal cord injury is so great.)

When I put my hands on Joseph's head, it felt like a rock. His weakened CRI only pulsated about one time a minute, nowhere near normal. His sutures were so jammed together, only my years of experience let me know where they were. It took me months to loosen the sutures in his skull and help his brain regain normal motion. His headaches didn't improve much. "But that disc problem in my low back is gone," he said. Treating his sacrum helped that.

Then I decided to focus on opening the channels where the venous blood leaves the skull, helping to decrease fluid backpressure in the skull. This is a powerful technique that William Sutherland invented toward the end of his life. Opening up the canals leading out of the skull first, I applied pressure gradually up and along the venous sinuses in an orderly manner. As I've come to understand, this is a crucial technique necessary for almost everyone who has had a brain injury, even twenty years earlier. After several sessions, Joseph's headaches lessened in severity and frequency, until they became an occasional annoyance rather than daily, excruciating pain.

As Joseph now realizes, he had had a number of concussions. "I had my bell rung a lot—but we didn't think anything of it then. I even remember being unconscious and waking up in the locker room after a particularly bad head blow. They sent me back into the game after halftime." He has some other signs of brain injury such as forgetfulness at times, but he and I are convinced that my cranial work has given him back his life and significantly diminished the consequences of his repeated brain injuries.

Ten Steps to Healing Chronic Brain Injury

My approach to treating the chronic effects of brain injury is very similar to how I treat an acute injury. However, when a condition is chronic, treatment generally takes longer. Many of the same healing modalities that work for recent brain injury (see page 283) are even more important for those suffering long-term damage to the brain. Here are my suggestions for your path to recovery:

1. *Find a physician skilled in cranial osteopathic treatment.* As Joseph's story demonstrates, osteopathic treatment can be critically important, no matter how much time has passed. Opening up the brain's fluid channels and removing mechanical stress patterns embedded in the membranes and/or brain can help improve brain health years after a brain injury. I've successfully treated many patients who came to see me months or even years after the injury. They have many different complaints: chronic headaches, mood problems and depression, obsessive water drinking, weight gain, fatigue, visual problems, and seizures. I have cured three cases of childhood epilepsy that resulted from traumatic brain injury. In all three cases, the children stopped having seizures. They also received homeopathic remedies. The two that had abnormal EEG changes before treatment had completely normal EEGs afterward.

2. *Continue to feed your brain a healing diet.* Antioxidant-rich, colorful fruits and vegetables are essential. Eat foods high in omega-3 fatty acids such as wild salmon, and use brain-healing fats like avocado and coconut oil to mend damaged membranes.

3. *Supplement your diet with good-quality vitamin and mineral supplements.* These should include vitamins A, B, C, D, E, and K2 and magnesium and zinc. Omega-3 supplements are probably the most important to take on an ongoing basis.

4. *Grow a bigger brain with meditation, yoga, tai chi, and exercise.* Bigger brains are healthier, have stronger fluid flow, and are more resilient. Meditation, yoga, tai chi, and exercise have all been shown to increase the brain's volume, in addition to their many other health benefits.

I have found both meditation and creative visualization extremely helpful for calming the nervous system, decreasing pain and mood disorders, and helping memory and cognition. While I have seen the powerful healing effects of these practices for years, studies are now demonstrating that meditation increases the density of axons in the brain, expands the myelin sheaths that cover them, increases cerebral blood flow, and reduces cortisol levels. It's already well established that meditation can decrease injury shock and inflammation, and I suspect that the same mechanisms are at work in healing the brain. I strongly recommend slowly beginning a meditation or creative-visualizations practice. There are books and DVDs about both, although having a teacher is generally best.

After some injuries, however, the brain pathways used to meditate seem to be compromised. Occasionally after a brain injury, a patient who has meditated for years will say to me, "I'm horrified. I can't meditate anymore. I can't drop into peace" or "When I try to meditate, I get a headache." If someone feels worse when meditating, they should temporarily stop. Talk to a meditation teacher about a different way to meditate or consider a different method, such as a walking meditation, or chanting and/or repeating a mantra. Tai chi, qigong, yoga, or breathing exercises may help some regain their connection to meditation.

If a person enjoyed a spiritual or religious practice before their injury, I encourage them not only to explore medical therapies but also to explore avenues of healing within the spiritual and/or religious context of their lives.

5. Consider homeopathy. I cannot recommend homeopathy strongly enough. In my thirty years of practice, I have seen it work wonders for all kinds of brain injuries, both chronic and acute. If I did not have homeopathy readily available to me, I would feel like I'm practicing medicine with one hand tied behind my back.

In 1999, Ted Chapman, MD, a physician from the Harvard Medical School, conducted a double-blind study on the use of homeopathy in the treatment of MTBI that had often occurred years earlier. The study, done at the Spaulding Rehabilitation Hospital, in Boston, found that "homeopathic treatment significantly reduced the intensity of patients' symptoms . . . and reduced difficulty in functioning."

Homeopathic treatment is based on accurately matching symptoms to remedies. Doctor Chapman picked eighteen of the most common brain-injury remedies for use in the study. Remedies were matched to the patient's unique symptoms; the patient took the medication every day. I recommend a patient undertake homeopathic treatment of MTBI only under the care of a qualified homeopathic practitioner.

6. *Explore Oriental medicine.* I often send people with significant brain injury to practitioners of Oriental medicine. A good herbalist can design a specific concoction for the individual patient's needs. Acupuncture can decrease pain and can increase blood flow to the brain and help with insomnia.

7. *Remember to exercise.* Exercise dampens continuing inflammation, awakens healing factors, and spurs brain repair. It is one of the most critical ways to heal the injured brain. Wait until you are cleared by your physician, however. Beginning exercise too early after a brain injury can actually be counterproductive.

Movement activities that require learning a new movement pattern, such as tai chi, dance, or a sport such as tennis, seem to reprogram brain pathways and facilitate healing. I discussed how playing basketball helped Phillip regain cognitive function. I have repeatedly seen tai chi, qigong, and dance therapy help repair brain function. This makes sense for many reasons. Not only does learning help build new cognitive patterns, but movement also helps with fluid flow within the brain.

8. *Utilize developmental optometry.* This is a branch of optometry that uses eye exercises and different kinds of glasses to address problems in the visual pathways. Children with visual-pathway problems often then have learning difficulties that can significantly diminish with developmental optometry. Similarly, brain injury that either temporarily or permanently injures the visual pathways can often be helped with customized eye exercises or special glasses, including prism glasses.

9. *Seek help from a supportive therapist.* A supportive psychotherapist can be extremely helpful for the family unit after one of its members suffers a brain injury. Brain injury often destabilizes the patient's sense of themselves. Family dynamics can change dramatically after a brain injury. Not only are the person's functions compromised, but they also usually look totally normal, further confusing the family. Therapy can help the patient and their family members understand and manage the new reality that MTBI brings to all of their lives.

After her husband sustained a brain injury in a motor vehicle accident, one of my patients told me she cried when she watched the movie *Regarding Henry*. In the movie, Henry, played by Harrison Ford, is shot in the head. Even though her husband's injury wasn't as severe as Henry's, the movie helped her understand how her husband had changed and how much he had to struggle to perform simple tasks. Luckily, with cranial osteopathy, homeopathy, clinical medicine, and psychological support, he made seemingly unimaginable improvement.

10. *Find encouragement with a brain-injury support group.* There are numerous brain-injury support groups throughout the country that provide invaluable information and support to patients and their families. The Brain Injury Association of America and similar groups have affiliates and local chapters throughout the United States.

Given how complex the brain is, I have only touched on the major modalities that I know augment healing; more are constantly being created and discovered. Keep exploring. Every day, researchers and ordinary people alike are discovering new ways to help the brain heal itself. The exploration itself can help you heal. Don't get discouraged. I have seen hundreds of victims of brain injury astound their friends, doctors, and family with the extent of their recovery. Whether your injury is new or old, please realize that the brain has a remarkable ability to heal, given a bit of a chance. Sometimes it just needs a little help.

23

The Pathways of Pain

Most of my patients come to see me because they are in physical pain. I help many of them by addressing problems in their musculoskeletal and nervous systems. As they begin to feel better, they find it easier to believe they can recover, and they feel able to add more nutritious foods to their meals and to move in healthier ways. Chances are, however, that if you are reading this chapter, you are still in pain and need further answers. So, let me summarize some of the common causes of pain I've discussed and mention a few others.

In the previous sections of this book, I have extensively covered how injury can cause pain in a specific area and radiate to nearby areas. I've discussed how strains in one region can pull on the kinetic chain and cause distant problems, such as a fall on the sacrum leading to headaches. I've also focused on the ways injury can cause diffuse, nonspecific pain when untreated injury shock disrupts the nervous system and compromises the whole body.

More generally, chronic pain from untreated injuries, the complaint of the majority of the people who come to me in pain, is the subject of this book. I have seen far too many people identified as chronic-pain patients when the real problem is that their injury remains unresolved. Treat the injury and, most of the time, the pain disappears.

Undiagnosed structural problems can also exacerbate an injury. I covered several of these in chapter 17. They can cause local pain or can ripple their effects throughout the body. Other, more easily diagnosable structural problems like scoliosis (curvature of the spine) also tend to compromise recovery from an injury and contribute to pain on their own. Structural problems respond well to the three cornerstones of treatment I've described: addressing injury shock and inflammation and restoring motion to restricted areas.

Medical conditions such as arthritis can be precipitated by trauma as well as aggravated by it. I cover some of the most frequently missed medical conditions that cause pain in chapter 28.

Closely allied with medical conditions that cause diffuse pain are environmental irritants such as mold and heavy metals like lead and mercury, which can attack the nervous system and inflame mucous membranes, fascia, and joints. Because environmental toxins are so ubiquitous, undiagnosed reactivity to these toxins is commonplace and puts an additional burden on a body already under stress from injury. There are exciting developments in the branch of medicine devoted to improving detoxification for individuals with compromised detoxification pathways. Of course, promoting lymphatic flow is an essential element in detoxification. It helps us to remember the simple phrase: health comes from the ability to bring good things in and take bad things out.

Pain can also persist because of problems within the nervous system itself, and that's what I cover next: the nervous system's role in chronic pain.

WHAT GOES WRONG

Pain is the 911 call to the brain that the body is in danger and we must act. Like inflammation, pain's twin, pain repeatedly saves our lives and is set up to be helpful, well regulated, and self-limited. Most of our tissues have pain nerves (nociceptors) that send pain signals into the spinal cord. In the spinal cord, the nociceptor nerve meets a nerve that speeds the pain information up into the brain—for it is in the brain, not in the actual tissue, that we experience pain.

Once the pain signal reaches the base of the brain, a part of the brain known as the thalamus decides where to direct the information. Generally, the thalamus shoots the pain information to multiple sections of the brain: the motor section causes a person with a shard of glass in their foot to lift up their foot, the thinking part of the brain has them remove the glass, and the emotional centers create concern about walking barefoot. Memory gets laid down to prevent future mishaps.

Given that these pain circuits are wise and potentially self-limiting, the brain sends down a countersignal to help decrease the pain sensation inside the spinal cord. Once the glass is removed, there is less irritation on the nerve, the body begins its repair process, and, over time, pain will diminish and dissolve.

But as with inflammation, there are a number of places where this process can go wrong and create chronic pain. I am going to break this down into three components: what can increase or diminish pain in the periphery, in the spinal cord, and in the brain.

The Periphery

Pain nerves in the periphery (the outside of the body—not the organs) are known as C fibers. These lack the fatty covering known as myelin that helps speed the transmission of information in the nerve. As nerves go, these C pain fibers are rather slow, and they are very sensitive to painful stimuli like inflammatory factors, histamine, substance P, and other by-products of injury. They have a unique characteristic: the more C fibers are stimulated, the more sensitive they become and the stronger the pain sensations they evoke. That is why if you keep walking on a shard of glass, your foot hurts more and more.

Nerves for sensation are different. They are larger, myelinated nerves that can have a number of other functions. They tell us where we are in space (proprioception), or they sense touch or vibration. Because they are myelinated, their information is transmitted quickly. We probably need sensory information to reach the brain fast so we can move through the world and keep our balance.

To stop the small C fibers from transmitting pain signals, the offending object, glass, nail, or splinter must be removed. It is also critical to quickly resolve inflammation. (I discussed factors influencing inflammation in section II.)

Unfortunately, when a small C pain fiber is seriously injured or dies, another kind of nerve, a myelinated sensory nerve like the ones for touch or proprioception, can try to pinch-hit. These large sensory nerves sprout new branches to fill in for the injured C fibers. These baby fibers need two to four months to grow, and then they take over for the damaged or dead C fibers. These newly sprouted nerves often have serious identity problems: since they began their mission in life as nerves designed to report touch, they are essentially hybrids. That means when something gently brushes them, they can report that touch as excruciating pain. A slight breeze—something that sensory nerves would normally transmit to the brain as a pleasant caress—is instead read as an excruciating signal that the arm just got stabbed.

Since these nerves take a while to grow, the person might hurt a lot for a week after a trauma, then not hurt very much until months later. Suddenly, they find themselves in agony from all of those pesky pinch-hitting nerves. This may be a partial explanation for the terrible problem we call complex regional pain syndrome (CRPS), which used to be called reflex sympathetic dystrophy (RSD). Because of this tendency for sensory nerves to fill in for pain nerves, I have not found killing pain nerves by burning them (rhizotomy) to be an effective treatment for chronic pain. It may provide temporary pain relief, only to lead to much more pain months later.

Problems in the spinal cord may also account for CRPS. This appears to be linked to an overreaction of the glial cells when they sense trauma to the very nerves they are designed to protect. The glial cells can become like helicopter parents, far too active, interfering with the nerves' function to their detriment. This is an area under active investigation by numerous researchers.

I have found that treating peripheral injuries quickly with manual medicine (hopefully, within seventy-two hours) helps prevent ongoing pain problems. It appears that addressing injury shock calms peripheral nerve irritation. Restoring motion to the periphery helps promote lymphatic flow, which removes toxic debris and diminishes inflammation. Nutritional support can also significantly promote healing and prevent ongoing pain.

The Spinal Cord

In the spinal cord, some factors diminish the pain sensation, while others increase the pain or facilitate it. Ongoing, persistent pain can change the shape and chemistry of nerves in the spinal cord in such a way that the spinal cord keeps sending a pain signal to the brain long after the peripheral injury has healed; in essence, a habit of pain is created. Because of this potentially disastrous scenario, once an injury has caught the body's attention, it is crucial to quickly quiet pain.

The nervous system has developed a number of ways to modulate the pain signal and keep it from becoming a pain habit. First, the large sensation fibers that have myelin coverings and the small pain fibers that have no myelin enter the spinal cord close to one another. Information from the large sensation fibers tends to be much bossier than that of the small pain fibers, generally demanding that the spinal cord pay attention to them first. That's why, if you rub your toe after stubbing it, you feel the rubbing more than the pain. This is thought to be the reason that when a vibrating transcutaneous electrical nerve stimulation (TENS) unit is placed in a region where peripheral pain arises and stimulates the myelinated fibers, the vibrations can often override the pain sensation.

The ability of the large sensation nerves to counteract the signal from the pain nerves is one of the many reasons we want to keep our myelin nerve coatings healthy and happy with nutritious oils. If we consume trans fats and toxic oils, we tend to compromise those membranes; the medical literature convinces me that consuming those toxic substances increases pain.

Second, neurons called interneurons also dock where the pain and sensation fibers dock. Interneurons are intermediary nerves that link to other nerves and can either increase or decrease the transmission of information. Lots of them exist in the spinal cord and the brain. Many of these interneurons are inhibitory; they sing reassuring lullabies to the overexcited pain nerves to keep them modulated. The central nervous system (the spine and the brain together) actually has ten times more inhibitory neurons (IN) than stimulating ones. Unfortunately, IN are far more delicate and therefore more easily injured than other nerves, so any injury that traumatizes the spinal cord and/or the brain is more likely to damage INs and increase the amount of pain someone suffers.

Trauma to the spinal cord can also cause pain originating there to be read by the brain as pain in the back or neck, depending on which part of the spinal cord got injured. Spinal cord injury can also create a pain pattern that expands up or down eight segments. Someone can injure their lower spinal cord when they are twenty years old and appear to have healed. Then, ten years later, a blow to their middle spine can not only create thoracic pain but also reawaken the hibernating lumbar pain. The new injury tends to resolve fairly quickly, but the old pain will generally take a lot longer to resolve.

I believe that unresolved injury shock has a hand in the nervous system's difficulty in fully healing from both spinal cord and brain injury. I suspect that by treating injury shock quickly, we help prevent pain memories from being laid down in the spinal cord and the brain. Treatment is still possible later; it just takes longer to break up the pain pathway. I generally have to use a combination of homeopathy and osteopathy; sometimes, I recommend people receive acupuncture treatment as well.

The spinal cord is not left alone to suffer. Along with inhibitory neurons to help diminish pain, it has receptors for the body's natural painkillers—endorphins and endocannabinoids—that the central nervous system sends down to help quiet pain. Opiates like morphine or opium are relatives of these naturally occurring narcotic compounds. Marijuana acts on the endocannabinoid receptors, and one recent study seems to indicate that osteopathic manual medicine helps relieve pain through the endocannabinoid receptors.

The Brain

Pain lives in the brain. The brain is also mission control for pain signals. Lonnie K. Zelter, MD, in her book *Conquering Your Child's Chronic Pain*, compares the pain signal to the volume control on a television set that can be turned up or down. A lot of pain-volume control occurs in the brain. We don't understand all the ways the brain manages this, but here is some of what we do understand:

Hormones play a large role in the volume of the pain signal. The pituitary gland provides and/or regulates most of the hormones in the body. Progesterone and cortisol are both known to decrease pain, so problems with the pituitary can certainly affect pain levels. I talked about the pituitary in both the sexual-healing and brain-injury chapters. Hormonal changes after menopause may account for the onset of migraines that some women experience.

The limbic system. The thalamus feeds into the brain's limbic system, which resembles the shell of an egg around the thalamus and the corpus callosum. The limbic system is responsible for processing positive and negative emotions and modulating their intensity. A critical part of the limbic system, the amygdala, lives toward the tips of the temporal lobes. This region of the temporal lobe, as you saw previously, is especially vulnerable to damage during rotational head injury. Sensory information for various pleasant and unpleasant emotional states feeds into the amygdala. (Learned fear is believed to be stored in the amygdala.)

It is well known that fear and anxiety can increase the intensity of pain sensations, whereas joy and pleasure can decrease suffering. Clearly, the amygdala–limbic system, which remembers and experiences pleasure and pain, plays a critical role in the amount of pain we experience. Research has shown that trauma and PTSD can inhibit the calming components of the nervous system and increase sympathetic outflow. PTSD is also believed to activate the amygdala–limbic system in such a way as to increase pain.

I have noticed that when areas containing the limbic system, like the temporal lobe, have been twisted by dural or bony distortions, people tend to be more fearful and anxious and to experience more pain. As I remove those dural and bony strains and take pressure off areas of the limbic system, their fear, anxiety, and pain tend to diminish. I therefore speculate that resolving dural strains that compromise the temporal lobes can help quiet amygdala excitation.

Cerebral spinal fluid. The periaqueductal grey matter is a part of the brain that surrounds two ponds of cerebral spinal fluid (CSF) in the brain (the third and fourth ventricles), as well as the cerebral aqueduct that connects them. In the brain-injury chapters, I discussed how the CSF flow provides needed nutrients to the brain and helps remove toxic debris. The CSF's ability to remove inflammatory debris may explain its apparent function in quieting pain. According to the Nobel prize–winning physician Eric Kandel, MD, stimulation of the periaqueductal grey region helps suppress pain. Since the area is uniquely situated around major ponds of CSF channels, I suspect that this region of the brain secretes substances into the CSF that inhibit pain. These circulate through the brain and then down into the spinal cord. Cranial osteopathy has long focused on a number of techniques to help promote CSF flow. These techniques, such as the compression of the fourth ventricle (CV4), are known to decrease inflammation in the body as well as to help calm the nervous system and decrease pain.

THE TREATMENT OF PAIN

Throughout this book, I have reviewed numerous ways to address injury shock, inflammation, and restricted motion to restore function and decrease or eliminate pain. I have encouraged movement, breathing exercises, sufficient sleep and rest, and finding pleasure. In the next section, I discuss how to take charge of your healing journey; all that I cover and will cover addresses pain and healing. Here, I want to mention once more several modalities that have a proven track record to reduce pain and are available to everyone:

Meditation. In 1982, Jon Kabat-Zinn, PhD, trained chronic-pain patients who had not been helped by traditional medicine in Mindfulness-Based Stress Reduction (MBSR). All of the enrolled patients complained of chronic pain lasting six months to forty-eight years. After being trained in and practicing mindfulness meditation, 88 percent perceived a decrease of pain of at least 50 percent. Patients reported significantly greater pain reduction with MBSR than they had achieved with morphine or other drugs. Brain scans showed that after practicing MBSR, they had quieted the regions in the brain usually associated with processing pain. Mindfulness meditation gently focuses on a detached observation of self while we are engaged in a practice such as following our breathing. MBSR trains people to use this detached observational state when physical and mental stressors arise. I suspect that other forms of meditation can also be very powerful. Mindfulness meditation has become successful not only because it is so effective but also because it is relatively easy to learn.

Creative visualization is a form of self-hypnosis similar to mindfulness meditation. It, too, helps patients diminish pain. In some instances, it helps patients address the pathology causing their pain. Both meditation and visualization also combat the destructive helplessness that chronic pain patients feel.

Acupuncture has been shown in studies to be able to decrease pain. I have seen it be quite effective in helping a number of my patients who are in pain due to trauma or to various medical conditions.

Homeopathy. I have repeatedly seen homeopathy significantly diminish pain. When my patients have used it after surgery, their surgeons have been surprised both by how little pain medication the patient needed and how quickly they recovered.

I found homeopathy invaluable when my mother was dying of cancer that had invaded her spine and her hip. Cancer in the bone tends to create terrible pain that morphine usually cannot completely control. My mother had watched her father die in agony from the same problem. I was determined to make sure that was not her fate.

I used some gentle osteopathy to help calm the irritability in her nervous system and decrease her pain. What I did was similar to the technique I use to treat injury shock. Despite the morphine and the osteopathy, however, she still had pain, so I gave her *Symphytum officinalis* (homeopathic comfrey), which wiped away all the remaining bone pain and kept her comfortable; it worked like a miracle. My mother took *Symphytum* twice a day during the last week of her life. I still miss my mom five years later. But I am glad I provided her comfort and some peace as she passed from the world. Having all her beloved children around her was also an essential aspect of her peaceful passage.

Most of us fear pain. My experiences have taught me that the body is wise and has countless ways to help us heal and diminish or eliminate pain. And when our body can't turn down the volume on its own, adding some powerful modalities like osteopathy, homeopathy, acupuncture, and meditation can often give our body the very assistance it needs.

V.

Participate in Your Healing Journey

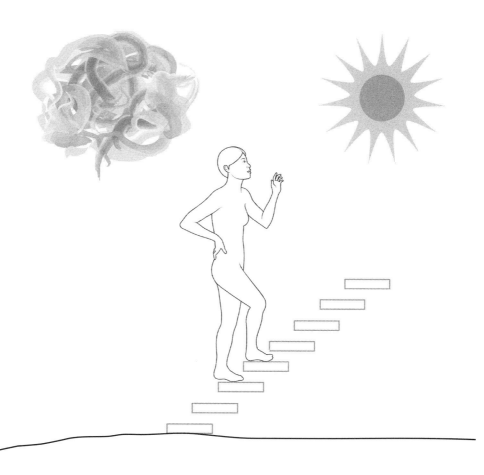

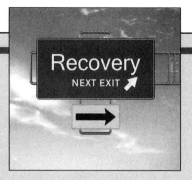

Rules of the Healing Marathon

1. Take three minutes a day to heal
2. Accept—and adapt
3. Set a goal
4. Chart your progress
5. Be consistent
6. Be patient
7. Listen to your body
8. Create joy
9. Embrace connection
10. Practice gratitude
11. Believe!

24

The Healing Marathon

*"To accomplish great things we must not only act, but
also dream, not only plan, but also believe."*
—Anatole France

In my thirty years of practice, I've discovered a magic pill that will help you
heal: your commitment to your own healing. So please read this chapter—
it's the most important in this book.

Healing from an injury can be like training for the marathon. It requires
patience and persistence, is often dull, and rarely produces instant results.

Your intention to heal is the most powerful healing force in the universe. It creates, supports, and lifts up your entire healing journey. The more
you repeat your intention, the more you will see what will help you and
the more you will act on it. Energy and action follow intent to an amazing
degree. The power of your intention to heal will change the trajectory of
your healing journey.

Whether your injuries are minor or major, *your chances for recovery
are vastly improved if you participate in the process.* To help you along, here
are my rules of the journey:

1 Take Three Minutes a Day to Heal

"A good intention clothes itself with sudden power." —Emerson

Before you even get up in the morning, give yourself three minutes to heal. Give yourself the tools to change the trajectory of your day.

Express to yourself your intention to get well.

As you prepare for the day, focus on three things you are grateful for in your life. Practicing gratitude is a powerful antidote to the feelings of helplessness and despair that can overwhelm us in the face of prolonged suffering.

Decide on one simple and readily achievable thing you will do today to aid your journey to health: stretching during the day. Taking a walk at noon. Connecting with a friend or family member.

Call forth the feelings you want to feel again: the joy of moving freely without pain, the elation of running or walking or thinking clearly again, the satisfaction of being able to work a full day with energy and focus. Experience and luxuriate in those feelings. They are a powerful motivator when things get hard.

2 Accept—and Adapt

"Adapt or die." —anonymous

Be flexible—do what works to help you heal.

The patients who make the most dramatic recoveries are the ones who can change their behavior on a dime. Because of their strong commitment to getting well, they are willing to accept that their injury has changed their lives, and they act accordingly to achieve their goals. They assess the situation as it is, not as they wish it were. If I tell them to stay home for three days, they stay home. If they can't take time off work, they look for ways to lighten their load. They ask a friend to make dinner. They renegotiate family duties to accommodate their new situation. They heal much faster and more completely.

Most people will not readjust their lives for the few weeks needed after an injury. They refuse to accept the reality of their injury and often won't rest even for a day. They muscle through and pay with months of pain. If only they had quickly changed course after an accident and rested, they might have had a relatively brief period of pain and an uneventful recovery.

Adaptability also means you may have to try out new healing modalities and open your mind to new possibilities. When I became very ill again with asthma in my twenties, my roommate told me of an acupuncturist who cured a friend of asthma. Though I was very skeptical of such a foreign and peculiar concept, I forced myself to go. After four treatments, I had no more asthma for many years. That experience opened my mind to other possibilities in medicine and helped pave my way to finding osteopathic medicine.

If some modality isn't working for you, move on. Try something else. Adapt.

3 Set a Goal

"When a man does not know what harbor he is making for, no wind is the right wind." —Lucius Annaeus Seneca

Setting a specific goal is even better than intention alone. Where do you want to be in three months? Thirty days? Tomorrow? Setting a goal—like decreasing your shoulder pain or getting more help at home—is the first step in your recovery. Choose something achievable. Take small steps at first and then congratulate yourself for having done what you've chosen. Remember that healing is not a sprint. No matter how modest the steps you choose, success breeds success.

Make a simple plan to achieve your goal. It's like drawing a map to getting well. Let's say you choose a five-minute stretching routine for your shoulder or asking your partner to do the grocery shopping. Whatever you choose, add *rest* and good nutrition to your list, because these are two of the most healing things you can do.

Buy a notebook. Write down your goal. Write down your plan. Then do it!

4 Chart Your Progress

"The palest ink is better than the best memory." —*Chinese proverb*

I once took a detailed history from a patient who came in with multiple problems. She was depressed, angry, fatigued, and unable to sleep, with back pain on a scale of seven out of ten. When she returned a month later, she gloomily told me she was not any better. So I read to her from the history I had taken. She was no longer angry or tired, her sleep had improved, and her pain was about a three. She was shocked. She sheepishly admitted she had blocked out how bad she had been. Once she realized how much better she had gotten, she became even more committed to her healing and eventually became completely well.

It's human nature: we forget how bad things were. Unfortunately, if you don't remember how bad your health was, you'll never appreciate how much progress you've made. You might get discouraged and quit just when your health is really improving. I see this every day. Keep track of improvements and setbacks in your notebook and use that information to tweak your plans.

When you write down what makes you feel better or worse, a fascinating thing happens. You will notice facts you've overlooked. You might realize that certain shoes cause your back to hurt, or that certain foods give you headaches. You might notice you crash every afternoon and that a twenty minute nap makes all the difference. Also be sure as well to write down what makes you *better*. You definitely want to keep track of that!

5 Be Consistent

"This one thing—choosing a goal and sticking to it—changes everything." —*Scott Reed*

"Victory belongs to the most persevering." —*Napoleon Bonaparte*

The ones who get better and stay better are the most consistent ones—the ones who regularly and faithfully do their program. The more consistent in your practice you are, the more your body will trust you, the more information your body will tell you, and the faster you will heal.

6 Be Patient

"How poor are they that have not patience! What wound did ever heal but by degrees?" —William Shakespeare

"Be not afraid of growing slowly; be afraid only of standing still." —Chinese proverb

No matter how deeply you want your body to hurry up and get better, healing takes time. Healing rarely goes in a straight line—it goes up and down. Healing often comes in big, sudden leaps after what seems like weeks of no improvement. Pushing yourself too hard or too fast is usually counterproductive.

Don't give up! Keep your eye on your goal: to play tennis again, ride up the mountain again, enjoy a supercharged brain again. When you get discouraged, remember how you want to feel when you are well. A few small steps every day will add up to big changes in a week or month.

7 Listen to Your Body

"There is more wisdom in your body than in your deepest philosophy." —Friedrich Nietzsche

I love to treat dancers, athletes, and people trained in yoga and the martial arts. These people usually have tremendous body awareness and a strong determination to recover. Not only are they highly attuned to what helps (or hurts) them, they are also focused and determined and they follow their body's clear instructions.

Your body is extremely smart. Even if you aren't an athlete, stop and listen! Once you start listening to your body, it will tell you lots of crucial things to help you get better. It may tell you to get up and stretch every hour, or that sitting in a certain chair makes your shoulder feel worse. It may tell you to take a nap, or that it's time to try something new and different. The more you do the things your body communicates to you it needs, the more clearly your body will talk to you and the faster you'll recover.

8 Create Joy

"Success is not the key to happiness; happiness is the key to success."
—Albert Schweitzer

Be creative. Create joy for yourself. Give your imagination free play to create a world where you can fly, swim, sing, and do the things you crave. In my early forties, when I was seriously ill, I felt great joy watching my children play on the jungle gym—or just enjoy the pancakes I made them. Sometimes we can luxuriate in other people's joy.

Since the brain and its wiring are critical factors in survival and recovery, nourish the brain with music, poetry, dance, computer games or mathematical puzzles, playing cards, or reading. Joy for you may be sitting by a waterfall, having a delicious meal, going to a museum, or taking a soothing bath. Learn to cherish your own pleasure. Luxuriate in sensual pleasures, including making love. Do whatever gives you joy. Never underestimate the crucial role of the happy brain in survival and recovery.

9 Embrace Connection

"All things are bound together. All things connect." —*Chief Seattle*

Injury or illness can be devastating to even the strongest person. Injury can destroy our sense of self, steal control of our lives, and take everything we thought we knew about ourselves and turn it upside down. Injury can make us selfish and isolated as we desperately try to reassert control over our lives. One of the curses of ill health is its tendency to tear away our connection to loved ones. Just at the time we need to reach out the most, injury can make us a stranger to even our closest friends.

Connection can come with family or friends. It may express itself by helping a stranger at a soup kitchen. It might come from walking in nature or through a spiritual practice. Embrace connection; it defeats the loneliness and isolation of illness by joining us with something greater than ourselves and reminding us that we matter.

10 Practice Gratitude

"Survivors take great joy from even their smallest success."
—Laurence Gonzales, from his book Deep Survival: Who Lives,
Who Dies, and Why

Gratitude really is the path to salvation.

When I started learning my craft forty years ago from two magnificent, wise osteopathic physicians, Howard and Rebecca Lippincott, they repeatedly emphasized the importance of gratitude. As I grew and developed, I came increasingly to understand why: gratitude creates an easing of the soul. It pulls you away from depression and despair.

Be grateful every day for being alive, for the parts of you that still work. Even if your legs can't dance yet, your hands can bathe and dance in warm water. If your brain feels muddled in the afternoon, feel grateful that you were able to plant your garden the way you wanted to in the morning. Celebrate each success. Only allow friends around who cheer you on.

11 Believe!

"Turn your face to the sun and the shadows fall behind you."
—Maori proverb

If you act like the tasks you've undertaken will help you, your belief will follow. If you act like you matter enough to make the effort, you will matter more to yourself. When you want something badly enough, you will do what you need to in order to get it. A friend of mine loved basketball so much, she shoveled snow off a basketball court in the dead of winter so she could practice her jump shot. Where there is a will, there is a way.

If you have an injured back, don't just say, "Oh, but it's my son's Little League game—two hours on those hard metal bleachers couldn't hurt me." Find another way. Have someone else carry a supportive chair in for you and set it up. What heals you must guide you and the choices you make.

Anything that takes practice means you'll make mistakes. Mistakes are fine. Learn from them. Never use your failures as another way to beat yourself up. Self-reproach slows down recovery. Move forward.

Isn't it awful that just when you least feel like doing anything hard, you must add mountains of inner strength to your core? Lock self-reproach away in a deep, dark prison. Like an athlete training for the Olympics, suck it up! Move beyond the humiliation you may feel asking someone to carry your clothes to the self-service laundry, or asking your assistant to carry your briefcase. There will be moments when you feel foolish as you heal. It comes with the territory. Who says life grants victors elegance? Keep your eye on the goal. You will find that the people who truly care about you are happy to lend a hand.

Praise yourself for each small success. Since this journey can be so difficult, you must acknowledge your triumphs. They may feel small, but they are *huge*. It takes great courage to heal.

Believe, because the bad times always come along with the good. Be persistent in the pursuit of your goal. Let moments of grace warm you. And know that all along, your body is your greatest ally, working with you and rewarding your success.

> *"Your own resolution to succeed is more important than any other one thing."* —Abraham Lincoln

25

Landmarks of Recovery

You would think that people would know when they are getting better, yet often they don't. Healing takes time, and in this fast-paced world, people tend be very impatient and forget how much they've suffered. This blindness to past pain led one theologian to claim that our erasing of memory is proof of God's grace and therefore of God's existence.

While I don't believe our forgetting of pain proves that God exists, I do believe it's a blessing. Unfortunately, this gracious dissolving of memory makes it harder for us to realize when we are getting better. That's why the following conversation with a patient is so typical.

SASHA was a thirty-eight-year-old mother of two who had fallen down the stairs two months ago while carrying a laundry basket. On her fifth visit, I asked her how she was doing.

Sasha: "I'm no better. I'm actually getting worse. My neck still hurts a lot."

Me: "How about your headaches?"

Sasha: "I don't have any headaches."

Me: "How is your sleep?"

Sasha: "I sleep fine. But when I wake up in the morning, my neck hurts."

Me: "What number would you put the pain at?"

Sasha: "A four."

Me: "And irritability?"

Sasha: "Was I irritable?"

Me: "Yes, when you first came in, you were yelling at your kids. You had trouble falling asleep. You woke up every two hours in pain. You had a constant headache, and you put your pain at an eight. You are a lot better."

Sasha: "But I want my neck pain gone."

Me: "It takes time."

Sasha: "I guess I am better."

It was hard for Sasha to discern improvement because she was still in pain. Yet pain, by itself, is usually a poor guideline for improvement. Sleep, energy level, emotional well-being, and digestive function are usually much more accurate indicators of progress. I call these the SEED guides for recovery.

SEEDS OF RECOVERY: Sleep, Energy, Emotions, Digestion

I look at sleep, energy, and emotion as indicators of a positive healing trajectory because they reflect the state of our neurological function. Digestive health is also a critical landmark in the complex process of healing.

Sleep. Injury shock can profoundly affect sleep patterns. Initially, most people are agitated and unable to sustain deep, prolonged sleep. They often fall asleep for an hour or two, then dream they've been tossed off a cliff or sustained some other terrible insult. They wake with a start, heart pounding.

This may reflect the nervous system's need to discharge the trauma through bad dreams, but that should only be temporary. Persistent nightmares tend to be a symptom of lingering injury shock. Injury shock can also have the opposite effect, as it can exhaust the nervous system. The patient sleeps too much and still wakes up exhausted. However, as the nervous system and the patient heals, sleep should improve. They sleep more deeply and for more restful periods. Sleep feels like a balm. People need a lot of sleep after a trauma, often ten to twelve hours a night. Embrace sleep after an injury. It's the greatest healer of all.

Energy. With the surge of adrenaline and cortisol that accompanies injury, patients often feel like Superman on speed. This dangerous energy helps them flee from danger despite broken bones. However, the constant bath of stress hormones eventually results in fatigue, insomnia, anxiety, depression, and slow healing. Extreme fatigue is also a very common problem after brain injury.

As the nervous system heals and digestion and sleep improve, healthy, balanced energy will gradually develop. At first, the patient may only be alert for three hours, then perhaps for five, gradually working their way back to handling a normal day. Remember, all healing goes up and down somewhat—two steps forward, then one step back. But as the patient heals, their energy and ability to cope with life will gradually improve. Improving, balanced energy is always a good sign of progress in healing.

Emotions. Mood and energy are intimately related to the health of the digestive and nervous systems. Stress hormones can interfere with mood-enhancing neurotransmitters in the brain, the chemicals we depend on for feeling happy. They also interfere with digestion, and poor digestion negatively affects brain chemistry, making us feel cranky and exhausted. As the nervous system heals, the parasympathetic nervous system wakes up and digestion improves. As digestion improves, so will mood. Improving mood is a good indicator that the nervous system and the gut are healing.

Digestion. Digestive function reflects the health of many areas of the body, from the brain to the nervous system. Like neurological improvement, gastrointestinal improvement reflects improving health and propels the body toward it. Proper GI function depends on a fully pumping diaphragm and a well-positioned and correctly moving sacrum, reflecting balance in the autonomic nervous system. The health of all of these systems is mirrored in the health of the gut. As the gut improves, general healing profoundly accelerates. The body is able to absorb nutrients and eliminate toxins. As toxins are eliminated, mood will improve, and so will sleep. Bowel movements will become fuller, better formed, and easier to produce, and not painful to eliminate.

All the components in SEED are interrelated, affecting each other and generally improving together. Each aspect of SEED may have its own trajectory, but as a patient reaches optimal healing, these critical indicators of health tend to cross the finish line together, holding hands.

THE BODY HEALS IN A LOGICAL MANNER

It will also help you understand your progress and be more patient with your healing knowing that the body tends to heal in a logical manner. The body wisely focuses its initial healing energy on mending the most life-sustaining functions and the most essential organs. That's why the heart and brain tend to heal first. Serious injuries tend to heal before less important ones.

Understanding these tendencies, early homeopathic physicians elucidated what they called laws of cure that reflect our body's inherent healing wisdom. These laws of cure follow a more consistent pattern when the body is coping with disease rather than with trauma, but even after trauma's more chaotic attack on the body, these laws remain helpful guidelines. Like most rules, they are never absolute:

The Laws of Cure

- *The body heals the most important organs first, less important tissues later.* The brain, nervous system, and heart will heal before a pulled muscle in the groin.

- *The body heals the most serious injuries first, less important last.* A puncture in the lung heals before a sprained ankle.

- *The body heals from the inside out.* Brain, cardiac, and digestive function will generally improve before a surface skin rash improves.

- *The body heals more recent injuries before chronic ones.*

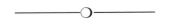

TONY couldn't understand why I was thrilled that he was sleeping for so long every night and his fingers were numb after a major car crash. Tony's case demonstrates how these guidelines can help me evaluate a patient's progress toward recovery.

Tony came to see me eight weeks after his Camry was broadsided by a pickup truck that ran a red light. The force whipsawed him around, throwing his head against the window before his car hit a pole and his airbag went off. He suffered second-degree burns on his forearms from the airbag.

For a few days after the accident, Tony didn't feel much pain. Then everything fell apart. His head and his ribs ached. He had searing pain down his left arm. He was exhausted. He couldn't think clearly. He had severe headaches—a level nine out of ten. He could sleep for only two hours before waking up. Only after I asked about his digestion did he admit to painful constipation. MRIs showed no evidence of a brain injury but revealed a mild disc protrusion in the lower part of his neck. I'm going to talk not about how I treated Tony, but about how I evaluated his progress toward recovery.

Tony's exhaustion, headaches, insomnia, and inability to focus were evidence of a mild traumatic brain injury (MTBI), probably sustained when his head struck the car window. The brain injury was his most serious medical problem. His constipation was my second concern, partly because it indicated

314

continuing problems with his nervous system and partly because his inability to eliminate toxins effectively compromised his healing. Next was the discrete cervical (neck) injury, which caused the weakness and pain in his left arm. Last were his burns, which, though painful, were not life threatening.

What did I want to see improve first? Tony's sleep. Sleep is a profound indication of nervous system health and essential for all healing.

At his third appointment, Tony came back irritated. "My arm is killing me," he said.

"Of course," I said sympathetically. Then I asked, "How's your sleep?"

"Terrible. I sleep for ten hours a night."

"Great! When you first came in, you could hardly sleep at all because your brain was too injured. Being able to sleep is major progress." The most critical injury—the brain injury—was healing first. Then I asked, "How's your gut?"

"Not perfect, but it's better."

Tony's improved gut function was the second thing I wanted to see get better. Happier bowel function indicated that his overactive sympathetic nervous system (SNS) was calming down and his nutritive parasympathetic nervous system (PNS), which controls digestion, had become much more active. As his gut healed, his bowels could more effectively eliminate the toxins that had been inflaming his mood and his intestines better absorb healing nutrients. Tony's most important organs—his brain, nervous system, and gut—were healing first.

"How's your arm?" I asked him.

"It's not so weak, but now my fingers feel pretty numb," he responded.

"Good," I said. "That means some of the pressure on the nerves to the arm has gone away. As your nerves continue to recover, the numbness should go away, too. Chances are you'll also have more pain for a while, then that should go away." As nerves heal, the pain generally leaves the extremities and returns to the original source, which in Tony's case was his neck. But I did not necessarily look to complete resolution of the disc injury until it could receive better nutrition and fuller neurological input from the healing gut and nervous system.

As Tony's sleep and digestion continued to get better, he began to feel less discouraged and more hopeful that he could recover. Tony's more positive attitude, including his belief that he could get better, reflected improvements in digestive and brain health. As the digestive system functions better, it can better eliminate toxins that poison the brain and affect emotions and mood.

What about the burns on Tony's arms? Given his other serious pathology, the burns were slow to heal and left some scars on his arms. This, too, followed the laws of cure. Although extensive burns certainly can be life threatening, when not seriously injured, the skin is often the slowest to heal. The body needs to focus its healing powers on the more essential organs—in this case, the nervous system and the gut.

If you are impatient with your recovery, remember the SEEDS of recovery and the laws of cure. During this difficult journey, watch for these guideposts so you will know when you are on your way back to health.

26

Sleep: The Greatest Healer

Put sleep on a pedestal and bow down before it. To truly heal, you must get enough sleep. Sleep may have more power to heal you than all the medications and expensive specialists you see after an injury. It is the greatest healer of all.

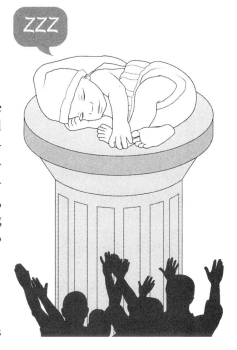

Sleep replenishes energy, boosts the immune system, rests the brain, improves memory, and decreases pain. Neurotransmitters and hormones critical to repairing injured tissues, particularly brain tissue, are released in great quantities during sleep. Sleep improves longevity, increases mental acuity, and enhances learning and creativity. Most healthy people need eight to nine hours of sleep a night. If you are injured, especially brain injured, you need a lot more.

Lack of sleep increases pain. It coaxes the sympathetic nervous system into overdrive and elevates levels of the stress hormone cortisol as well as interfering with the production of key hormones that regulate the repair of injured tissues. It impairs memory and learning and increases inflammation. It affects the body's ability to metabolize glucose and can lead to symptoms that look like diabetes. Lack of sleep has been linked to shortened life span, impaired cognitive function, mood disorders, and heart disease. It alters the level of hormones affecting hunger and weight gain and

A Soliloquy on Naps

Naps are very healing. You may need a twenty-minute or a two-hour nap every afternoon. Studies show that if you don't do it too late in the day, napping doesn't interfere with nighttime sleep. During World War II, sixty-six-year-old Winston Churchill stayed up until 2 a.m. and took four-hour afternoon naps. While I don't recommend such a late bedtime, naps can be especially critical in times of stress.

increases your appetite for junk food. People who don't rest enough are generally thirty-five pounds heavier than the people who sleep enough and well. You cannot heal without sleep.

Sleep problems after trauma are very common. Pain can disturb your sleep or force you to sleep in a position you hate. Pain medications can interfere with sleep. Brain injury, including mild traumatic brain injury, causes significant sleep disturbances. You may be too agitated to fall into restful sleep if your fight-or-flight sympathetic nervous system (SNS) is still on high alert.

Don't panic if you have sleeping problems after an injury. A few changes in habits, some basic supplements, relaxing sound technology, and a few restorative poses may give you all the help you need to return to deep, restful sleep without the need for drugs. Even if your clumsy and sleep-deprived brain has trouble figuring out what to do, this chapter will tell you many ways to improve your sleep.

A good night's sleep begins as soon as you wake up in the morning. Exposure to natural light, exercise, good food, and nutritional supplements can have a powerful influence on the quality of your sleep. In the evening, most people will at some point feel a wave of fatigue, which I call the sleep wave. Learn to catch the wave, and you are much more likely to have restful sleep. This chapter will give you lots of suggestions on how to do that.

FIVE STEPS TO IMPROVING YOUR SLEEP

1 Establish Healthy Sleep Routines

Your body likes a regular bedtime routine. You will relax more easily into sleep if you have one:

- Pick a regular bedtime and be faithful to it.
- Budget eight hours for sleep after an injury. If you sustained a brain injury, you will need much more.
- Forty-five minutes to one hour before your bedtime, stop doing things that rev you up. Get your must-do list done well before your bedtime—brush

your teeth, organize tomorrow's stuff, wash the dishes—so you can catch the sleep wave.

- The closer you are to bedtime, the smaller and lighter your meals should be. Big meals consumed too close to bedtime, particularly ones high in fat and complex protein, can interfere with sleep.

- Avoid foods and drinks that interfere with sleep. Alcohol may make you sleepy, but it does not foster restful sleep. Avoid it right before bedtime. If you're jittery at bedtime, maybe you are drinking coffee or tea too late in the day. Move that last cup of caffeine earlier in the day, or eliminate it. Take a brief reviving nap in the afternoon instead.

- Foods high in sleep-inducing tryptophan (bananas, milk, and turkey when eaten with carbohydrates) can make you drowsy and make good bedtime snacks. Foods that provide magnesium also help with sleep. These include cheese, almonds, and bananas. Cherries are one of the few natural sources of melatonin, and any source of calcium will help regulate the production of sleep-promoting melatonin.

- Do what relaxes you. Play sudoku. Take a warm bath with Epsom salt or essential oils. Meditate. Do yoga. Read. That's what I do every night in bed before I sleep. Some purists say no reading in bed, but as long as you are not having neck or other problems that make it difficult to read in bed without pain, I think reading in bed is great. Learn what kind of reading suits you. Reading thrillers before bed may not be the most relaxing.

2 Create a Comfortable Sleep Environment

- Make sure your bedroom temperature is comfortable for you, and you have the right blankets for your nature. I like a cold room and lots of blankets weighing down on me.

- Sleep in complete darkness. The absence of light is one of the most powerful triggers for the brain to initiate sleep. Even the light from a clock radio can influence our internal clock through specialized cells in the retina of our eyes that tell the brain it's daytime. This can disrupt

Snooze Foods
Bananas
Milk
Almonds
Cherries
Turkey and crackers

Insomniac Foods
Alcohol
Caffeine
Nicotine
Foods high in fat
Complex protein

the pineal gland's circadian rhythm and interfere with sleep. If you can't block light with shades or curtains, consider a sleep mask. Numerous patients have told me sleep masks really helped them regain deep, healing sleep.

- Noise disrupts restful sleep. If you live in a noisy environment, a white-noise generator, a fan, or an air purifier can provide a constant, low level of sound that effectively drown out most unwanted noise.

- Sound can powerfully alter brain waves and promote sleep. When I take my daily nap, I put on my headphones and play the meditative Holosync wave technology (www.centerpointe.com), which seems to relax my nervous system. Several of my patients also report good results using this technology. Other well-regarded sound technologies include the Insight CD of the Immrama Institute (www.immramainstitute.com) and the sound technologies based on the work of Joshua Leeds, author of *The Power of Sound* (www.sound-remedies.com).

3 Exercise During the Day

Exercise has both sleep-inducing and sleep-impairing properties. Moving and exercising during the day will help you sleep. A walk in the morning that exposes you to natural light can dramatically improve your sleep by resetting your body's sleep-wake cycle. Try it for ten minutes the next few days and see if it improves your sleep.

Vigorous exercise too late in the evening, on the other hand, is very stimulating to the body and may interfere with sleep. You have to know how exercise affects you and adapt accordingly.

4 Decrease Pain by Having Proper Support

Your mattress should be comfortable. Men tend to prefer harder beds. Because of our hips and butts, women usually need softer beds. Either way, your bed must offer good support. If your bed suddenly feels too soft, I recommend putting a piece of exterior-grade plywood (it has fewer toxins than interior grade) between the mattress and the box spring to make it firmer.

I generally don't recommend that my injured patients purchase a new mattress. Many people find their immune systems much more vulnerable after an injury, and new mattresses can be a virtual font of toxic chemicals. At all times, avoid new mattresses with flame-retardant toxins. Some mattress manufacturers, including McRoskey Mattress Company and European Sleep Works, avoid using them, and more chemical-free mattresses are becoming available.

It's often very hard to get comfortable after an injury, so here is some advice on how to lessen the strain on your injured parts.

Most spinal injuries require you to lie on your back. You can make that position more comfortable by putting a pillow or wedge under your knees and a small towel under each elbow to take the weight of the arms off the shoulders and neck. When lying on their backs, most people need a small pillow under their head and maybe some support under their necks. A small rolled towel or washcloth will work.

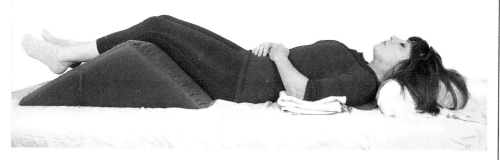

If you sleep on your side, put one or two pillows between your knees, which will take strain off your pelvis. Under your head, put a higher pillow than you would normally use when sleeping on your back so your neck stays level. Try propping up your upper arm with a pillow, or rest it on a body pillow.

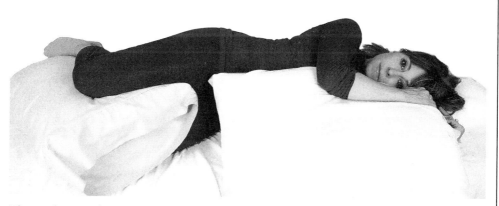

Please do not sleep on your stomach after an injury, as that can strain the neck.

5 Calm the Nervous System with Restorative Practices

Now that you are going to bed at a semiregular time, have taken a daytime walk, have cut out your afternoon caffeine, have relaxed in a nice warm bath, and have a good book to read in a comfortable, dark, and quiet room, you are ready to sleep! What do you do if the sleep wave still won't cooperate? Use the resources in chapter 7 and the companion DVD to calm and rebalance your agitated nervous system. The breathing practices and restorative poses are designed for just that purpose and are extremely powerful tools in helping you fall asleep. Pick one or two that you like and use them when you need that extra boost. A ten-minute meditation practice, closing the eyes and focusing on your breathing, can work wonders for calming the mind and body.

SUPPLEMENTS THAT HELP YOU SLEEP

When you lack critical amino acids and minerals, your body can have trouble dropping into sleep. You become like a hungry predator desperately searching for what's missing. Here I list some key nutritive components critical for sleep. While it is always preferable to get these nutrients from food, sometimes we need some extra help. Like any sleep aid, these supplements—particularly the amino acids and hormones—are meant for acute episodes of insomnia rather than for ongoing, chronic sleep problems. If you are taking antidepressants, always check with your physician first before adding any of them to your sleep regimen:

Your constitutional homeopathic remedy in a low dose (9C–12C) before bed often helps sleep. For those not on a constitutional remedy, a homeopathic combination remedy for sleep, such as Hyland's Insomnia, can be helpful.

Vitamin B complex is critical for brain, nerve, and adrenal function. Vitamin B3 has been shown to increase REM sleep and increase the effectiveness of tryptophan, a precursor to the manufacture of melatonin. Melatonin is the master hormone that regulates our circadian rhythms and controls the many hormones involved in sleeping and waking. Vitamin B6 is essential for production of serotonin, which calms the body before sleep. B5 deficiency has been linked to sleep disturbance, and folic acid deficiency to insomnia. Because it can be a stimulant, take a vitamin B complex in the morning. The supplement should have at least 50 mg of B5, B6, and niacinamide (or niacin), and 100 mg of inositol.

Vitamin D helps regulate the pineal gland's secretion of melatonin. Recent studies also suggest that vitamin D acts directly on areas of the brain involved in sleep. Though vitamin D is manufactured naturally by the skin after exposure

Supplements for Sleep

	WHAT IT DOES	WHEN TO TAKE	TYPICAL DOSE	COMMENTS
Vitamin B complex	Critical for nerve, brain, and adrenal function	Morning	At least 50 mg of B5, B6, and niacin, and 100 mg of inositol	Can be stimulating, so take early in the day
Vitamin D3	Assists in the production of melatonin	Morning or mid-day only with fat-containing meals	Between 2000 and 5000 IU per day	Can interfere with sleep if taken too late in the day; take with vitamin A and K2; use lab test to check levels
Calcium	Assists in the production of melatonin	With meals	500 mg	Take with vitamin D and magnesium but not with vitamin C
Magnesium	Helps the body use calcium; helps quiet SNS	45 minutes before bed	600 mg	Natural Calm magnesium powder is a good source
L-theanine amino acid supplement	Helpful to some patients	Right before bed	200 mg	Dr. Whitaker's Restful Night Essentials is a good form of this
Melatonin hormone supplement	Helps regulate the sleep-wake cycle; works extremely well for some, does nothing for others	45 minutes before bed	500 mg	Only use occasionally; melatonin spray is quickly absorbed
Bach Flower Rescue Remedy				Many patients find this helpful

to sunlight, most of us aren't getting nearly enough (thirty minutes per day) of natural sunlight.

Take the vitamin D3 (cholecalciferol) form of vitamin D, and be sure to take it with vitamins A and K2. Because these supplements are fat-soluble, take them only with a meal containing dietary fat in some form. Good-quality fish-oil supplements are excellent sources of vitamins A and D. Vitamin D can interfere with sleep if taken too late in the day, so take it by midday. I typically recommend 2,000–5,000 IU a day, depending on the patient's lab results.

Calcium helps the brain use the amino acid tryptophan. It also appears to help with REM sleep. Take 250 mg in the morning and again in the evening with 125 mg of magnesium.

Magnesium helps regulate the sympathetic nervous system, increases deep sleep, and shortens the time required to drop into sleep. It is also essential for the metabolism of calcium.

Natural Calm is a good version of magnesium that you put in hot water and can drink before bed. (However, too much magnesium can cause loose stools or diarrhea.) Nutritional Breakthroughs offers a compound called Sleep Minerals that also can be helpful.

L-theanine is an amino acid found in green tea that has shown strong antistress effects in the body, lowering blood pressure, reducing the concentrations of stress hormones, and increasing dopamine and serotonin production. Julian Whitaker, MD, a respected nutritional physician, has a product called Restful Night Essentials, available at www.drwhitaker.com.

Melatonin is a hormone that helps regulates the sleep-wake cycle in the brain. It is produced primarily in darkness, and its production is inhibited by light. Supplementation seems to work extremely well for some but does nothing for others. Jacob Teitelbaum, MD, author of *From Fatigued to Fantastic*, recommends 1/2 mg taken within two hours of bedtime. If used repeatedly, melatonin may inhibit the body's own production of this critical sleep hormone. The sublingual, liquid form of the supplement is absorbed more quickly.

Pharmacological Medications

With a combination of osteopathy, homeopathy, some advice about sleep, and the restorative practices in chapter 7 on calming the nervous system, I find most patients can sleep. But every so often, after trauma, I have to add 10 mg of Elavil at bedtime. My patients use it for a few weeks and then generally don't need it any more. I recommend if you need to go further on the path toward medication that you speak with a physician who is cautious about medication and up to date. Medication changes and evolves so quickly that by the time you read this, there will probably be new, helpful pharmaceuticals on the market. I generally find that neurologists and psychiatrists best understand the relationship between pharmaceuticals and sleep.

Sleep Apnea

If you still have trouble sleeping, you may need to be evaluated for sleep apnea. Sleep apnea occurs when you are not getting enough oxygen at night. The lack of oxygen wakes you or stops you from dropping into deep sleep. You may have been fine before your injury, but an accident may have changed the position of your tongue in your mouth, the relationship of your neck to your head, or the position of your nose or sinuses—all of which can cause sleep apnea. If the apnea began with an injury, once you restore proper position and function to these regions with manual medicine and appropriate movement therapy, the sleep apnea should resolve. However, you may need a sleep study and the proper nighttime-breathing apparatus to treat the apnea.

Ultimately, remind yourself yet again to worship sleep—the best and least expensive cure of all.

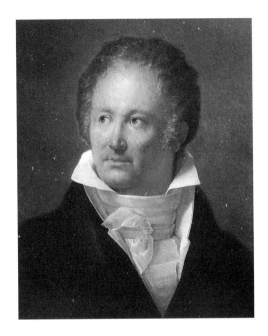

Dr. Samuel Hahnemann

In the late 1700s, a brilliant young physician and scholar named Samuel Hahnemann became disillusioned with the barbaric and ineffective medical practices of his day, which included bloodletting and the use of powerful amalgams of poisons like mercury and arsenic. Hahnemann gave up the practice of medicine, believing that medicine did more harm than good. After years of rigorous experimentation, Hahnemann determined that a substance that provokes a symptom in a large dose is capable of curing it in an infinitesimal dose. This is the insight on which Hahnemann ultimately built the system of homeopathy.

27

Homeopathy for Pain and Injury

Homeopathy is one of the most profound healing modalities I have encountered, curing or significantly improving conditions ranging from deep psychological and physical problems to ailments such as bronchitis, asthma, heart arrhythmias, herpes, ear infections, epilepsy, headaches, and menstrual problems. I have found its powerful healing properties invaluable in treating trauma, including herniated discs, sprains, strains, fractures, and brain injuries.

After I finished medical school, the last thing I wanted to do was learn the complex and demanding practice of homeopathic medicine. Besides, I thought homeopathy too bizarre and inexplicable. But I was intrigued by what appeared to be homeopathy's ability to cure seemingly incurable conditions. I mentioned earlier that I studied karate with a young woman who had suffered from epilepsy for over a decade until cured by an Indian homeopath she saw in New York. A number of my brilliant osteopathic mentors were also committed homeopathic practitioners. Viola Frymann, who is both an MD and a DO, had trained in England, where homeopathy is much more widely accepted. Eliott Blackman, DO, who practices in San Francisco, is also achieving remarkable success with homeopathy as well as osteopathy.

Early in my practice, I saw a young woman with serious, persistent infections that responded to neither antibiotics nor osteopathic manual medicine. After her homeopathic physician gave her a remedy, within hours her infections ceased. They did not return during the years I knew her. My patient's positive response to homeopathic treatment made me rethink my bias against homeopathy. I began to explore this remarkable healing modality so that I could be the best doctor possible for my patients.

Some parts of homeopathy are relatively easy to learn and use, such as giving patients *Arnica montana,* a form of the daisy flower, for bruising and bleeding. But treating a serious condition usually depends on a deeper understanding of the patient and homeopathic remedies themselves, as the next case will show.

MARIA's daughter Paula had been seeing me faithfully for more than a year, so when I heard her panicked voice canceling the day's appointment, I knew something was terribly wrong. "What happened?" I asked.

"Four days ago, Mother stepped on a rattlesnake that had been under her bed," she said. "The bite turned her leg yellow and black, and the doctors at the hospital are talking about amputation."

"Before you go to the hospital, stop at the homeopathic pharmacy," I said. "Pick up *Crotalus horridus*—homeopathic rattlesnake venom—and with her doctor's permission give your mother a dose."

People bitten by a snake typically don't need the homeopathic remedy made from snake's venom. I knew, however, from listening to Paula's stories about her mom that *Crotalus horridus* was her mother's constitutional remedy, the remedy that best matched the essence of her nature. Since *Crotalus horridus* also happened to be the most appropriate remedy for her mother's physical pathology, it had the best chance of preventing amputation.

What was it that Paula had said in the time she'd been my patient that made me know that this was the right remedy for her mother? Paula had described Maria's violent attacks on her when she was a child. She had slammed eight-year-old Paula's head with a hairbrush and was repeatedly physically abusive. This horrific behavior, hard as it was to hear about, later helped me discern the appropriate remedy for Maria. Something else also keyed me in to Maria's nature. Paula told me that when she and her children visited Maria in her rustic home in the hills of northern Los Angles County, she had to check the closet and look under the beds for rattlesnakes. Then she would remove them before she allowed the children in the house. When Paula told her mother, "Mom, if you would only keep your patio doors closed, the snakes couldn't slither in," her mother would reply, "They were on the land before I arrived, so they have more of a right to be here than I do. I can't keep them from their home."

Clearly, rattlesnakes were Maria's children that she protected and cared for more than her own grandchildren. Given Maria's propensity for collecting her brethren, it was inevitable that one night, as Maria climbed out of bed to go to the bathroom, she would step on a rattlesnake.

Maria's doctor, thinking the homeopathic remedy pointless but benign, told Paula she could give it to her mother. Within a day of receiving her remedy, Maria's leg began to heal. Talk of amputation ceased. Far more remarkable, the day Maria received *Crotalus horridus,* she turned to her daughter and said, "Where have you been all my life?" And for the first time ever, Maria told her daughter, "I love you."

After fully recuperating, Maria revealed herself as a concerned mother. Thereafter, when she displayed some abusive quality, Paula would tell her mother to take her remedy. Upon complying, Maria once more became the caring mother she could be.

DR. HAHNEMANN'S INSIGHT

In the late 1700s, a brilliant young physician and scholar named Samuel Hahnemann became disillusioned with the barbaric and ineffective medical practices of his day, which included bloodletting and the use of powerful amalgams of poisons like mercury and arsenic. Hahnemann gave up the practice of medicine, believing that medicine did more harm than good. To supplement his income, he translated medical treatises into German, always searching for a sound, rational principle of medicine. During the course of his work, he amassed an encyclopedic and far-ranging knowledge of medical history and the use and potential therapeutic effects of drugs and herbs, covering centuries of medical history written in at least eight languages.

In the course of his translations, Hahnemann came across a medical treatise by a Scottish physician named William Cullen. Cullen noted that the drug cinchona, which was used to treat malaria, could cause malaria-like symptoms in a healthy person if taken in a large dose. (Cinchona is derived from Peruvian tree bark and is a source of quinine, which is still used today to treat malaria.)

Skeptical of Cullen's explanation for the efficacy of cinchona, Hahnemann experimented on himself. He systematically ingested an overdose of cinchona and carefully noted his symptoms. His extremities became cold, his heart rate increased, and he noted anxiety, shivering, fever, and thirst—symptoms similar to those caused by malaria. This result—that a substance can cure the very same symptoms it causes—was the insight on which Hahnemann ultimately built the system of homeopathy. Calling this principle the law of similars, a tenet stretching all the way back to Hippocrates, Hahnemann made the substances he used much safer by drastically diluting them into infinitesimal doses. Surprisingly, he found that the more he diluted the substances, the more powerfully curative they became, and that they further increased in effectiveness if they were shaken up repeatedly, a process called potentizing.

After years of rigorous experimentation, Hahnemann published his seminal work based on the law of similars—the ancient principle that like cures like.

Homeopathy was so successful in treating the diseases, plagues, and ailments of the 1800s that its use rapidly spread throughout Europe and America. The Hahnemann Medical College in Philadelphia, still in existence today, was established in 1848 to train American homeopathic physicians. Homeopathy proved its mettle before the advent of antibiotics and other drugs, when it was often the successful treatment of choice for conditions such as bacterial infections, typhoid, and yellow fever, as well as the sequelae of trauma.

Examples of the law of similars can be seen in the use of three commonly prescribed homeopathic remedies: homeopathic coffee (*Coffea cruda*), homeopathic belladonna (*Belladonna*), and homeopathic onion (*Allium cepa*). Homeopathic coffee is used to treat high fevers and some forms of insomnia. Homeopathic belladonna, made from the deadly nightshade plant, is used to treat some forms of headaches, queasiness, and vomiting. Homeopathic onion is used to treat colds marked by burning nasal discharge and dry coughs.

Homeopathic remedies are made from plants, animals, minerals, poisons, and disease substances themselves. Many of the original remedies came from plants with medicinal qualities—compounds like quinine, used to treat malaria. Its homeopathic form (*China* or *Cinchona officinalis*) can be effective in the treatment not only of malaria but also of other infectious diseases. The herb comfrey (also known as boneset) is the source of the homeopathic remedy *Symphytum*. Comfrey leaf has been used for thousands of years to promote the healing of bones and wounds. It is the remedy I gave my mom to decrease her bone pain. Homeopathically, it is also used for treating trauma to the eye, as in Jasmine's case below, and for healing bone fractures after the fracture has been properly set.

Other remedies come from minerals, like *Calcarea carbonica,* which is made from the middle layer of seashells. *Calc carb* is often helpful for back spasm caused by heavy lifting. Remedies like Maria's *Crotalus horridus* come from animals: venom from snakes, milk from mammals, or feathers from birds. *Lac felinum* (cat's milk) is often helpful for eye problems. Hahnemann's original eighty remedies have now become more than six thousand.

The use of poisons, for better and worse, has been part of medicine for thousands of years. Homeopathy uses them to heal conditions similar to what the poison would cause in larger doses. The process of diluting these substances to an infinitesimal concentration, of course, has made homeopathy very safe. These remedies are some of the most effective for treating common conditions like food poisoning and serious neurological conditions like epilepsy.

A RESPECTED HEALING MODALITY

More than a hundred million people throughout the planet use homeopathy regularly, some as their main source of treatment. Its efficacy has been demonstrated in more than two hundred carefully proven, rigorously performed scientific studies done by major medical centers.

To explain how Switzerland and many other countries have come to recognize homeopathy's profound effectiveness and safety, I mention just a few of the studies that stand out.

In 1998, the government of Switzerland commissioned a health-technology assessment (HTA) of the effectiveness of homeopathic treatment. The HTA exhaustively reviewed the clinical research in homeopathy. The report included a summary of twenty-two systematic reviews of clinical trials, twenty of which revealed the positive direction of clinical evidence for homeopathy. The authors, Doctor Gudrun Bornhöft and Professor Peter Matthiesen, concluded that there was sufficient evidence for the clinical efficacy of homeopathy and for its safety and economy compared with conventional treatment. In 2012, homeopathic treatment was included in Switzerland's national health service, joining England, New Zealand, and India as nations that include homeopathic treatment in their national health care systems.

In 2003, Doctor J. Jacobs published the results of three randomized, double-blind, placebo-controlled trials using homeopathy as an adjunct in the treatment of children with severe diarrhea. The children also received oral rehydration fluids. Her studies, reported in *The Pediatric Infectious Disease Journal,* confirmed that individualized homeopathic treatment decreased the duration of acute childhood diarrhea. Some of the studies were done in developing nations, where uncontrolled diarrhea commonly causes death.

A six-year observational study conducted at the Bristol Homeopathic Hospital, in England, found that more than 70 percent of patients with severe, chronic disease showed positive health changes after receiving homeopathic remedies prescribed by their physician. The health conditions included migraines (74% showing clinical improvement), irritable bowel syndrome (71%), menopausal symptoms (77%), arthritis (70%), and depression (71%). The greatest improvements were reported among children, where more than 89 percent of children under the age of sixteen reported improvement of their asthma, and 82 percent of eczema patients under the age of sixteen reported improvement. The study involved an analysis of more than 23,000 outpatient consultations, representing more than 6,500 individual patients.

A German study published in 2010 showed that patients with a history of chronic migraines (ten to fifteen years) showed relevant improvements that persisted for the observed twenty-four-month period of the study. In 2009, the same authors had published a study that demonstrated that classic homeopathic treatment markedly decreased the severity of low-back pain and significantly improved the patients' quality of life during the two years of the study.

As I mentioned in the section on brain injury, a study done at a Harvard-affiliated hospital in 1999 found significant improvement in the ten most common symptoms of mild traumatic brain injury among patients who received an individually chosen homeopathic medication. The patients had, on average, suffered from symptoms of traumatic brain injury lasting about three years.

Numerous studies have shown the effectiveness in trauma of homeopathic *Arnica montana* to limit bleeding, swelling, and bruising, including one recently done at the University of California, San Francisco with face-lift patients. Patients receiving the *Arnica* regimen had significantly less postoperative bruising.

TREATING TRAUMA WITH HOMEOPATHIC REMEDIES

I have found homeopathy to be an extremely useful adjunct to other therapies when treating trauma. Please remember that a visit to a medical professional is always the first step in treating acute trauma, and homeopathy is not a substitute for that care. However, homeopathy can play an important role in treating trauma, and if medical care is not immediately available, it can be invaluable.

The most common traumatic injuries that I treat result from low-speed rear-end vehicle collisions. Having treated hundreds of patients injured in this all-too-common event, I've developed protocols that help patients heal more rapidly.

Let's assume the patient has not sustained serious injuries. (Numbness, severe pain or headache, mental disorientation, leaking bowel or urine, and abdominal pain are some of the potentially serious symptoms that demand immediate transport to the emergency room.) In a typical accident in which the patient has sustained neck or back injury, homeopathic *Arnica* and *Aconitum* are generally my first line of homeopathic treatment.

I recommend that my patients take one dose (four to five pellets) of *Arnica* in a strength of 1M. In fact, I recommend one dose of *Arnica* after almost any significant trauma. *Arnica* is from a medicinal plant in the daisy family and is useful to treat almost all blows, bangs, and bumps. Though you may not see any bruises on your body, a car accident often causes hidden bleeding or bruising.

If there are no contraindications (such as worsening of symptoms, an underlying bleeding problem, or a patient on blood thinners), I continue the

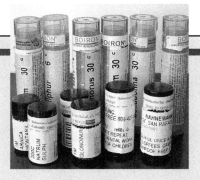

Homeopathic Dosing

Homeopathic remedies, like all pharmaceuticals, are made in licensed pharmacies and come in different strengths or potencies. A homeopathic remedy is designated by a number and a letter such as 6C or 1M. The number refers to the amount of times the remedy has been diluted—the more it has been diluted, the stronger it is. A 30C is stronger, for example, than a 6C. The letter, which is actually a Roman numeral, refers to the proportion of original substance to liquid in the dilution. C, which denotes 100, represents a dilution of one part substance to 99 parts liquid. M, which denotes 1,000, represents a dilution of one part substance to 999 parts liquid. A 10M remedy is much stronger than a 10C.

Many health food stores carry homeopathic remedies in potencies of 6C or 12C. These strengths are relatively weak but generally quite safe because they have less punch than the higher doses and can still be helpful after trauma. Even with such a low dose, however, if you get worse taking a remedy, **stop taking it.**

Higher-strength remedies such as 1M, 10M, and up have a lot more power and can sometimes cause problems when taken inappropriately. Only licensed practitioners can obtain and/or prescribe these higher doses. Homeopathic medications generally have fewer and much less dangerous side effects than pharmaceutical and over-the-counter drugs.

Arnica 1M, one dose twice a day for three days. Usually, the bruises reduce much more quickly, and they have less pain and muscle spasm than someone who didn't take *Arnica*. After three days, I occasionally switch remedies, based on the patient's improvement. I switch sooner if the *Arnica* isn't helping enough.

Patients also commonly experience injury shock after an injury or accident when their sympathetic nervous system (SNS) is in overdrive and cannot calm down. They may feel disoriented, off balance, or anxious. They may be scared to get in a car for fear of being in another injury or accident. That injury shock state usually calls for homeopathic *Aconitum*. Aconite is from a monkshood plant whose roots and juice are so toxic that they have been used as a poison on arrows. But don't worry: the substance is so diluted in the remedy that it is no longer toxic. I typically dispense one dose (4–5 pellets) of *Aconitum* in a strength of 1M. The 200C potency of *Aconitum,* available at many health food stores, can also be quite helpful in treating injury shock.

Classical homeopathic physicians like me typically prescribe only one remedy at a time, and wait to see how a patient reacts before repeating or changing the remedy. But after an injury or accident, *Arnica* and *Aconitum* can be so helpful that I often prescribe both together.

ERIC. My son Eric is a championship springboard diver. When he was in college, he missed a dive off a 3-meter board and landed hard on his chest. He began to cough up blood. After he was released from an overnight stay in the hospital, he saw a local osteopathic physician to restore motion to his chest and body. She gave him homeopathic *Arnica*, the remedy of choice after trauma. Then, after consultation with me, she added a second remedy in the same plant family, homeopathic yarrow (*Achillea millefolium*), known as the warrior's remedy and made from the yarrow plant, once known as allheal and bloodwort. *Achillea millifolium* is specific for chest trauma that leads to lung hemorrhage. Yarrow's medicinal use to staunch bleeding has been known as far back as the *Iliad* of Homer, where Achilles, for whom it is named, used it to treat his fallen comrades. Eric quickly made a full recovery and successfully returned to diving.

Once a layperson has developed some basic acquaintance with homeopathy and some of the more common remedies, they can often treat a whole range of common ailments successfully. I'll describe how some of my patients have used homeopathy to treat acute injuries:

MARSHALL. When a car suddenly pulled out in front of her, Jillian slammed on her brakes. Her eight-year-old son was perched in the passenger seat when his seat belt failed. Marshall flew forward; his head hit the windshield so hard that the windshield cracked. Jillian pulled over immediately and attended to her crying son. A large lump had already begun to form on his forehead. She grabbed the bottle of *Arnica* 1M that she kept in the glove compartment and gave him a dose, then raced to the emergency room. The emergency room physician examined Marshall about thirty minutes later. His forehead was smooth, with no trace of swelling. He was chipper and alert, with no apparent symptoms of a head injury. All of the tests were negative. When Jillian explained that her son's head had cracked the windshield, the doctor suggested that the windshield had been defective.

Over the next few days, Jillian observed her son carefully, but he exhibited no symptoms of head or brain injury. Three days later, I evaluated his cranial motion and found nothing to indicate he had sustained a significant injury.

DERRICK, the neighborhood football star, had saved his money for a whole year so he could go to football camp. Derrick was going into the eighth grade and was full of enthusiasm for his favorite sport. One evening, he was showing off his running technique to his neighborhood pals when his foot caught on a raised piece of sidewalk and he went flying, wrenching his right ankle.

Derrick's mom took him to the family doctor, who told him it was a severe sprain and ordered him to stay off his ankle for three weeks. The football camp was less than a week away, and Derrick was devastated. With his mom's okay, Derrick hobbled over to Marlene's house with his ankle swollen and bruised. He was trying to be a tough guy, but he was in tears as he told her he couldn't go to the camp. He had heard from kids in the neighborhood that she had these amazing pills that helped all kinds of things. Was there anything she could do?

With a long history as a basketball player and coach, Marlene knew a lot about ankle sprains, and had even taken a course on treating them. After Derrick lay down on her sofa, she gently worked to undo the twist in the leg caused by the sprain. Ankle sprains typically twist the long bone on the outside of the leg (the fibula). For the ankle to heal, the fibula has to be gently untwisted or the ankle will keep being reinjured. But she also gave Derrick a dose of homeopathic *Ruta* (rue), the remedy of choice for sprained ligaments. She had only a low dose on hand from her little kit, so she told him to take it three times a day for three days and to check in with her each day.

By the third day, the swelling in the ankle had almost disappeared, and Derrick's ankle was becoming less tender every day. By the fourth day, he said it felt fine. His mom took him back to the family doctor, who was quite amazed at his rapid recovery. Derrick was cleared to go to camp that weekend, where he performed like a star.

JASMINE was driving on the freeway when a pebble from an overloaded gravel truck shot off the pavement and bounced through her open side window, striking her in the left eye. A tiny piece of stone lodged under her eyelid; every time she blinked, the stone scratched her eye. Jasmine pulled over and was able to sweep the stone out of her eye, but she felt like someone had stabbed her in the eye with a knife.

Fearing a serious injury, she decided to drive herself to the hospital. By sheer coincidence, she had a kit of homeopathic remedies in the car that she had just purchased at my office. She called me to ask if there was anything she could take. The eye can heal quickly, but eye injuries can also be extremely serious and must be attended to quickly. I advised her to continue to the hospital but to take a dose of homeopathic *Symphytum*. Five minutes later, she called back, saying that the pain had gotten much worse, and her eye now felt like it was on fire. I advised her to continue on to the emergency room.

By the time Jasmine arrived at the hospital ten minutes later, the pain was gone. Her vision had cleared. She started to walk to the emergency room, but she decided that there was nothing to tell them anymore and went home. Her eye did not bother her again.

While the following two cases do not strictly deal with trauma, they illustrate how homeopathy makes brilliant use of the varied substances in the homeopathic tool chest to deal with common problems.

ANGELINES. As any film buff knows from the movie *Arsenic and Old Lace*, arsenic poisoning results in vomiting, diarrhea, and stomach pains. Homeopathic *Arsenicum album,* made from diluted and potentized arsenic, can be dramatically curative in cases of food poisoning or stomach flu where the symptoms resemble food poisoning.

Angelines started violently throwing up ten hours after eating a chicken salad sandwich that hadn't been properly refrigerated. I told her to put two pellets of homeopathic *Arsenicum* 30C from her homeopathic kit into a small glass of water, stir a few times, and take a sip every few minutes. After four sips (the equivalent of four doses), her vomiting ceased and the nausea had eased. I instructed her to take a sip once an hour for three more hours and then stop. She could take several more sips later if the symptoms returned. But she needed only one more sip, and the next day, aside from being a bit exhausted, she felt fine.

TOBIAS. Five-year-old Tobias had fits of rage that led him to slam doors, scribble on the walls, and yell and scream. He also had terrible nightmares and fears of the dark. His frantic parents left his lights on at night, but nothing seemed to help. After taking a complete history, I gave Tobias homeopathic *Stramonium.* The plant datura stramonium, from which the remedy is made, also known as devil's apple and jimson weed, is a highly poisonous plant that causes hallucinations and blocks a key neurotransmitter in the central nervous system. Stramonium poisoning is marked by a combination of fear and rage. After Tobias took homeopathic *Stramonium,* his rages markedly diminished, as did his nightmares and fears. He no longer needed the light on in his room.

Why was Tobias so frightened and rageful? That I cannot say. Many children can be full of fears. Had his behavior persisted, I would have recommended psychotherapy for him or perhaps his entire family.

Matching the Patient and Remedy

Homeopathy is one of the most intensely patient-centered healing modalities in existence. All great homeopaths must be careful observers and listeners, for in homeopathy, paying attention to the whole human being is paramount. Those of us who are physicians might test, X-ray, or listen to the patient's heart and examine the rest of their body after taking a homeopathic history, but the most important component of the patient's visit is our careful observation of what someone says and how they express themselves. Are they shy and embarrassed, or gregarious and exuberant? In homeopathy, two patients with similar physical symptoms but totally different fears and temperaments generally require different remedies. The psychological makeup of a patient is as critical to determining the appropriate remedy as their main physical complaint.

When I take an initial full homeopathic history, the patient is usually very surprised by how long and quirky it is. I learn not only about their pain but also about their moods, their food preferences, the type of weather and geography they prefer, the times of day they like, and their dreams. Their attitude toward their suffering also helps me home in on the right remedy. For example, if a patient with an obvious, severe injury tells me there is nothing wrong, I would immediately prescribe *Arnica,* which I call the tough-guy remedy. A patient who is irascible and just impossible to be around after a trauma makes me suspect homeopathic *Chamomila* might be effective. The person who always fears they left the stove burners on suggests the remedy *Argentum nitricum.* The patient whose symptoms change by the hour suggests *Pulsatilla,* the wildflower that bends in the wind. On the other hand, if that patient is thirsty, the remedy is most likely not *Pulsatilla,* because *Pulsatilla* patients almost never experience thirst. It is amazing how these details reveal the keys that lead us to the proper prescription. As in all healing modalities, determining the right homeopathic remedy requires both rigorous analysis and a trained intuition.

Homeopathic physicians used to depend on large tomes to catalogue the symptoms and ailments that lead us to particular remedies. Now we are lucky to have complex computer programs and over a gigabyte of data to help us home in on the right prescription. This accessible knowledge base is available to all practitioners of homeopathy. Some of the most important work in homeopathy has come from countries such as England and India, which have homeopathic medical schools and homeopathic hospitals. While the United States once had many of each, we have no hospitals and only one full-time medical school, located in Arizona. Hopefully, more will come.

I always encourage my patients, family, and friends—as well as you, my reader—to take as much charge of their own health care as possible. We are fortunate that there are excellent resources available that make homeopathy for acute care understandable and more accessible to everyone. I recommend Doctors Judyth Reichenberg-Ullman and Robert Ullman's wonderful book *Homeopathic Self-Care* for everyday prescribing. For musculoskeletal problems, I also recommend Doctor Asa Hershoff's book *Homeopathy for Musculoskeletal Healing.*

The care of a good homeopathic practitioner can have profound positive effects on your health. See the Resources (page 358) for information on finding a certified, licensed homeopathic practitioner in your area. For practitioners of homeopathy, further notes on my choice of remedy in a particular situation can be found at www.healingpainandinjury.com.

28

Hidden Medical Obstacles to Cure

Trauma can damage the body in subtle and unexpected ways. Untreated injury shock, inflammation, and motion restriction can tax the body's integrity so severely that dormant medical problems, such as Lyme disease or arthritis, take advantage of the poor body and burst forth. Trauma can alter the body's chemistry, causing new allergies and endocrine problems to arise. Finally, subtle, under-the-radar injuries to glands and organs can cause lingering problems. I have found that injury to the thyroid gland, the gut, and the liver can happen after trauma and be the source of untold misery. When a medical problem starts after trauma, I look for injuries to the most vulnerable organs and glands that can cause a smorgasbord of baffling symptoms. Many of my patients' unresolved and mysterious symptoms can be traced to one of these sources and treated.

Here are a few of the medical obstacles to cure that can prevent a return to health after trauma.

1 Thyroid Problems and Other Hormonal Imbalances

Symptoms:

- Fatigue
- Dry skin
- Weight gain or loss
- Depression
- Hair loss
- Sensitivity to cold
- Joint pain
- Painful menstrual periods
- Loss of outside third of eyebrows
- Cardiac problems
- Digestive problems
- Poor recovery from injury or illness

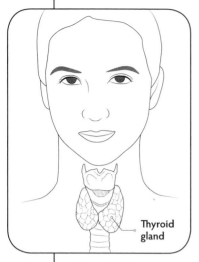

Thyroid gland

The thyroid gland is a butterfly-shaped gland perched around the windpipe in front of the neck. It is the body's master gland of energy production. Every cell in the body depends on the hormones produced by the thyroid gland to regulate its metabolism. Thyroid hormones affect energy levels, heart rate, body weight, mood, muscle strength, digestion, reproductive health, and cardiac function and are critical in dealing with inflammation.

The thyroid gland's exposed position in front of the windpipe makes it extremely vulnerable to trauma. A blow to the neck or back can cause the thyroid to strike the cartilaginous trachea on which it perches, damaging the thyroid and compromising its function. Low thyroid levels dramatically slow healing. Even without a direct blow to the thyroid, trauma can injure the thyroid by placing excess demands on it.

Fatigue, weight gain, dry skin, brain fog, depression, hair loss, low blood pressure, and sensitivity to cold are some of the more common symptoms of low thyroid production. Low thyroid can also impair digestion, aggravate heart conditions, and cause reproductive problems such as abnormal menstrual periods and infertility. Women are at higher risk for thyroid problems than are men.

To find out if you are low in thyroid, start by getting a lab test. Standard thyroid tests check the levels of two thyroid hormones that circulate in the blood: free T3 and free T4. It's also important, however, to check blood levels of a third hormone, called thyroid-stimulating hormone. TSH is produced not by the thyroid but by the pituitary—the master gland. It's a polite message from the pituitary to the thyroid, telling the thyroid how much hormone (T3 and T4) the body needs. When the pituitary starts getting complaints from the body's cells that they need more thyroid hormones, the pituitary increases TSH levels, yelling at the thyroid to shape up and start producing more hormones. But chances are that the thyroid is doing the best it can. We call that weakened condition hypothyroidism.

You would expect that blood levels of T3 and T4 would be lower than normal when the pituitary's high TSH production is scolding the thyroid to produce more hormones. But sometimes levels of T3 and T4 can be normal but still not high enough. Why? Cells can become partially resistant to thyroid hormones, similar to the way they can become resistant to insulin or cortisol. When that happens, the cells are unable to take in enough of the circulating thyroid hormone to meet their needs and the person may need supplemental thyroid. Temporarily adding thyroid medication can give the thyroid gland a rest so it can heal until the cells' resistance fades. All this should be done under proper medical supervision.

Measuring early-morning body temperature with a glass basal body thermometer, available at some drugstores, is also a fairly accurate measure of thyroid function. The night before, shake the thermometer down. (If you shake the thermometer in the morning, that effort will raise your temperature and create an inaccurate reading.) For ten minutes, first thing in the morning (before you move), hold the thermometer in your armpit. Record your temperature for five days in a row. If you are menstruating, you need to start the second day of menstruation. For men and postmenopausal women, it makes no difference when you take the temperature. If your early morning temperature is below the range of 97.8–98.2 degrees, you may be hypothyroid.

Low levels of iodine, another widespread problem, can compromise thyroid function. A few years ago, I tested the iodine levels of twelve of my California patients. The healthiest one had 60 percent of the recommended level of iodine. Though my patients tend to eat fish, which has some iodine, they also generally eat sea salt, which does not contain iodine.

Despite the absence of iodine in sea salt, it is generally a healthy form of salt. If someone is deficient in iodine, they may need to find other ways to supplement it (e.g., kelp or an iodine supplement). Iodine is critical for many reasons, including its role in thyroid and reproductive health. However, some people are allergic to iodine, and in some cases its supplementation has been implicated in potentially dangerous overactive thyroid activity. If you suspect you are iodine-deficient, talk to your health care provider about a urine test and possible iodine supplementation.

Other hormonal imbalances tend to be rarer than thyroid problems, but they do occur. The problems that key me in to potential hormonal imbalance are unexplained weight gain, diminished sex drive, vaginal dryness, recalcitrant pain, fatigue, digestive problems, severe insomnia, mood swings, memory problems, weakness, and anxiety. When a patient continues to suffer with problems that indicate hormonal imbalance even after I've addressed the pituitary gland, and homeopathy hasn't given me the results I expect, I refer the patient to a physician or other practitioner who is knowledgeable about hormone imbalances and is well versed in the use of natural hormones.

341

2 Autoimmune Diseases

Symptoms:

- Joint pain
- Muscle pain
- Weakness
- Dry eyes
- Headaches

- Extreme fatigue
- Hair loss
- Weakness
- Anemia
- Stiffness and swelling in extremities

Continuing, chronic inflammation can incite or flare rheumatoid or other forms of arthritis as well as other autoimmune diseases. These are diseases in which the body attacks itself. In multiple sclerosis (MS), the autoimmune disease attacks the fatty myelin covering of the nerves. With rheumatoid arthritis (RA), the disease attacks the cartilage covering the joints. Stevens-Johnson syndrome, which attacks the mucous membranes, can occur after a course of antibiotics. Autoimmune diseases can attack almost any part of the body. Some autoimmune diseases, like MS and RA, are relatively easy to diagnose with the appropriate testing. Other autoimmune diseases can be very difficult to determine. If you still have unexplained symptoms that don't make sense to you, such as joint pain, fever, dizziness, or fatigue, or you keep catching every disease that passes by, ask your physician to check for autoimmune disease.

Rheumatologists and immunologists are the specialists most adept at diagnosing these problems and treating them. But once again, I will stress that removing the shock of injury, decreasing inflammation, and restoring motion to the body's fluid pathways and restricted areas can significantly restore the body's vitality. With that, a person has a much better chance of putting these conditions into remission and sometimes even curing them. I have seen homeopathy effectively treat autoimmune diseases. I have also seen several patients misdiagnosed with autoimmune disease when they actually had Lyme disease, which I discuss next.

3 Lyme Disease and Its Co-Infections

Symptoms:

- Joint pain and swelling
- Fatigue
- Brain fog
- Digestive disorders
- Balance problems
- Fevers

- Heart problems
- Headaches
- Unusually stiff and painful muscles
- Multiple sclerosis–like symptoms, including numbness and weakness

Lyme disease and its co-infections are chameleons. Their symptoms are numerous and systemic (the list of symptoms above is by no means complete) and can masquerade as many other conditions and diseases. For that reason, health care practitioners frequently miss these conditions.

Lyme disease is carried by the deer tick. These tiny creatures hitch a ride on pets, shoes, grass, and tree leaves. Most Lyme tick bites do not cause a bull's-eye rash—people can be bitten by one of these tiny ticks and never know it. In fact, there may be no initial symptoms. Pet owners are especially vulnerable, because pets go outside, bring in ticks, and drop them on the carpet or furniture. Hours or days later, the tick can bite them without their knowing it. Lyme disease has been with the human race for thousands of years. DNA analysis of Otzi, the five-thousand-year-old Iceman found in the Tyrolean Alps, showed infection by the Lyme spirochete.

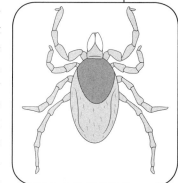

Like rheumatologic and immune system disorders, Lyme disease and its common co-infections, like ehrlichiosis and babesiosis, can lie dormant for years until trauma insults the body. Infectious organisms such as viruses and bacteria are clever and opportunistic. When the immune system is overwhelmed from dealing with trauma, these infectious organisms rush in to take advantage of the stressed body. Lyme disease can cause unexplained fevers, pericarditis, and other heart problems. Spasticity and weakness resembling Parkinson's disease or MS can occur. Anyone suffering from unexplained headaches and/or joint pain, neurological problems such as trouble swallowing or problems with balance, or brain fog and memory problems that are resistant to all other forms of treatment should consider Lyme disease and its co-infections. Those who spend a lot of time outdoors, such as hunters and hikers, are particularly at risk for Lyme. Several of my patients got Lyme disease by removing ticks from their dogs with bare hands. Always use tweezers, and do not touch the tick.

I have found a relatively inexpensive test called the CD 57, from LabCorp, to be a fairly good initial screening test for Lyme. Most recently, we have an even more accurate culture from Advanced Laboratory Services, which actually cultures the Lyme spirochete. If a person suspects that they may suffer from this disease or its co-infections, it is critical to see a practitioner who is knowledgeable about them. But please realize that Lyme and its co-infections are very clever, especially if they've been in the body for a while. They find good hiding places deep in the cells, with the result that many Lyme tests miss them, even the culture. In the end, no test is as accurate as good clinical judgment.

4 Infected Teeth

Symptoms:

- Headaches
- Fevers
- Sinusitis
- Joint pain
- Facial pain
- Jaw pain
- Allergies
- Susceptibility to infection or flu

An infected tooth can slowly poison the body. Much of the time, a person feels the discomfort of an infected tooth and gets it treated promptly, but sometimes teeth hold hidden infections. Though we generally think of teeth as solid, there are dozens of small channels intersecting the nerve roots running through the teeth. Any of these channels, especially at the root of the tooth, can hold a pocket of infection that can brew for years and seed the body with poison. Root canals, especially old ones, can hide an infection. The tools a skilled root canal specialist currently uses are much better at successfully cleaning out the tooth and ridding it of potential infection.

These hidden infections are hard to diagnose and can lead to serious systemic problems, including generalized achiness, constant bacterial and viral infections, allergies, and headaches. Chronic sinus infections may be a warning sign of an infection in a tooth.

Some dentists and physicians think all root canals are dangerous because of the potential for hidden infection, but I don't. If a person is healthy, there is probably no need to worry about a possible root canal infection. However, I've seen a number of patients who did not get well until they had their tooth infection cured, their root canal redone, or the tooth removed. If you suspect an infected tooth, the newer I-CAP dental X-rays can visualize the roots of the teeth much more accurately than previous X-rays and better discern an infection.

5 Parasites

Symptoms:

- Unexplained anxiety
- Weight loss
- Nausea and vomiting
- Digestive problems
- Diarrhea
- Asthma
- Allergies
- Generalized inflammation

CINDY. Two decades ago, a young woman in her late twenties named Cindy came to see me. She was bone-thin and nauseated. Doctors had worked her up for digestive problems, but the lab tests had turned up nothing. Despite her insistence that she was eating a lot, they decided she was anorexic and suffering from an anxiety disorder. They referred her to a psychiatrist. The psychiatrist agreed she was anorexic. Desperate, she came to see me.

I listened to her complaints about her gut and how much it hurt. I asked her if they had checked her for parasites. She said yes, but since she hadn't been out of the country, they had done a standard stool test that had come back negative for worms and parasites. I took out my stethoscope and listened to her abdomen. Her intestines were gurgling way too much. I put my hands on her belly and listened with my hands. I felt significant gut irritation. The history she gave and the physical diagnosis convinced me she had parasites.

I ordered a much more comprehensive stool test from a specialized lab to tell me what antibiotics her parasite would best respond to. The test confirmed she had amoebic dysentery. After a course of Flagyl, she recovered completely. She gained weight and no longer suffered from the anxiety that led doctors to conclude she had mental problems.

Again and again, I've found that gut disorders cause anxiety. I suspect this results from undigested food products that become toxic in the body, or the poorly performing gut's inability to obtain the proper nutrients.

There is a myth that people get parasites only from travel to exotic locations in Africa, Asia, or Latin America, but American food is quite capable of transmitting parasites. Of course, we do get a certain amount of our food from elsewhere, such as Central and South America. In Cindy's case, the parasites probably came from her camping trip in the Shasta lake region of California, where she swam in the lake.

I don't do a great deal of parasite testing, but when I do, I use specialized labs like Doctor's Data, Genova Diagnostics, or Meridian Laboratory. Their labs not only look for parasites but also evaluate the physiologic condition of the gut. Evaluating the general health of the gut is important, as no lab can test for all the thousands of possible worms and parasites. Lab tests can even miss the common ones if the bugs are in their hibernating cycle and don't show up for their audition.

Time after time, I've seen physicians miss parasites. Since the digestive tract is one of the keys to health, when it is inflamed, not only do patients complain of gut pain or dysfunction, but they can also have allergies such as asthma and eczema. If the problem is severe enough, the whole body, including the brain, can be inflamed. Patients with stubborn digestive problems after an accident or injury may be suffering from a parasite or gut infection that their immune system had previously been able to keep under control. Once we know the gut is infected, we can begin treatment.

To prevent ingesting live parasites, I cook my vegetables. If I plan to eat raw vegetables or salad, I soak them for ten to fifteen minutes in water with several drops of grapefruit seed extract, which I rinse off before I consume them. There are other products on the market for cleaning off vegetables but none provide absolute safety. I am totally opposed to irradiating food as a way to deal with pathogens.

6 Allergies and Gluten Intolerance

Symptoms:

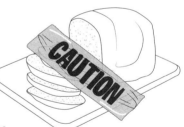

- Headaches
- Eczema
- Joint pain
- Inflammation
- Sinus problems
- Brain fog
- Asthma
- Gut problems
- Fatigue
- Allergies
- Bronchitis
- Irritable bowel
- Breathing problems
- Boggy tissues
- Constant infections
- Low-back and sacral pain
- "Raccoon" eyes
- General malaise

Jim had been an energetic nineteen-year-old college student who loved to run track and play the trumpet, until he was struck with debilitating headaches on the left side. After six months of agony, he found his way to me. Like so many of the people who arrive at my office, he could not associate his pain with a trauma or event, but when I put my hand on his head and felt his sutures welded solid, I knew something profound was locking up his head—I just didn't know what.

I made him trace back to the year prior to his pain and learned two critical factors. One year earlier, he'd fallen backward and hit his head; two months prior, he'd had his wisdom teeth extracted. All the pulling and yanking of the tooth extractions had distorted the bones in and around the tooth, including the temporal bone.

I went to work opening up the compressed sutures in his head, especially the critical occipitomastoid suture in the back, one of the troublemakers that causes headaches. I had more trouble than usual getting his locked-up skull to release. I also took his homeopathic case and gave him a constitutional remedy. By his third treatment, he felt much better and could return to a distant school and function well. He continued his osteopathic case with a talented colleague of mine.

His concerned parents wisely counseled him to avoid sports that could involve head injury, and he dutifully complied. Luckily, track was quite safe, and he thought sailing was, too, until a careless classmate let the boom fly and it crashed into the side of his head. His headaches exploded again. Cranial osteopathy helped but could no longer completely remove the pain. Then my colleague tested Jim for gluten intolerance with a new test developed by Cyrex Laboratories. Indeed, Jim had severe gluten intolerance. Within weeks of eliminating all gluten, he had no more headaches.

Jim's cranial restrictions now made much more sense to me. Of course, the blows to his head and his dental extractions had compromised his cranial motion and helped create his initial headaches. But trauma doesn't usually cause all the sutures to lock up the way they had with Jim. I suspect the gluten intolerance he'd always had had tightened his scalp and the underlying dura, ratcheting a vise around the bones of the skull. The subsequent head injuries became the proverbial straws that broke the camel's back.

I've found in my decades of practice that allergies can tighten up everything in the body. Since an allergic reaction tends to provoke systemic inflammation, it makes sense that much of the body tightens up. Furthermore, the body's all-encompassing fascial web contains the mast cells—cells that react to allergens by releasing inflammatory histamine. It's no wonder that the main controller of our structural integrity, the fascia, tightens up with allergies.

Gluten intolerance is often missed because it can cause systemic symptoms, not just digestive problems. As with Jim, gluten intolerance can have no gut symptoms at all. The lower-back and sacral areas are especially likely to be affected by gluten intolerance because nerves from the gut come into the spinal cord at those regions. A person suffering from these symptoms for no apparent reason might do well to explore the possibility of gluten allergy with their health care practitioner.

Why has gluten intolerance become so common? Agriculture introduced a new type of wheat approximately forty years ago, which now makes up almost all wheat consumed in the world. This dwarf wheat grows much more quickly and is made up of some very different chromosomes than the ones the human race had spent 10,000 years digesting. So for many people, instead of being nourishing, wheat attacks the gut and causes the myriad of problems linked to gluten intolerance. I suspect some of our increased sensitivity to gluten also comes from the many preservatives and genetically modified products all of us have consumed. As we keep forcing damaging substances on our bodies, we get more and more sensitive and it takes less and less to irritate the digestive track.

Other food allergies can cause similar symptoms. To make matters more confusing, the person may not have had allergies until trauma restricted their lymphatic system's ability to rid the body of allergens. Restoring the free flow of the lymphatic channels, particularly in the gut, can be critical in enabling the gut to heal and allergies to diminish.

Given that the symptoms can be so vague, how do people know if they have food allergies? Allergy testing can often indicate which foods cause an allergic reaction. Specialty labs like Meridian Valley Labs and Doctor's Data have blood tests to discern the airborne and food products that people may be reacting to. Skin tests, thought by many allergists to be the most accurate way to diagnose allergies, give the allergist the information they need to design allergy drops or shots that, over time, can help desensitize people to allergies.

These are but a snapshot of medical problems that trauma can unleash or that can significantly slow down recovery from injury. Their often-confusing and misleading symptoms demand that you, the patient, as well as your practitioner, keep a hungry mind. If the patient can just trust themselves and listen to whatever peculiar suspicions arise, they usually have an inherent sense of what caused the problem. Know that no matter how confusing or elusive the underlying problem, if you address trauma's three critical components and promote the function of the five unsung heroes of health, you will almost always improve, no matter what the nature of your problem. Take charge, be curious, be persistent, believe in the body's healing process, and *never give up*.

29

How I Treat

My training as an osteopathic physician has deeply affected how I approach a patient, for I have learned that the attitude a practitioner brings to the treatment has a profound effect on their ability to create healing. Most people think osteopathy—as well as all manual medicine—is all about technique. Technique is important, but it is only part of what's necessary to help people's bodies move toward health. That's why when I treat, I imagine that I am sitting on a metaphorical three-legged stool of listening, awe, and technique.

When a child or adult first sees me, they enter a bright room with open skylights and pictures of colorful landscapes. A small child often plays with toys first. I listen to the patient's or parent's tales and watch the child. Watching is a kind of listening.

Once my patient is comfortable with me, I observe them move and then examine them standing and sitting. Do their hands turn in or out? Is one hip or shoulder lower than the other? As the patient bends forward, do all of their vertebrae move down evenly, or is there a hitch in the movement, indicating that two or more vertebrae are jammed together? I pay special attention to the patient's feet and make sure the Achilles tendon runs straight down and doesn't bow to one side or the other.

All this watching is rather hard on me because I'm not very visual. Though both my parents are painters, most visual cues are lost on me. I'm dyslexic, so I've worked hard to be able to perceive visual differences. My sensory wisdom lies elsewhere. Since childhood, I have been about touch: how clay feels and how to mold it. Growing up, I thought I'd be a sculptor. My patients tell me I am a sculptor of bodies.

Given my propensity toward touch, I had a bit of an advantage when I decided to use touch to help people's bodies heal. But touch is unique among the human senses. Not everyone can become a gifted painter, musician, or chef (using the senses of sight, sound, and taste), but almost everyone can become talented at touch.

I have spoken elsewhere about the extensive medical training osteopathic physicians have; that training is important. Our scientific background grounds us and gives us a profound base of knowledge. That perspective is the platform of the stool on which we sit. It allows us to sit back and not get pulled into the patient's possible despair or frustration with their condition. That knowledge gives us the tools to differentiate a potentially fatal abdominal aneurysm from a painful but not life-threatening episode of back pain. When I suspect a serious pathology, I order an MRI or other appropriate evaluation.

Being grounded and calm within is an essential part of our profession, since it allows clarity. It enables me to really and truly listen to my patient, both to their words and, with my hands, to the wisdom of their body and what it is trying to tell me. Since much of medical diagnosis comes from paying attention to the patient's words and tone, listening with my hands adds depth to that accuracy.

Over the years, as I deepened my ability to perceive with my fingers, not only could I feel the restrictions in the patient's tissues and the body's living pulsations, but I also learned to look for the health that lights up their tissues. By doing that, I gained a powerful tool in helping them heal and gained a sense of their unique and personal blueprint for health. Each of us has our own set of instructions for how our parts fit together and should move.

The wondrous sense of health that exists in every living person's tissues increases the sense of awe I have for the person's unique healing ability. I found that the more reverence I have for the patient's unique healing ability, the more powerful their own healing force becomes and the faster and more completely they recover.

That's why I say that awe is the second critical component of the three-legged stool. Coming to the patient with a sense of awe helps wash away preconceived ideas of how I might impose my doctor's will to remake the body. Awe washes away any judgment I might have for how they've addressed their problems.

My touch transmits my reverence for the patient's unique healing power. And, feeling respected, the patient's body allows me to make the mechanical changes that correspond with their blueprint for optimal health. I believe it is my sense of awe for their life force that allows their nervous system to accept the mechanical changes I make in their joints, fascia, muscles, lymphatic system, and organs—indeed, every part of the body. Once my work is accepted, then the body incorporates these changes as its own. This is part of my answer as to why such gentle work has such profound effects. My techniques also work because they are performed in harmony with the patient's needs and in concert with the rhythms within their body. As I make the mechanical changes that their blueprint for health is asking of me, I am simultaneously listening for guidance from the rhythms deep in their tissues.

I have mentioned before that there are a number of currents flowing through our bodies. A healthy ebb and flow of the cranial rhythmic impulse (CRI), which pulsates through the whole nervous system and can be felt everywhere in the body, occurs six to fourteen times a minute. There is also what Russian scientists have discerned as a "slow tide" that courses about three times a minute through the body. As I work, I feel my fingers surfing on these currents. If the currents are becoming choppier, more erratic, I'm making matters worse and I must back off. When I'm helping, the currents smooth and become more powerful. I can teach this individually to other practitioners much more easily than I can explain it.

Technique is pretty straightforward. Each practitioner needs to find techniques that are not only the most effective for treating the patient but are also the best fit for the practitioner. For example, I have relatively small fingers, so I have learned to use people's arms and legs as levers to make changes at the spine or rib attachments. I especially like facilitated positional release (FPR), a technique invented by my mentor Stanley Schiowitz, DO, FAAO. FPR is precise and uses a lot of levers to create immediate structural change. I also have worked for thirty-five years to perfect my ability to affect the nervous system through cranial osteopathy. And I use fascial-release techniques throughout the body to address everything from problems affecting the organs to the critical lymphatic system.

Once I'm sitting on my three-legged stool of listening, awe, and technique, how do I approach a patient? Here are some guidelines I initially give the patient:

- You will probably need three to five treatments before you feel a significant change.

- The first change may not be the exact one you want. For example, you may seek treatment to diminish your back pain, but your mood, energy, digestion, or head pain may improve first. The body tends to heal in the manner that I discuss in chapter 25 on the laws of cure.

- I ask most people to return in two weeks. If their condition is acute or serious, I may see them twice a week and then, after they have improved significantly, every two weeks. As they continue to improve, I gradually spread out the treatments. My goal is that people only need a twice-a-year tune-up.

When I was first in practice I tended to overtreat patients, doing too much in one visit. Overtreating can overwhelm the patient's body and ultimately cause it to reject many of the changes. Here, less is often more, and it creates much better results. I have learned to limit my treatments to about twenty-five minutes and focus mainly on three to five areas, which usually include the sacrum, diaphragm, and head. I also often spend time treating critical vertebral restrictions and some brief time on legs, arms, and feet.

I find that it is important to leave some work for the patient's body to do on its own, so I generally stop when I feel that the treatment is 85 percent complete. A psychiatrist friend told me that she, too, was trained to stop her patients' therapy sessions at 85 percent to allow the person's own healing to take over. If the patient's body is encouraged to complete the healing on their own, the result is much more profound. After severe trauma or illness or with young children, however, the body is generally unable to initially take over the healing, and then I have to finish the treatment myself.

I am always being advised by the patient's own healing force. I feel what the remarkable Rebecca Lippincott, DO, articulated to me when I was a third-year medical student: "When a part of the body has been treated enough, it expands like a balloon and pushes you off." So, when I sense that gentle nudge, I move on to the next region. I usually end my treatment with the head. When the skull gently and symmetrically pushes me away, usually the treatment is done. I then remove my hands and trust the patient's healing to continue on its own. The treatment session is only the beginning of the process. Most of the improvement occurs over the next two to five weeks as the body integrates the changes set in motion by the treatment.

Before the patient leaves, I tell them they may feel very sore for twenty-four to forty-eight hours after the first visit, and to call me if a problem arises or soreness lasts more than forty-eight hours. I warn them that some of the old symptoms of the trauma may temporarily reappear, only to quickly disappear. If I have felt their vital force pick up—which I almost always do—I assure them that I believe they will get better. I am continually surprised by people's ability to heal.

Osteopathy—my work—does not cure everyone, but it almost always

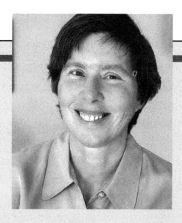

Your Health Care Team

We all need someone to watch over us when we are hurt or ill. In the aftermath of trauma, your primary health care practitioner should provide a thorough evaluation of your injuries and immediately treat any severe or life-threatening symptoms. Once that is done, removing injury shock, calming inflammation, and restoring motion to restricted tissues are the critical next steps in your healing.

Osteopathic and allopathic physicians trained in manual medicine can address both of these needs, but there aren't very many of us. Most likely, you will need to put together your own team of healers to help you recover your health. Your team members can be physicians, yoga teachers, acupuncturists, Pilates instructors, physical therapists—whoever can help you with your particular situation.

Each situation and problem demands a different team. When auditioning your health care team, you'll want to find practitioners who are knowledgeable about the neurological and musculoskeletal systems, who take time with their patients, and who believe in the innate intelligence of the body. It is always wise to find out their level of training and experience as well. I have put together information and resources to help you determine which are the best modalities for you and what to look for in a practitioner. These are posted at **www.healingpainandinjury.com**. Healing is much easier when you have good guides along the way!

helps. I am always ready to make referrals to other talented professionals for the rare person I don't help or the person I don't feel like I'm helping enough. As this book shows, people can benefit from many different approaches. Each person needs to find for themselves the best instruments or the best orchestra of practitioners for their healing.

For me, being an osteopathic physician has been a joyous and humbling journey. I stand on the shoulders of giants, and my hands are linked with thousands of osteopathic colleagues who, like me, know that the body has a remarkable ability to heal. I thank all the marvelous patients who have inspired me with their courage and curiosity and have honored me with their trust.

I wrote this book because it pains me to see how much needless suffering consumes people's lives. I wanted you, the reader, to be able to bathe in the warmth of the knowledge passed down to me. I hope as you read this book that you found many ways to help yourself heal. You now know how hard your body is working to be your greatest ally. Please follow in the footsteps of the patients who have graced us with their stories—be curious, practice awe, mix in a little patience and persistence, and your own miraculous ability to heal will astound you.

Acknowledgments

I have been blessed to have so many people provide me so many gifts on this journey. First, my mother Joann, who believed I could be a writer even though I couldn't spell and kept putting words in the wrong order. Of course, she couldn't spell either. My stepfather, Leopold, who carried me up and down the hall when I couldn't breathe from asthma. With his patient, energetic kindness, he helped keep me alive during those dark nights.

And then there were all the magnificent osteopathic physicians who showed me that brilliance could also have hearts so large that they filled the room: Muriel Chapman, Stanley Schiowitz, Howard and Rebecca Lippincott, Herbert Miller, Ann Wales, Ernest Bernhardi, Robert Fulford, Joyce Vetterlein, Eliott Blackman, Tony Chila, and many more. I live amongst a group of generous people who give not just the shirts off their backs but their very souls to help patients.

I also thank the brilliant homeopathic practitioners who helped me learn and practice this amazing form of medicine: Roger Morrison, MD, whose heart matches his genius, Nancy Herrick, Lou Klein, and Melissa Fairbanks as well as David Warkentin, whose computer program helps make homeopathic prescription much more accurate and effective. And I express my gratitude to my colleague Dr. Yat Ki Lai, whose work embodies on a daily basis the remarkable healing power of Oriental medicine.

Laura Lovett has done a remarkable job of designing the inside and outside of the book so that the words and images are enticing. But she did far more than that. She shepherded the book through the maze of difficuties inevitable in the process, gave me encouragement, and set necessary deadlines, or the book would never have been finished.

I found my amazing illustrator, Sarah Chen, just two days after she graduated from scientific illustration school. Thank you, Sarah, for making my ideas live with such humor and style. Now, off to medical school at U.C. Davis! If you don't wow them all, I'll have to give them a piece of my mind. Thanks to Rachel Ann Owen for taking over and providing the last few wonderful drawings.

My publisher, David Cole, mixed wisdom with kindly patience. I promise I will get the next book in on time.

And, of course, the wise Patricia Sullivan who created an amazing amalgam of healing movements using yoga, qigong, tai chi, and Egoscue. Life is motion and she is proof of that in so many ways.

Numerous people have read parts of this book, offering invaluable comments and picking up errors. Editor Janet Goldstein helped us focus the book—although she wanted it to be three hundred pages, not closer to the four hundred it is. Without her help, it would have been five hundred. My best friend from medical school, Maryanne Cucchiarelli, DO, PMR, went above and beyond for months helping make the book so much better. Chloe Haimson, my niece, and Amy Bloom offered invaluable insights as the book neared conclusion on its fifteenth or twentieth draft. Donald Hankinson, DO, Sean Maloney, DO, Lucette Nadle, DO, David Hagie, DO, Meg Fitzgerald, my son William Gordh, Steve Carmichael, and John Melnichek, DHom, all gave helpful feedback. But any errors or misstatements are mine.

Given my dyslexia, when I type it looks like a language yet to be invented, so I have many typists to thank: my son Daniel Vincent Gordh, Lindsay Adams, Jeremy Rice, Shirlene Brass, Kate Banner, Kathryn Thorne, and many others, no doubt, over the eight-year genesis of this book.

And, ultimately, I must thank Adrienne Larkin, my partner of twenty-seven years. With her lawyer's sharp mind and philosopher's genius, she saw the holes in the logic my restless mind created at every opportunity. Many a night she'd grill me at 10:30 p.m. and force me to think in an orderly fashion so she could reframe my concepts coherently. I am so lucky that she has a master's degree in the philosophy of science. This is as much her book as mine. But she prefers, like water and astrocytes, to work in the background.

Then there are my patients, the gracious people who have placed their trust in my hands and my knowledge. I thank you for all you have allowed me. A number of your experiences enrich this book—disguised, of course. I hope I have done you justice. Thank you for letting me tell your stories.

Some brilliant and kind people helped me hone my skills as a writer. Janet Lewis Winters and Mary Jane Moffat taught me at Stanford and continued to believe in me. We stayed friends until their deaths. I still miss their wise presence.

It has been an amazedly blessed journey. I am most proud of the section on traumatic brain injury. Those few pages have powerful suggestions that can offer help for so many struggling with this devastating condition. I hope to carry this work forward into a book on healing traumatic brain injury.

Resources

FIND PRACTITIONERS

The American Academy of Osteopathy (www.academyofosteopathy.org) has an online guide for locating practitioners near you who practice osteopathic manipulative therapy.

To find practitioners trained in cranial osteopathy, visit the Cranial Academy's website: www.cranialacademy.org.

To find a practitioner of homeopathy, see the Center for Homeopathic Certification's website: www.homeopathicdirectory. com. Also see the National Center for Homeopathy's list of practitioners at www.nationalcenterforhomeopathy.org.

To learn more about Patricia Sullivan's workshops and retreats, visit www. patriciasullivanyoga.com. To purchase the companion DVD by Patricia, see www.healingpainandinjury.com.

FURTHER READING

D'Adamo, Peter and Catherine Whitney. *Eat Right 4 (for) Your Type: The Individualized Diet Solution to Staying Healthy, Living Longer & Achieving Your Ideal Weight*. New York: G.P. Putnam & Sons, 1996.

Egoscue, Pete, with Roger Gittines. *Pain Free: A Revolutionary Method for Stopping Chronic Pain*. New York: Bantam Books, 1998.

Emmons, Henry. *The Chemistry of Calm: A Powerful, Drug-Free Plan to Quiet Your Fears and Overcome Your Anxiety*. New York: Simon & Schuster, 2010.

Fallon, Sally, with Mary G. Enig. *Nourishing Traditions: The Cookbook that Challenges Politically Correct Nutrition and the Diet Dictocrats*. Washington, DC: Newtrends Publishing, 1999.

Enig, Mary and Sally Fallon. "The Oiling of America." The Weston A. Price Foundation. January 2000. www. westonaprice.org/know-your-fats/the-oiling-of-america.

Fields, R. Douglas. *The Other Brain*. New York: Simon & Schuster, 2011.

Fulford, Robert, with Gene Stone. *Dr. Fulford's Touch of Life: The Healing Power of the Natural Life Force*. New York: Pocket Books, 1996.

Gershon, Michael D. *The Second Brain: A Groundbreaking New Understanding of Nervous Disorders of the Stomach and Intestine*. New York: HarperCollins, 1998.

Goldstein, Joel. *No Stone Unturned: A Father's Memoir of His Son's Encounter With Traumatic Brain Injury*. Washington, DC: Potomac Books, 2012.

Gonzales, Laurence. *Deep Survival: Who Lives, Who Dies, and Why*. New York: W.W. Norton & Co., 2004.

Herbert, Martha R. and Karen Weintraub. *The Autism Revolution: Whole-Body Strategies for Making Life All It Can Be*. New York: Ballantine Books, 2012.

Hershoff, Asa. *Homeopathy for Musculoskeletal Healing*. Berkeley, CA: North Atlantic Books, 1996.

Hitzmann, Sue. *The Melt Method: A Breakthrough Self-Treatment System to*

Eliminate Chronic Pain, Erase the Signs of Aging, and Feel Fantastic in Just 10 Minutes a Day! New York: HarperOne, 2013.

Hyman, Mark. *The UltraMind Solution: Fix Your Broken Brain by Healing Your Body First.* New York: Scribner, 2008.

Johnson, Larry. *Energetic Tai Chi Chuan.* San Francisco, CA: White Elephant Monastery, 1989.

Kabat-Zinn, Jon. *Mindfulness for Beginners: Reclaiming the Present Moment—and Your Life.* Boulder, CO: Sounds True, 2012.

———. *Wherever You Go, There You Are.* New York: Hyperion, 2005.

Leeds, Joshua. *The Power of Sound: How to Be Healthy and Productive Using Music and Sound.* Rochester, VT: Healing Arts Press, 2010.

Levine, Peter A., with Ann Frederick. *Waking the Tiger: Healing Trauma.* Berkeley, CA: North Atlantic Books, 1997

Lewis, John. *A.T. Still: From the Dry Bone to the Living Man.* Gwynedd, Wales: Dry Bone Press, 2012.

McCall, Timothy. *Yoga as Medicine: The Yogic Prescription for Health and Healing.* New York: Bantam Books, 2007.

Nathan, Neil. *On Hope and Healing: For Those Who Have Fallen Through the Medical Cracks.* Little Rock, AR: Et Alia Press, 2010.

Newport, Mary T. *Alzheimer's Disease: What If There Was a Cure?* Laguna Beach, CA: Basic Health Publications, 2013.

Scaer, Robert C. *The Trauma Spectrum: Hidden Wounds and Human Resiliency.* New York: W. W. Norton & Co., 2005.

Sears, Barry. *The Anti-Inflammation Zone: Reversing the Silent Epidemic That's Destroying Our Health.* New York: William Morrow, 2005.

Spurlock, Morgan. *Super Size Me.* Directed by Morgan Spurlock. Distributed by Roadside Attractions, Samuel Goldwyn Films, Showtime Independent Films. Released May 7, 2004.

Ullman, Robert and Judyth Reichenberg-Ullman. *Homeopathic Self-Care: The Quick and Easy Guide for the Whole Family.* Edmonds, WA: Three Rivers Press, 2012.

Weil, Andrew. *Spontaneous Healing: How to Discover and Enhance Your Body's Natural Ability to Maintain and Heal Itself.* New York: Random House, 2000.

OTHER USEFUL LINKS

Holosync Sound technology: www.centerpointe.com

M.E.L.T. fascial release method: www.meltmethod.com

There are many excellent resources for survivors of MTBI. The Betty Clooney Center has a list of TBI support groups (www.bcftbi.org). Also see Brainline (www.brainline.org) and Brain Injury Association of America (www.biausa.org). To explore alternatives for treating PTSD: tapping or EFT therapy (www.emofree.com) and EMDR (www.emdr.com).

There are also many excellent resources on meditation available. Good places to start are UCLA's Mindful Awareness Research Center (www.marc.ucla.edu), the conscious life (www.theconsciouslife.com) and Jon Kabat-Zinn's interview on YouTube (http://youtu.be/3nwwKbM_vJc).

Current guidelines on returning to play after a concussion can be found at the American Academy of Neurology's website: www.aan.com/concussion.

The National Center for Complementary and Alternative Medicine provides an overview of the benefits of tai chi and qigong at nccam.nih.gov/health/taichi and nccam.nih.gov/taxonomy/term/249.

Notes

For a more extensive bibliography of scholarly materials used in researching this book, see www.healingpainandinjury.com.

MEDICAL TEXTS

Chila, Anthony G. and American Osteopathic Association. *Foundations of Osteopathic Medicine*. 3rd ed. Philadelphia: Wolters Kluwer Health/Lippincott Williams & Wilkins, 2011.

DiGiovanna, Eileen L., Stanley Schiowitz, and Dennis J. Dowling. *An Osteopathic Approach to Diagnosis and Treatment*. 3rd ed. Philadelphia: Lippincott Williams & Wilkins, 2005.

Guyton, Arthur C. and John E. Hall. *Textbook of Medical Physiology*. 10th ed. Philadelphia: W.B. Saunders, 2000.

Kandel, Eric R. *Principles of Neural Science*. 5th ed. New York: McGraw-Hill, 2013.

Kapandji, I. A. *The Physiology of the Joints* [Physiologie articulaire.]. 6th English ed. Edinburgh; New York: Churchill Livingstone, 2007.

Kuchera, Michael L. and William A. Kuchera. *Osteopathic Considerations in Systemic Dysfunction*. Kirksville, MO: M.L. and W.A. Kuchera, 1990; 1991.

Magoun, Harold I. *Osteopathy in the Cranial Field*. 3rd ed. The Cranial Academy: 1976.

Murray, John F. and Robert J. Mason. *Murray and Nadel's Textbook of Respiratory Medicine*. 5th ed. Philadelphia: Saunders/Elsevier, 2010.

Seffinger, Michael A. and Raymond J. Hruby. *Evidence-Based Manual Medicine*. Philadelphia: Saunders/Elsevier, 2007.

Standring, Susan and Henry Gray. *Gray's Anatomy*. 40th anniversary ed. Edinburgh: Churchill Livingstone/Elsevier, 2008.

Weaver, Charlotte. *Charlotte Weaver: Pioneer in Cranial Osteopathy*. Edited by Margaret Sorrel. Indianapolis, IN: Cranial Academy Press, 2010.

Wheater, Paul R. *Basic Histopathology: A Colour Atlas and Text*. 2nd ed. Edinburgh; New York: Churchill Livingstone, 1991.

PART 1: REMOVING INJURY SHOCK

Agren, T., J. Engman, A. Frick, J. Bjorkstrand, E. M. Larsson, T. Furmark, and M. Fredrikson. "Disruption of Reconsolidation Erases a Fear Memory Trace in the Human Amygdala." *Science (New York, N.Y.)* 337, no. 6101 (Sep 21, 2012): 1550–52.

Bhavanani, A. B., Madanmohan, Z. Sanjay, and I. V. Basavaraddi. "Immediate Cardiovascular Effects of Pranava Pranayama in Hypertensive Patients." *Indian Journal of Physiology and Pharmacology* 56, no. 3 (Jul–Sep, 2012): 273–78.

Busillo, J. M. and J. A. Cidlowski. "The Five Rs of Glucocorticoid Action during Inflammation: Ready, Reinforce, Repress, Resolve, and Restore." *Trends in Endocrinology and Metabolism: TEM* 24, no. 3 (Mar, 2013): 109–119.

Cohen, S., D. Janicki-Deverts, W. J. Doyle, G. E. Miller, E. Frank, B. S. Rabin, and R. B. Turner. "Chronic Stress, Glucocorticoid Receptor Resistance, Inflammation, and Disease Risk." *Proceedings of the National Academy of Sciences of the United States of America* 109, no. 16 (Apr 17, 2012): 5995–99.

Field, T., M. Diego, and M. Hernandez-Reif. "Tai chi/yoga Effects on Anxiety, Heartrate, EEG and Math Computations." *Complementary Therapies in Clinical Practice* 16, no. 4 (Nov, 2010): 235–8.

Finnerty, C. C., N. T. Mabvuure, A. Ali, R. A. Kozar, and D. N. Herndon. "The Surgically Induced Stress Response." *Journal of Parenteral and Enteral Nutrition* 37, no. 5 Suppl (Sep–Oct, 2013): 21S–9S.

Jahnke, R., L. Larkey, C. Rogers, J. Etnier, and F. Lin. "A Comprehensive Review of Health Benefits of Qigong and Tai Chi." *American Journal of Health Promotion: AJHP* 24, no. 6 (Jul–Aug, 2010): e1–e25.

Kirby, E. D., A. C. Geraghty, T. Ubuka, G. E. Bentley, and D. Kaufer. "Stress Increases Putative Gonadotropin Inhibitory Hormone and Decreases Luteinizing Hormone in Male Rats." *Proceedings of the National Academy of Sciences of the United States of America* 106, no. 27 (Jul 7, 2009): 11324–29.

Kohn, David. *"Mindfulness and Meditation Training Could Ease PTSD Symptoms, Researchers Say."* www.washingtonpost.com, February 18, 2013.

McIntyre, C. K. and B. Roozendaal. "Adrenal Stress Hormones and Enhanced Memory for Emotionally Arousing Experiences." *Neural Plasticity and Memory: From Genes to Brain Imaging.* Edited by Bermudez-Rattoni, F. Boca Raton, FL: Taylor & Francis Group, 2007.

Mohamed, A., G. Wilson, W. Johnson, M. Tucci, J. A. Cameron, Z. Cason, and H. Benghuzzi. "The Effects of Sustained Delivery of Corticosterone on the Adrenal Gland of Male and Female Rats." *Biomedical Sciences Instrumentation* 49, (2013): 94–100.

Mori, H., H. Yamamoto, M. Kuwashima, S. Saito, H. Ukai, K. Hirao, M. Yamauchi, and S. Umemura. "How Does Deep Breathing Affect Office Blood Pressure and Pulse Rate?" *Hypertension Research: Official Journal of the Japanese Society of Hypertension* 28, no. 6 (Jun, 2005): 499–504.

Pena, D. F., N. D. Engineer, and C. K. McIntyre. "Rapid Remission of Conditioned Fear Expression with Extinction Training Paired with Vagus Nerve Stimulation." *Biological Psychiatry* 73, no. 11 (Jun 1, 2013): 1071–77.

Rees, B. "Overview of Outcome Data of Potential Meditation Training for Soldier Resilience." *Military Medicine* 176, no. 11 (Nov, 2011): 1232–42.

Shin, L. M. and I. Liberzon. "The Neurocircuitry of Fear, Stress, and Anxiety Disorders." *Neuropsychopharmacology: Official Publication of the American College of Neuropsychopharmacology* 35, no. 1 (Jan, 2010): 169–91.

Sinha, A. N., D. Deepak, and V. S. Gusain. "Assessment of the Effects of Pranayama/Alternate Nostril Breathing on the Parasympathetic Nervous System in Young Adults." *Journal of Clinical and Diagnostic Research: JCDR* 7, no. 5 (May, 2013): 821–23.

van Dixhoorn, J. and A. White. "Relaxation Therapy for Rehabilitation and Prevention in Ischaemic Heart Disease: A Systematic Review and Meta-Analysis." *European Journal of Cardiovascular Prevention and Rehabilitation: Official Journal of the European Society of Cardiology, Working Groups on Epidemiology & Prevention and Cardiac Rehabilitation and Exercise Physiology* 12, no. 3 (Jun, 2005): 193–202.

van Dixhoorn, J. J. and H. J. Duivenvoorden. "Effect of Relaxation Therapy on Cardiac Events After Myocardial Infarction: A 5-Year Follow-Up Study." *Journal of Cardiopulmonary Rehabilitation* 19, no. 3 (May–Jun, 1999): 178–85.

PART II: INFLAMMATION AND HEALING

Anglund, D. C. and M. K. Channell. "Contribution of Osteopathic Medicine to Care of Patients with Chronic Wounds." *The Journal of the American Osteopathic Association* 111, no. 9 (Sep, 2011): 538–42.

Bellingan, G. J., H. Caldwell, S. E. Howie, I. Dransfield, and C. Haslett. "In Vivo Fate of the Inflammatory Macrophage during the Resolution of Inflammation: Inflammatory Macrophages do Not Die Locally, but Emigrate to the Draining Lymph Nodes." *Journal of Immunology (Baltimore, MD: 1950)* 157, no. 6 (Sep 15, 1996): 2577–85.

Butterfield, T. A., T. M. Best, and M. A. Merrick. "The Dual Roles of Neutrophils and Macrophages in Inflammation: A Critical Balance between Tissue Damage and Repair." *Journal of Athletic Training* 41, no. 4 (Oct–Dec, 2006): 457–65.

Choi, I., S. Lee, and Y. K. Hong. "The New Era of the Lymphatic System: No Longer Secondary to the Blood Vascular System." *Cold Spring Harbor Perspectives in Medicine* 2, no. 4 (Apr, 2012): a006445.

Das, U. N. "Is Multiple Sclerosis a Proresolution Deficiency Disorder?" *Nutrition (Burbank, CA)* 28, no. 10 (Oct, 2012): 951–58.

Dhabhar, F. S., W. B. Malarkey, E. Neri, and B. S. McEwen. "Stress-Induced Redistribution of Immune Cells—from Barracks to Boulevards to Battlefields." *Psychoneuroendocrinology* 37, no. 9 (Sep, 2012): 1345–68.

Dixon, J. B. "Lymphatic Lipid Transport: Sewer Or Subway?" *Trends in Endocrinology and Metabolism: TEM* 21, no. 8 (Aug, 2010): 480–87.

Egger, G. "In Search of a Germ Theory Equivalent for Chronic Disease." *Preventing Chronic Disease* 9, (2012): E95.

Freire, M. O. and T. E. Van Dyke. "Natural Resolution of Inflammation." *Periodontology 2000* 63, no. 1 (Oct, 2013): 149–64.

Garcia-Romo, G. S., S. Caielli, B. Vega, J. Connolly, F. Allantaz, Z. Xu, M. Punaro, et al. "Netting Neutrophils are Major Inducers of Type I IFN Production in Pediatric Systemic Lupus Erythematosus." *Science Translational Medicine* 3, no. 73 (Mar 9, 2011): 73ra20.

Hodge, L. M., M. K. Bearden, A. Schander, J. B. Huff, A. Williams Jr, H. H. King, and H. F. Downey. "Lymphatic Pump Treatment Mobilizes Leukocytes from the Gut Associated Lymphoid Tissue into Lymph." *Lymphatic Research and Biology* 8, no. 2 (Jun, 2010): 103–10.

Huggenberger, R., S. S. Siddiqui, D. Brander, S. Ullmann, K. Zimmermann, M. Antsiferova, S. Werner, K. Alitalo, and M. Detmar. "An Important Role of Lymphatic Vessel Activation in Limiting Acute Inflammation." *Blood* 117, no. 17 (Apr 28, 2011): 4667–78.

Jaillon, S., M. R. Galdiero, D. Del Prete, M. A. Cassatella, C. Garlanda, and A. Mantovani. "Neutrophils in Innate and Adaptive Immunity." *Seminars in Immunopathology* 35, no. 4 (Jul, 2013): 377–94.

Jones, B. M. "Changes in Cytokine Production in Healthy Subjects Practicing Guolin Qigong: A Pilot Study." *BMC Complementary and Alternative Medicine* 1, (2001): 8.

Kashiwagi, S., K. Hosono, T. Suzuki, A. Takeda, E. Uchinuma, and M. Majima. "Role of COX-2 in Lymphangiogenesis and Restoration of Lymphatic Flow in Secondary Lymphedema." *Laboratory Investigation; a Journal of Technical Methods and Pathology* 91, no. 9 (Sep, 2011): 1314–25.

Kataru, R. P., K. Jung, C. Jang, H. Yang, R. A. Schwendener, J. E. Baik, S. H. Han, K. Alitalo, and G. Y. Koh. "Critical Role of CD11b+ Macrophages and VEGF in Inflammatory Lymphangiogenesis, Antigen Clearance, and Inflammation Resolution." *Blood* 113, no. 22 (May 28, 2009): 5650–59.

Kumar, R K, and D Wakefield. "Inflammation: Chronic." *Encyclopedia of Life Sciences.* John Wiley & Sons Ltd, Chichester. September 2010.

Lawrence, T. and D. W. Gilroy. "Chronic Inflammation: A Failure of Resolution?" *International Journal of Experimental Pathology* 88, no. 2 (Apr, 2007): 85–94.

Lech, M. and H. J. Anders. "Macrophages and Fibrosis: How Resident and Infiltrating Mononuclear Phagocytes Orchestrate all Phases of Tissue Injury and Repair." *Biochimica Et Biophysica Acta* 1832, no. 7 (Jul, 2013): 989–97.

Li, Q. Z., P. Li, G. E. Garcia, R. J. Johnson, and L. Feng. "Genomic Profiling of Neutrophil Transcripts in Asian Qigong Practitioners: A Pilot Study in Gene Regulation by Mind-Body Interaction." *Journal of Alternative and Complementary Medicine (New York, N.Y.)* 11, no. 1 (Feb, 2005): 29–39.

Lin, C. L., C. P. Lin, and S. Y. Lien. "The Effect of Tai Chi for Blood Pressure, Blood Sugar, Blood Lipid Control for Patients with Chronic Diseases: A Systematic Review." *Hu Li Za Zhi: the Journal of Nursing* 60, no. 1 (Feb, 2013): 69–77.

Marwick, J. A., D. A. Dorward, C. D. Lucas, K. O. Jones, T. A. Sheldrake, S. Fox, C. Ward, et al. "Oxygen Levels Determine the Ability of Glucocorticoids to Influence Neutrophil Survival in Inflammatory Environments." *Journal of Leukocyte Biology* (Aug 20, 2013).

Mittal, A., V. Ranganath, and A. Nichani. "Omega Fatty Acids and Resolution of Inflammation: A New Twist in an Old Tale." *Journal of Indian Society of Periodontology* 14, no. 1 (Jan, 2010): 3–7.

Musk, P. "Unfulfilled Inflammatory Resolution Leads to Chronic Inflammatory Diseases." *Discovery Medicine* 4, no. 22 (Jun, 2004): 191-193.

Narahari, S. R., T. J. Ryan, K. S. Bose, K. S. Prasanna, and G. M. Aggithaya. "Integrating Modern Dermatology and Ayurveda in the Treatment of Vitiligo and Lymphedema in India." *International Journal of Dermatology* 50, no. 3 (Mar, 2011): 310–34.

Podgrabinska, S., O. Kamalu, L. Mayer, M. Shimaoka, H. Snoeck, G. J. Randolph, and M. Skobe. "Inflamed Lymphatic Endothelium Suppresses Dendritic Cell Maturation and Function Via Mac-1/ICAM-1-Dependent Mechanism." *Journal of Immunology (Baltimore, MD: 1950)* 183, no. 3 (Aug 1, 2009): 1767–79.

Rydell-Tormanen, K., L. Uller, and J. S. Erjefalt. "Direct Evidence of Secondary Necrosis of Neutrophils during Intense Lung Inflammation." *The European Respiratory Journal* 28, no. 2 (Aug, 2006): 268–74.

Saggio, G., S. Docimo, J. Pilc, J. Norton, and W. Gilliar. "Impact of Osteopathic Manipulative Treatment on Secretory Immunoglobulin A Levels in a Stressed Population." *The Journal of the American Osteopathic Association* 111, no. 3 (Mar, 2011): 143–47.

Savill, J. and V. Fadok. "Corpse Clearance Defines the Meaning of Cell Death." *Nature* 407, no. 6805 (Oct 12, 2000): 784–88.

Serhan, C. N. "Resolution Phase Lipid Mediators of Inflammation: Agonists of Resolution." *Current Opinion in Pharmacology* 13, no. 4 (Aug, 2013): 632–40.

Serhan, C. N. and J. Savill. "Resolution of Inflammation: The Beginning Programs the End." *Nature Immunology* 6, no. 12 (Dec, 2005): 1191–97.

Silva, M.T. "When Two is Better than One: Macrophages and Neutrophils Work in Concert in Innate Immunity as Complementary and Cooperative Partners of a Myeloid Phagocyte System." *Journal of Leukocyte Biology* 87, no. 1 (Jan, 2010): 93–106.

Silva, M. T. and M. Correia-Neves. "Neutrophils and Macrophages: The Main Partners of Phagocyte Cell Systems." *Frontiers in Immunology* 3, (2012): 174.

Wang, Y. and G. Oliver. "Current Views on the Function of the Lymphatic Vasculature in Health and Disease." *Genes & Development* 24, no. 19 (Oct 1, 2010): 2115–26.

Zgraggen, S., A. M. Ochsenbein, and M. Detmar. "An Important Role of Blood and Lymphatic Vessels in Inflammation and Allergy." *Journal of Allergy* 2013, (2013): 672381.

Zhou, Q., R. Guo, R. Wood, B. F. Boyce, Q. Liang, Y. J. Wang, E. M. Schwarz, and L. Xing. "Vascular Endothelial Growth Factor C Attenuates Joint Damage in Chronic Inflammatory Arthritis by Accelerating Local Lymphatic Drainage in Mice." *Arthritis and Rheumatism* 63, no. 8 (Aug, 2011): 2318–28.

PART II: FOOD IS THE BEST MEDICINE

Alexander, J. C. "Chemical and Biological Properties Related to Toxicity of Heated Fats." *Journal of Toxicology and Environmental Health* 7, no. 1 (Jan, 1981): 125–38.

Barnett, M. P., J. M. Cooney, Y. E. Dommels, K. Nones, D. T. Brewster, Z. Park, C. A. Butts, W. C. McNabb, W. A. Laing, and N. C. Roy. "Modulation of Colonic Inflammation in Mdr1a(-/-) Mice by Green Tea Polyphenols and their Effects on the Colon Transcriptome and Proteome." *The Journal of Nutritional Biochemistry* 24, no. 10 (Oct, 2013): 1678–90.

Bray, G. A. "Soft Drink Consumption and Obesity: It is All About Fructose." *Current Opinion in Lipidology* 21, no. 1 (Feb, 2010): 51–57.

Bruunsgaard, H. "Physical Activity and Modulation of Systemic Low-Level Inflammation." *Journal of Leukocyte Biology* 78, no. 4 (Oct, 2005): 819–35.

de Koning, L., V. S. Malik, M. D. Kellogg, E. B. Rimm, W. C. Willett, and F. B. Hu. "Sweetened Beverage Consumption, Incident Coronary Heart Disease, and Biomarkers of Risk in Men." *Circulation* 125, no. 14 (Apr 10, 2012): 1735–41, S1.

Drewnowski, A. and C. D. Rehm. "Energy Intakes of US Children and Adults by Food Purchase Location and by Specific Food Source." *Nutrition Journal* 12, (May 8, 2013): 59-2891-12-59.

Ebbeling, C. B., J. F. Swain, H. A. Feldman, W. W. Wong, D. L. Hachey, E. Garcia-Lago, and D. S. Ludwig. "Effects of Dietary Composition on Energy Expenditure during Weight-Loss Maintenance." *JAMA: The Journal of the American Medical Association* 307, no. 24 (Jun 27, 2012): 2627–34.

Enig, M. G., S. Atal, M. Keeney, and J. Sampugna. "Isomeric Trans Fatty Acids in the U.S. Diet." *Journal of the American College of Nutrition* 9, no. 5 (Oct, 1990): 471–86.

Hamburg, N. M., C. J. McMackin, A. L. Huang, S. M. Shenouda, M. E. Widlansky, E. Schulz, N. Gokce, N. B. Ruderman, J. F. Keaney Jr, and J. A. Vita. "Physical Inactivity Rapidly Induces Insulin Resistance and Microvascular Dysfunction in Healthy Volunteers." *Arteriosclerosis, Thrombosis, and Vascular Biology* 27, no. 12 (Dec, 2007): 2650–56.

Jonnalagadda, S. S., L. Harnack, R. H. Liu, N. McKeown, C. Seal, S. Liu, and G. C. Fahey. "Putting the Whole Grain Puzzle Together: Health Benefits Associated with Whole Grains." *The Journal of Nutrition* 141, no. 5 (May, 2011): 1011S–22S.

Kohli, R., M. Kirby, S. A. Xanthakos, S. Softic, A. E. Feldstein, V. Saxena, P. H. Tang, et al. "High-Fructose, Medium Chain Trans Fat Diet Induces Liver Fibrosis and Elevates Plasma Coenzyme Q9 in a Novel Murine Model of Obesity and Nonalcoholic Steatohepatitis." *Hepatology (Baltimore, MD)* 52, no. 3 (Sep, 2010): 934–44.

La Berge, A. F. "How the Ideology of Low Fat Conquered America." *Journal of the History of Medicine and Allied Sciences* 63, no. 2 (Apr, 2008): 139–77.

Levitan, E. B., N. R. Cook, M. J. Stampfer, P. M. Ridker, K. M. Rexrode, J. E. Buring, J. E. Manson, and S. Liu. "Dietary Glycemic Index, Dietary Glycemic Load, Blood Lipids, and C-Reactive Protein." *Metabolism: Clinical and Experimental* 57, no. 3 (Mar, 2008): 437–43.

Lin, W. T., H. L. Huang, M. C. Huang, T. F. Chan, S. Y. Ciou, C. Y. Lee, Y. W. Chiu, et al. "Effects on Uric Acid, Body Mass Index and Blood Pressure in Adolescents of Consuming Beverages Sweetened with High-Fructose Corn Syrup." *International Journal of Obesity (2005)* 37, no. 4 (Apr, 2013): 532–39.

Morris, M. S., L. Sakakeeny, P. F. Jacques, M. F. Picciano, and J. Selhub. "Vitamin B-6 Intake is Inversely Related to, and the Requirement is Affected by, Inflammation Status." *The Journal of Nutrition* 140, no. 1 (Jan, 2010): 103–10.

Poudyal, H., S. K. Panchal, L. C. Ward, J. Waanders, and L. Brown. "Chronic High-Carbohydrate, High-Fat Feeding in Rats Induces Reversible Metabolic, Cardiovascular, and Liver Changes." *American Journal of Physiology. Endocrinology and Metabolism* 302, no. 12 (Jun 15, 2012): E1472–82.

Shaik-Dasthagirisaheb, Y. B., G. Varvara, G. Murmura, A. Saggini, A. Caraffa, P. Antinolfi, S. Tete, et al. "Role of Vitamins D, E and C in Immunity and Inflammation." *Journal of Biological Regulators and Homeostatic Agents* 27, no. 2 (Apr-Jun, 2013): 291–95.

Spreadbury, I. "Comparison with Ancestral Diets Suggests Dense Acellular Carbohydrates Promote an Inflammatory Microbiota, and may be the Primary Dietary Cause of Leptin Resistance and Obesity." *Diabetes, Metabolic Syndrome and Obesity: Targets and Therapy* 5, (2012): 175–89.

Swithers, S. E. "Artificial Sweeteners Produce the Counterintuitive Effect of Inducing Metabolic Derangements." *Trends in Endocrinology and Metabolism: TEM* 24, no. 9 (Sep, 2013): 431–41.

Vanhees, K., I. G. Vonhogen, F. J. van Schooten, and R. W. Godschalk. "You Are What You Eat, and So Are Your Children: The Impact of Micronutrients on the Epigenetic Programming of Offspring." *Cellular and Molecular Life Sciences: CMLS* (Jul 27, 2013).

PART III: RESTORING MOTION

Baltazar, G. A., M. P. Betler, K. Akella, R. Khatri, R. Asaro, and A. Chendrasekhar. "Effect of Osteopathic Manipulative Treatment on Incidence of Postoperative Ileus and Hospital Length of Stay in General Surgical Patients." *The Journal of the American Osteopathic Association* 113, no. 3 (Mar, 2013): 204–9.

Burra, P. "Liver Abnormalities and Endocrine Diseases." *Best Practice & Research. Clinical Gastroenterology* 27, no. 4 (Aug, 2013): 553–63.

Cacioppo, S., F. Bianchi-Demicheli, C. Frum, J. G. Pfaus, and J. W. Lewis. "The Common Neural Bases between Sexual Desire and Love: A Multilevel Kernel Density fMRI Analysis." *The Journal of Sexual Medicine* 9, no. 4 (Apr, 2012): 1048–54.

Carlsson, A., A. Linder, J. Davidsson, W. Hell, S. Schick, and M. Svensson. "Dynamic Kinematic Responses of Female Volunteers in Rear Impacts and Comparison to Previous Male Volunteer Tests." *Traffic Injury Prevention* 12, no. 4 (Aug, 2011): 347-357.

Croft, A. C. and M. D. Freeman. "Correlating Crash Severity with Injury Risk, Injury Severity, and Long-Term Symptoms in Low Velocity Motor Vehicle Collisions." *Medical Science Monitor: International Medical Journal of Experimental and Clinical Research* 11, no. 10 (Oct, 2005): RA316–21.

Foreman, Stephen M. and Arthur C. Croft. *Whiplash Injuries: The Cervical Acceleration/Deceleration Syndrome*, 3rd ed. Philadelphia: Lippincott Williams & Wilkins, 2002.

Franke, H. and K. Hoesele. "Osteopathic Manipulative Treatment (OMT) for Lower Urinary Tract Symptoms (LUTS) in Women." *Journal of Bodywork and Movement Therapies* 17, no. 1 (Jan, 2013): 11–18.

Giles, P. D., K. L. Hensel, C. F. Pacchia, and M. L. Smith. "Suboccipital Decompression Enhances Heart Rate Variability Indices of Cardiac Control in Healthy Subjects." *Journal of Alternative and Complementary Medicine (New York, N.Y.)* 19, no. 2 (Feb, 2013): 92–96.

Ivancic, P. C. and M. Xiao. "Cervical Spine Curvature during Simulated Rear Crashes with Energy-Absorbing Seat." *The Spine Journal: Official Journal of the North American Spine Society* 11, no. 3 (Mar, 2011): 224–33.

Kolar, P., J. Sulc, M. Kyncl, J. Sanda, O. Cakrt, R. Andel, K. Kumagai, and A. Kobesova. "Postural Function of the Diaphragm in Persons with and without Chronic Low Back Pain." *The Journal of Orthopaedic and Sports Physical Therapy* 42, no. 4 (Apr, 2012): 352–62.

Kramp, M. E. "Combined Manual Therapy Techniques for the Treatment of Women with Infertility: A Case Series." *The Journal of the American Osteopathic Association* 112, no. 10 (Oct, 2012): 680–84.

Licciardone, J. C. and S. Aryal. "Prevention of Progressive Back-Specific Dysfunction during Pregnancy: An Assessment of Osteopathic Manual Treatment Based on Cochrane Back Review Group Criteria." *The Journal of the American Osteopathic Association* 113, no. 10 (Oct, 2013): 728–36.

Licciardone, J. C., C. M. Kearns, and D. E. Minotti. "Outcomes of Osteopathic Manual Treatment for Chronic Low Back Pain According to Baseline Pain Severity: Results from the Osteopathic Trial." *Manual Therapy* (Jun 8, 2013).

Lundberg, P. O. and B. Hulter. "Sexual Dysfunction in Patients with Hypothalamo-Pituitary Disorders." *Experimental and Clinical Endocrinology* 98, no. 2 (1991): 81–88.

Marx, S., U. Cimniak, M. Rutz, and K. L. Resch. "Long-Term Effects of Osteopathic Treatment of Chronic Prostatitis with Chronic Pelvic Pain Syndrome: A 5-Year Follow-Up of a Randomized Controlled Trial and Considerations on the Pathophysiological Context." *Der Urologe.Ausg.A* 52, no. 3 (Mar, 2013): 384–90.

Noll, D. R., J. H. Shores, R. G. Gamber, K. M. Herron, and J. Swift Jr. "Benefits of Osteopathic Manipulative Treatment for Hospitalized Elderly Patients with Pneumonia." *The Journal of the American Osteopathic Association* 100, no. 12 (Dec, 2000): 776–82.

Parker, J., K. P. Heinking, and R. E. Kappler. "Efficacy of Osteopathic Manipulative Treatment for Low Back Pain in Euhydrated and Hypohydrated Conditions: A Randomized Crossover Trial." *The Journal of the American Osteopathic Association* 112, no. 5 (May, 2012): 276–84.

Richmond, T. S., J. D. Amsterdam, W. Guo, T. Ackerson, V. Gracias, K. M. Robinson, and J. E. Hollander. "The Effect of Post-Injury Depression on Return to Pre-Injury Function: A Prospective Cohort Study." *Psychological Medicine* 39, no. 10 (Oct, 2009): 1709–20.

Riley, G. W. "Osteopathic Success in the Treatment of Influenza and Pneumonia, 1919." *The Journal of the American Osteopathic Association* 100, no. 5 (May, 2000): 315–19.

Rowland, D. L. "Neurobiology of Sexual Response in Men and Women." *CNS Spectrums* 11, no. 8 Suppl 9 (Aug, 2006): 6–12.

Schwerla, F., A. K. Kaiser, R. Gietz, and R. Kastner. "Osteopathic Treatment of Patients with Long-Term Sequelae of Whiplash Injury: Effect on Neck Pain Disability and Quality of Life." *Journal of Alternative and Complementary Medicine (New York, N.Y.)* 19, no. 6 (Jun, 2013): 543–49.

Smith, M. D., A. Russell, and P. W. Hodges.. "The Relationship between Incontinence, Breathing Disorders, Gastrointestinal Symptoms, and Back Pain in Women: A Longitudinal Cohort Study." *The Clinical Journal of Pain* (Mar 12, 2013).

Stemper, B. D., N. Yoganandan, F. A. Pintar, and D. J. Maiman. "The Relationship between Lower Neck Shear Force and Facet Joint Kinematics during Automotive Rear Impacts." *Clinical Anatomy (New York, NY)* 24, no. 3 (Apr, 2011): 319–26.

Thomas, L. C., D. A. Rivett, G. Bateman, P. Stanwell, and C. R. Levi. "Effect of Selected Manual Therapy Interventions for Mechanical Neck Pain on Vertebral and Internal Carotid Arterial Blood Flow and Cerebral Inflow." *Physical Therapy* (Jun 27, 2013).

Tozzi, P., D. Bongiorno, and C. Vitturini. "Fascial Release Effects on Patients with Non-Specific Cervical or Lumbar Pain." *Journal of Bodywork and Movement Therapies* 15, no. 4 (Oct, 2011): 405–16.

Vleeming, A., A. L. Pool-Goudzwaard, D. Hammudoghlu, R. Stoeckart, C. J. Snijders, and J. M. Mens. "The Function of the Long Dorsal Sacroiliac Ligament: Its Implication for Understanding Low Back Pain." *Spine* 21, no. 5 (Mar 1, 1996): 556–62.

Willard, F. H., A. Vleeming, M. D. Schuenke, L. Danneels, and R. Schleip. "The Thoracolumbar Fascia: Anatomy, Function and Clinical Considerations." *Journal of Anatomy* 221, no. 6 (Dec, 2012): 507–36.

PART IV: HEALING BRAIN INJURY

Aguzzi, A., B. A. Barres, and M. L. Bennett. "Microglia: Scapegoat, Saboteur, or Something Else?" *Science (New York, NY)* 339, no. 6116 (Jan 11, 2013): 156–61.

Amenta, P. S., J. I. Jallo, R. F. Tuma, and M. B. Elliott. "A Cannabinoid Type 2 Receptor Agonist Attenuates Blood-Brain Barrier Damage and Neurodegeneration in a Murine Model of Traumatic Brain Injury." *Journal of Neuroscience Research* 90, no. 12 (Dec, 2012): 2293–2305.

Annweiler, C., B. Brugg, J. M. Peyrin, R. Bartha, and O. Beauchet. "Combination of Memantine and Vitamin D Prevents Axon Degeneration Induced by Amyloid-Beta and Glutamate." *Neurobiology of Aging* (Sep 4, 2013).

Arbogast, K. B., A. D. McGinley, C. L. Master, M. F. Grady, R. L. Robinson, and M. R. Zonfrillo. "Cognitive Rest and School-Based Recommendations Following Pediatric Concussion: The Need for Primary Care Support Tools." *Clinical Pediatrics* 52, no. 5 (May, 2013): 397–402.

Arenth, P. M., K. C. Russell, J. M. Scanlon, L. J. Kessler, and J. H. Ricker. "Corpus Callosum Integrity and Neuropsychological Performance After Traumatic Brain Injury: A Diffusion Tensor Imaging Study." *The Journal of Head Trauma Rehabilitation* (Apr 3, 2013).

Babikian, T., P. Satz, K. Zaucha, R. Light, R. S. Lewis, and R. F. Asarnow. "The UCLA Longitudinal Study of Neurocognitive Outcomes Following Mild Pediatric Traumatic Brain Injury." *Journal of the International Neuropsychological Society* 17, no. 5 (Sep, 2011): 886–95.

Bailes, J. E., A. L. Petraglia, B. I. Omalu, E. Nauman, and T. Talavage. "Role of Subconcussion in Repetitive Mild Traumatic Brain Injury." *Journal of Neurosurgery* (Aug 23, 2013).

Barkhoudarian, G., D. A. Hovda, and C. C. Giza. "The Molecular Pathophysiology of Concussive Brain Injury." *Clinics in Sports Medicine* 30, no. 1 (Jan, 2011): 33–48, vii-iii.

Barreto, G. E., J. Gonzalez, Y. Torres, and L. Morales. "Astrocytic-Neuronal Crosstalk: Implications for Neuroprotection from Brain Injury." *Neuroscience Research* 71, no. 2 (Oct, 2011): 107–13.

Bigler, E. D. "Neuroinflammation and the Dynamic Lesion in Traumatic Brain Injury." *Brain: A Journal of Neurology* 136, no. Pt 1 (Jan, 2013): 9–11.

Bouzat, P., N. Sala, J. F. Payen, and M. Oddo. "Beyond Intracranial Pressure: Optimization of Cerebral Blood Flow, Oxygen, and Substrate Delivery After Traumatic Brain Injury." *Annals of Intensive Care* 3, no. 1 (Jul 10, 2013): 23-5820-3-23.

Chen, G., L. Go, and B. Mao. "Biomechanical Mechanism of Diffuse Axonal Injury." *Sheng Wu Yi Xue Gong Cheng Xue Za Zhi (Journal of Biomedical Engineering)* 19, no. 3 (Sep, 2002): 500–04.

Chovanes, G. I. and R. M. Richards. "The Predominance of Metabolic Regulation of Cerebral Blood Flow and the Lack of 'Classic' Autoregulation Curves in the Viable Brain." *Surgical Neurology International* 3, (2012): 12-7806.92185. Epub 2012 Jan 21.

Clapham, R., E. O'Sullivan, R. O. Weller, and R. O. Carare. "Cervical Lymph Nodes are Found in Direct Relationship with the Internal Carotid Artery: Significance for the Lymphatic Drainage of the Brain." *Clinical Anatomy (New York, NY)* 23, no. 1 (Jan, 2010): 43–47.

Clarke, C. B., M. R. Suter, and R. D. Gosselin. "Glial Cells and Chronic Pain: From the Laboratory to Clinical Hope." *Revue Medicale Suisse* 9, no. 392 (Jun 26, 2013): 1342–45.

Du, B., A. Shan, Y. Zhang, X. Zhong, D. Chen, and K. Cai. "Zolpidem Arouses Patients in Vegetative State After Brain Injury: Quantitative Evaluation and Indications." *The American Journal of the Medical Sciences* (Mar 4, 2013).

Finnie, J. W. "Neuroinflammation: Beneficial and Detrimental Effects After Traumatic Brain Injury." *Inflammopharmacology* 21, no. 4 (Aug, 2013): 309–20.

Flygt, J., A. Djupsjo, F. Lenne, and N. Marklund. "Myelin Loss and Oligodendrocyte Pathology in White Matter Tracts Following Traumatic Brain Injury in the Rat." *The European Journal of Neuroscience* 38, no. 1 (Jul, 2013): 2153–65.

Gatson, J. W., V. Warren, K. Abdelfattah, S. Wolf, L. S. Hynan, C. Moore, R. Diaz-Arrastia, J. P. Minei, C. Madden, and J. G. Wigginton. "Detection of Beta-Amyloid Oligomers as a Predictor of Neurological Outcome After Brain Injury." *Journal of Neurosurgery* 118, no. 6 (Jun, 2013): 1336–42.

Gillette-Guyonnet, S., M. Secher, and B. Vellas. "Nutrition and Neurodegeneration: Epidemiological Evidence and Challenges for Future Research." *British Journal of Clinical Pharmacology* 75, no. 3 (Mar, 2013): 738–55.

Hellewell, S. C. and M. C. Morganti-Kossmann. "Guilty Molecules, Guilty Minds? The Conflicting Roles of the Innate Immune Response to Traumatic Brain Injury." *Mediators of Inflammation* 2012, (2012): 356494.

Hernandez-Ontiveros, D. G., N. Tajiri, S. Acosta, B. Giunta, J. Tan, and C. V. Borlongan. "Microglia Activation as a Biomarker for Traumatic Brain Injury." *Frontiers in Neurology* 4, (2013): 30.

Hessen, E., V. Anderson, and K. Nestvold. "MMPI-2 Profiles 23 Years After Paediatric Mild Traumatic Brain Injury." *Brain Injury* 22, no. 1 (Jan, 2008): 39–50.

Ho, A. J., C. A. Raji, J. T. Becker, O. L. Lopez, L. H. Kuller, X. Hua, I. D. Dinov, et al. "The Effects of Physical Activity, Education, and Body Mass Index on the Aging Brain." *Human Brain Mapping* 32, no. 9 (Sep, 2011): 1371–82.

Huston, J. M. "The Vagus Nerve and the Inflammatory Reflex: Wandering on a New Treatment Paradigm for Systemic Inflammation and Sepsis." *Surgical Infections* 13, no. 4 (Aug, 2012): 187–93.

Iliff, J. J., H. Lee, M. Yu, T. Feng, J. Logan, M. Nedergaard, and H. Benveniste. "Brain-Wide Pathway for Waste Clearance Captured by Contrast-Enhanced MRI." *The Journal of Clinical Investigation* 123, no. 3 (Mar 1, 2013): 1299–1309.

Iliff, J. J. and M. Nedergaard. "Is there a Cerebral Lymphatic System?" *Stroke; a Journal of Cerebral Circulation* 44, no. 6 Suppl 1 (Jun, 2013): S93–5.

Iliff, J. J., M. Wang, Y. Liao, B. A. Plogg, W. Peng, G. A. Gundersen, H. Benveniste, et al. "A Paravascular Pathway Facilitates CSF Flow through the Brain Parenchyma and the Clearance of Interstitial Solutes, Including Amyloid Beta." *Science Translational Medicine* 4, no. 147 (Aug 15, 2012): 147ra111.

Johanson, C. E., J. A. Duncan 3rd, P. M. Klinge, T. Brinker, E. G. Stopa, and G. D. Silverberg. "Multiplicity of Cerebrospinal Fluid Functions: New Challenges in Health and Disease." *Cerebrospinal Fluid Research* 5, (May 14, 2008): 10-8454-5-10.

Johnson, V. E., J. E. Stewart, F. D. Begbie, J. Q. Trojanowski, D. H. Smith, and W. Stewart. "Inflammation and White Matter Degeneration Persist for Years After a Single Traumatic Brain Injury." *Brain: A Journal of Neurology* 136, no. Pt 1 (Jan, 2013): 28–42.

Johnson, V. E., W. Stewart, and D. H. Smith. "Axonal Pathology in Traumatic Brain Injury." *Experimental Neurology* 246, (Aug, 2013): 35–43.

Kao, C., J. A. Forbes, W. J. Jermakowicz, D. A. Sun, B. Davis, J. Zhu, A. H. Lagrange, and P. E. Konrad. "Suppression of Thalamocortical Oscillations Following Traumatic Brain Injury in Rats." *Journal of Neurosurgery* 117, no. 2 (Aug, 2012): 316–23.

Koh, L., G. Nagra, and M. Johnston. "Properties of the Lymphatic Cerebrospinal Fluid Transport System in the Rat: Impact of Elevated Intracranial Pressure." *Journal of Vascular Research* 44, no. 5 (2007): 423–32.

Lam, L. C., R. C. Chau, B. M. Wong, A. W. Fung, V. W. Lui, C. C. Tam, G. T. Leung, et al. "Interim Follow-Up of a Randomized Controlled Trial Comparing Chinese Style Mind Body (Tai Chi) and Stretching Exercises on Cognitive Function in Subjects at Risk of Progressive Cognitive Decline." *International Journal of Geriatric Psychiatry* 26, no. 7 (Jul, 2011): 733–40.

Laman, J. D. and R. O. Weller. "Drainage of Cells and Soluble Antigen from the CNS to Regional Lymph Nodes." *Journal of Neuroimmune Pharmacology: The Official Journal of the Society on NeuroImmune Pharmacology* 8, no. 4 (Sep, 2013): 840–56.

Lewis, M., P. Ghassemi, and J. Hibbeln. "Therapeutic use of Omega-3 Fatty Acids in Severe Head Trauma." *The American Journal of Emergency Medicine* 31, no. 1 (Jan, 2013): 273.e5-273.e8.

Lewis, M. D. and J. Bailes. "Neuroprotection for the Warrior: Dietary Supplementation with Omega-3 Fatty Acids." *Military Medicine* 176, no. 10 (Oct, 2011): 1120–27.

Lim, S. W., C. C. Wang, Y. H. Wang, C. C. Chio, K. C. Niu, and J. R. Kuo. "Microglial Activation Induced by Traumatic Brain Injury is Suppressed by Postinjury Treatment with Hyperbaric Oxygen Therapy." *The Journal of Surgical Research* 184, no. 2 (Oct, 2013): 1076–84.

Lobanov, O. V., F. Zeidan, J. G. McHaffie, R. A. Kraft, and R. C. Coghill. "From Cue to Meaning: Brain Mechanisms Supporting the Construction of Expectations of Pain." *Pain* (Sep 17, 2013).

Lopez, N. E., M. J. Krzyzaniak, T. W. Costantini, J. Putnam, A. M. Hageny, B. Eliceiri, R. Coimbra, and V. Bansal. "Vagal Nerve Stimulation Decreases Blood-Brain Barrier Disruption After Traumatic Brain Injury." *The Journal of Trauma and Acute Care Surgery* 72, no. 6 (Jun, 2012): 1562–66.

Masel, B. E. and D. S. DeWitt. "Traumatic Brain Injury: A Disease Process, Not an Event." *Journal of Neurotrauma* 27, no. 8 (Aug, 2010): 1529–40.

McPartland, J.M. "The Endocannabinoid System: An Osteopathic Perspective." *The Journal of the American Osteopathic Association* 108 no. 10 (Oct. 2008): 586–600.

Men, W., D. Falk, T. Sun, W. Chen, J. Li, D. Yin, L. Zang, and M. Fan. "The Corpus Callosum of Albert Einstein's Brain: Another Clue to His High Intelligence?" *Brain: A Journal of Neurology* (Sep 24, 2013).

Mollanji, R., R. Bozanovic-Sosic, I. Silver, B. Li, C. Kim, R. Midha, and M. Johnston. "Intracranial Pressure Accommodation is Impaired by Blocking Pathways Leading to Extracranial Lymphatics." *American Journal of Physiology–Regulatory, Integrative and Comparative Physiology* 280, no. 5 (May, 2001): R1573–81.

Monti, J. M., M. W. Voss, A. Pence, E. McAuley, A. F. Kramer, and N. J. Cohen. "History of Mild Traumatic Brain Injury is Associated with Deficits in Relational Memory, Reduced Hippocampal Volume, and Less Neural Activity Later in Life." *Frontiers in Aging Neuroscience* 5, (Aug 22, 2013): 41.

Mortimer, J. A., D. Ding, A. R. Borenstein, C. DeCarli, Q. Guo, Y. Wu, Q. Zhao, and S. Chu. "Changes in Brain Volume and Cognition in a Randomized Trial of Exercise and Social Interaction in a Community-Based Sample of Non-Demented Chinese Elders." *Journal of Alzheimer's Disease* 30, no. 4 (2012): 757–66.

Nedergaard, M. "Neuroscience. Garbage Truck of the Brain." *Science (New York, NY)* 340, no. 6140 (Jun 28, 2013): 1529–30.

Orsu, P., B. V. Murthy, and A. Akula. "Cerebroprotective Potential of Resveratrol through Anti-Oxidant and Anti-Inflammatory Mechanisms in Rats." *Journal of Neural Transmission (Vienna, Austria: 1996)* 120, no. 8 (Aug, 2013): 1217–23.

Peng, P. W. "Tai Chi and Chronic Pain." *Regional Anesthesia and Pain Medicine* 37, no. 4 (Jul–Aug, 2012): 372–82.

Perry, E. and M. J. Howes. "Medicinal Plants and Dementia Therapy: Herbal Hopes for Brain Aging?" *CNS Neuroscience & Therapeutics* 17, no. 6 (Dec, 2011): 683–98.

Piao, C. S., B. A. Stoica, J. Wu, B. Sabirzhanov, Z. Zhao, R. Cabatbat, D. J. Loane, and A. I. Faden. "Late Exercise Reduces Neuroinflammation and

Cognitive Dysfunction After Traumatic Brain Injury." *Neurobiology of Disease* 54, (Jun, 2013): 252–63.

Pomschar, A., I. Koerte, S. Lee, R. P. Laubender, A. Straube, F. Heinen, B. Ertl-Wagner, and N. Alperin. "MRI Evidence for Altered Venous Drainage and Intracranial Compliance in Mild Traumatic Brain Injury." *PloS One* 8, no. 2 (2013): e55447.

Pop, V. and J. Badaut. "A Neurovascular Perspective for Long-Term Changes After Brain Trauma." *Translational Stroke Research* 2, no. 4 (Dec 1, 2011): 533–45.

Rangroo Thrane, V., A. S. Thrane, B. A. Plog, M. Thiyagarajan, J. J. Iliff, R. Deane, E. A. Nagelhus, and M. Nedergaard. "Paravascular Microcirculation Facilitates Rapid Lipid Transport and Astrocyte Signaling in the Brain." *Scientific Reports* 3, (Sep 4, 2013): 2582.

Sabet, A. A., E. Christoforou, B. Zatlin, G. M. Genin, and P. V. Bayly. "Deformation of the Human Brain Induced by Mild Angular Head Acceleration." *Journal of Biomechanics* 41, no. 2 (2008): 307–15.

Sharma, S., Z. Ying, and F. Gomez-Pinilla. "A Pyrazole Curcumin Derivative Restores Membrane Homeostasis Disrupted After Brain Trauma." *Experimental Neurology* 226, no. 1 (Nov, 2010): 191–99.

Shiramizu, H., A. Masuko, H. Ishizaka, M. Shibata, H. Atsumi, M. Imai, T. Osada, Y. Mizokami, T. Baba, and M. Matsumae. "Mechanism of Injury to the Corpus Callosum, with Particular Reference to the Anatomical Relationship between Site of Injury and Adjacent Brain Structures." *Neurologia Medico-Chirurgica* 48, no. 1 (Jan, 2008): 1–7.

Sofroniew, M. V. "Multiple Roles for Astrocytes as Effectors of Cytokines and Inflammatory Mediators." *The Neuroscientist: A Review Journal Bringing Neurobiology, Neurology and Psychiatry* (Oct 8, 2013).

Stern, R. A., D. O. Riley, D. H. Daneshvar, C. J. Nowinski, R. C. Cantu, and A. C. McKee. "Long-Term Consequences of Repetitive Brain Trauma: Chronic Traumatic Encephalopathy." *PM & R: The Journal of Injury, Function, and Rehabilitation* 3, no. 10 Suppl 2 (Oct, 2011): S460-7.

Sun, B. L., Z. L. Xia, Z. W. Yan, Y. S. Chen, and M. F. Yang. "Effects of Blockade of Cerebral Lymphatic Drainage on Cerebral Ischemia After Middle Cerebral Artery Occlusion in Rats." *Clinical Hemorheology and Microcirculation* 23, no. 2-4 (2000): 321–25.

Sword, J., T. Masuda, D. Croom, and S. A. Kirov. "Evolution of Neuronal and Astroglial Disruption in the Peri-Contusional Cortex of Mice Revealed by in Vivo Two-Photon Imaging." *Brain: A Journal of Neurology* 136, no. Pt 5 (May, 2013): 1446–61.

Szmydynger-Chodobska, J., N. Strazielle, J. R. Gandy, T. H. Keefe, B. J. Zink, J. F. Ghersi-Egea, and A. Chodobski. "Posttraumatic Invasion of Monocytes Across the Blood-Cerebrospinal Fluid Barrier." *Journal of Cerebral Blood Flow and Metabolism* 32, no. 1 (Jan, 2012): 93–104.

Tang, H., F. Hua, J. Wang, I. Sayeed, X. Wang, Z. Chen, S. Yousuf, F. Atif, and D. G. Stein. "Progesterone and Vitamin D: Improvement After Traumatic Brain Injury in Middle-Aged Rats." *Hormones and Behavior* 64, no. 3 (Aug, 2013): 527–38.

Wang, X. M. and S. L. Yang. "The Effect of Acupuncture in 90 Cases of Sequelae of Brain Concussion." *Chung i Tsa Chih Ying Wen Pan (Journal of Traditional Chinese Medicine)* 8, no. 2 (Jun, 1988): 127–28.

Weinstein, E., M. Turner, B. B. Kuzma, and H. Feuer. "Second Impact Syndrome in Football: New Imaging and Insights into a Rare and Devastating Condition." *Journal of Neurosurgery: Pediatrics* 11, no. 3 (Mar, 2013): 331–34.

Weller, R. O., M. Subash, S. D. Preston, I. Mazanti, and R. O. Carare. "Perivascular Drainage of Amyloid-Beta Peptides from the Brain and its Failure in Cerebral Amyloid Angiopathy and Alzheimer's Disease." *Brain Pathology (Zurich, Switzerland)* 18, no. 2 (Apr, 2008): 253–66.

Whedon, J. M. and D. Glassey. "Cerebrospinal Fluid Stasis and its Clinical Significance." *Alternative Therapies in Health and Medicine* 15, no. 3 (May–Jun, 2009): 54–60.

Willard, Frank. "*Pathways of Acute and Chronic Pain*." Presentation at the Sutherland Cranial Teaching Foundation, Continuing Studies Conference, Portland, ME; October 15, 2010.

Yoganandan, N., J. Li, J. Zhang, F. A. Pintar, and T. A. Gennarelli. "Influence of Angular Acceleration-Deceleration Pulse Shapes on Regional Brain Strains." *Journal of Biomechanics* 41, no. 10 (Jul 19, 2008): 2253–62.

Zaben, M., W. El Ghoul, and A. Belli. "Post-Traumatic Head Injury Pituitary Dysfunction." *Disability and Rehabilitation* 35, no. 6 (Mar, 2013): 522–25.

Zeidan, F., K. T. Martucci, R. A. Kraft, N. S. Gordon, J. G. McHaffie, and R. C. Coghill. "Brain Mechanisms Supporting the Modulation of Pain by Mindfulness Meditation." *The Journal of Neuroscience: The Official Journal of the Society for Neuroscience* 31, no. 14 (Apr 6, 2011): 5540–48.

Zhang, B. L., X. Chen, T. Tan, Z. Yang, D. Carlos, R. C. Jiang, and J. N. Zhang. "Traumatic Brain Injury Impairs Synaptic Plasticity in Hippocampus in Rats." *Chinese Medical Journal* 124, no. 5 (Mar, 2011): 740–45.

Zhou, Y., M. P. Milham, Y. W. Lui, L. Miles, J. Reaume, D. K. Sodickson, R. I. Grossman, and Y. Ge. "Default-Mode Network Disruption in Mild Traumatic Brain Injury." *Radiology* 265, no. 3 (Dec, 2012): 882–92.

Zipp, F. and O. Aktas. "The Brain as a Target of Inflammation: Common Pathways Link Inflammatory and Neurodegenerative Diseases." *Trends in Neurosciences* 29, no. 9 (Sep, 2006): 518–27.

PART V: YOUR HEALING JOURNEY

Bornhoft, G., U. Wolf, K. von Ammon, M. Righetti, S. Maxion-Bergemann, S. Baumgartner, A. E. Thurneysen, and P. F. Matthiessen. "Effectiveness, Safety and Cost-Effectiveness of Homeopathy in General Practice—Summarized Health Technology Assessment." *Forschende Komplementarmedizin (2006)* 13 Suppl 2, (2006): 19-29.

Broker, M. "Following a Tick Bite: Double Infections by Tick-Borne Encephalitis Virus and the Spirochete Borrelia and Other Potential Multiple Infections." *Zoonoses and Public Health* 59, no. 3 (May, 2012): 176-180.

Chapman, E. H., R. J. Weintraub, M. A. Milburn, T. O. Pirozzi, and E. Woo. "Homeopathic Treatment of Mild Traumatic Brain Injury: A Randomized, Double-Blind, Placebo-Controlled Clinical Trial." *The Journal of Head Trauma Rehabilitation* 14, no. 6 (Dec, 1999): 521–42.

Col, N. F., M. I. Surks, and G. H. Daniels. "Subclinical Thyroid Disease: Clinical Applications." *JAMA: The Journal of the American Medical Association* 291, no. 2 (Jan 14, 2004): 239–43.

Cote, K. A., C. M. McCormick, S. N. Geniole, R. P. Renn, and S. D. MacAulay. "Sleep Deprivation Lowers Reactive Aggression and Testosterone in Men." *Biological Psychology* 92, no. 2 (Feb, 2013): 249–56.

Danciger, Elizabeth. *Homeopathy: From Alchemy to Medicine.* Rochester, VT; New York: Healing Arts/Harper and Row, 1988.

Ferrie, J. E., M. Kivimaki, T. N. Akbaraly, A. Singh-Manoux, M. A. Miller, D. Gimeno, M. Kumari, G. Davey Smith, and M. J. Shipley. "Associations between Change in Sleep Duration and Inflammation: Findings on C-Reactive Protein and Interleukin 6 in the Whitehall II Study." *American Journal of Epidemiology* 178, no. 6 (Sep 15, 2013): 956–61.

Grandner, M. A., N. Jackson, J. R. Gerstner, and K. L. Knutson. "Sleep Symptoms Associated with Intake of Specific Dietary Nutrients." *Journal of Sleep Research* (Sep 2, 2013).

Jacobs, J., W. B. Jonas, M. Jimenez-Perez, and D. Crothers. "Homeopathy for Childhood Diarrhea: Combined Results and Metaanalysis from Three Randomized, Controlled Clinical Trials." *The Pediatric Infectious Disease Journal* 22, no. 3 (Mar, 2003): 229–34.

Kean, W. F., S. Tocchio, M. Kean, and K. D. Rainsford. "The Musculoskeletal Abnormalities of the Similaun Iceman ("OTZI"): Clues to Chronic Pain and Possible Treatments." *Inflammopharmacology* 21, no. 1 (Feb, 2013): 11–20.

Kireev, R. A., E. Vara, and J. A. Tresguerres. "Growth Hormone and Melatonin Prevent Age-Related Alteration in Apoptosis Processes in the Dentate Gyrus of Male Rats." *Biogerontology* 14, no. 4 (Aug, 2013): 431–42.

LeGates, T. A., C. M. Altimus, H. Wang, H. K. Lee, S. Yang, H. Zhao, A. Kirkwood, E. T. Weber, and S. Hattar. "Aberrant Light Directly Impairs Mood and Learning through Melanopsin-Expressing Neurons." *Nature* 491, no. 7425 (Nov 22, 2012): 594–98.

Mah, C. D., K. E. Mah, E. J. Kezirian, and W. C. Dement. "The Effects of Sleep Extension on the Athletic Performance of Collegiate Basketball Players." *Sleep* 34, no. 7 (Jul 1, 2011): 943–50.

Markwald, R. R., E. L. Melanson, M. R. Smith, J. Higgins, L. Perreault, R. H. Eckel, and K. P. Wright Jr. "Impact of Insufficient Sleep on Total Daily Energy Expenditure, Food Intake, and Weight Gain." *Proceedings of the National Academy of Sciences of the United States of America* 110, no. 14 (Apr 2, 2013): 5695–5700.

Merikanto, I., T. Lahti, R. Puusniekka, and T. Partonen. "Late Bedtimes Weaken School Performance and Predispose Adolescents to Health Hazards." *Sleep Medicine* (Aug 11, 2013).

Morrison, Roger. *Desktop Companion to Physical Pathology*. Nevada City, CA: Hahnemann Clinic Publishing, 1998.

Ritter, S. M., M. Strick, M. W. Bos, R. B. van Baaren, and A. Dijksterhuis. "Good Morning Creativity: Task Reactivation during Sleep Enhances Beneficial Effect of Sleep on Creative Performance." *Journal of Sleep Research* 21, no. 6 (Dec, 2012): 643–47.

Seeley, B. M., A. B. Denton, M. S. Ahn, and C. S. Maas. "Effect of Homeopathic Arnica Montana on Bruising in Face-Lifts: Results of a Randomized, Double-Blind, Placebo-Controlled Clinical Trial." *Archives of Facial Plastic Surgery* 8, no. 1 (Jan–Feb, 2006): 54–59.

Spence, D. S., E. A. Thompson, and S. J. Barron. "Homeopathic Treatment for Chronic Disease: A 6-Year, University-Hospital Outpatient Observational Study." *Journal of Alternative and Complementary Medicine (New York, NY)* 11, no. 5 (Oct, 2005): 793–98.

Sterniczuk, R., O. Theou, B. Rusak, and K. Rockwood. "Sleep Disturbance is Associated with Incident Dementia and Mortality." *Current Alzheimer Research* 10, no. 7 (Sep, 2013): 767–75.

Stricker, R. B. and L. Johnson. "Borrelia Burgdorferi Aggrecanase Activity: More Evidence for Persistent Infection in Lyme Disease." *Frontiers in Cellular and Infection Microbiology* 3, (2013): 40.

———. "Lyme Disease: The Next Decade." *Infection and Drug Resistance* 4, (2011): 1–9.

Totonchi, A. and B. Guyuron. "A Randomized, Controlled Comparison between Arnica and Steroids in the Management of Postrhinoplasty Ecchymosis and Edema." *Plastic and Reconstructive Surgery* 120, no. 1 (Jul, 2007): 271–74.

Veasey, S. C., J. Lear, Y. Zhu, J. B. Grinspan, D. J. Hare, S. Wang, D. Bunch, P. A. Doble, and S. R. Robinson. "Long-Term Intermittent Hypoxia Elevates Cobalt Levels in the Brain and Injures White Matter in Adult Mice." *Sleep* 36, no. 10 (Oct 1, 2013): 1471–81.

Vermeulen, Frans. *Prisma: The Arcana of Materia Medica Illuminated*. Haarlem, the Netherlands: Emyrss by Publishers, 2002.

Witt, C. M., R. Ludtke, and S. N. Willich. "Homeopathic Treatment of Patients with Migraine: A Prospective Observational Study with a 2-Year Follow-Up Period." *Journal of Alternative and Complementary Medicine (New York, N.Y.)* 16, no. 4 (Apr, 2010): 347–55.

Witt, C. M., R. Ludtke, R. Baur, and S. N. Willich. "Homeopathic Treatment of Patients with Chronic Low Back Pain: A Prospective Observational Study with 2 Years Follow-Up." *The Clinical Journal of Pain* 25, no. 4 (May, 2009): 334–39.

Xie, L., H. Kang, Q. Xu, M. J. Chen, Y. Liao, M. Thiyagarajan, J. O'Donnell, et al. "Sleep Drives Metabolite Clearance from the Adult Brain." *Science (New York, NY)* 342, no. 6156 (Oct 18, 2013): 373–77.

QUOTES

P. 149: I am indebed to Lia Lazar's wonderful article on alternet.org for the love triangle metaphor: www.alternet.org/10-fascinating-facts-about-men-sex-and-testosterone.

P. 259: Quotation from Scott Reed used with permission

P. 306: Quotation from Dr. Maiken Nedergaard used with permission.

P. 308: Quotation on happiness and success is usually attributed to Albert Schweitzer but is not found in any of his published writings.

P. 309: Quotation from *Deep Survival: Who Lives, Who Dies, and Why*. New York: W.W. Norton & Co., 2003. Used with permission from Laurence Gonzalez.

Index

sleep problems
   case material, 141–42,
      167, 311–12, 314–15
   PTSD and, 52
   sleep apnea, 325
   trauma and, 27, 312
sleeping position, 135, 193,
   321
   pillow between knees, 214
smoking, 199
snoring, 201
soldiers, 33, 51, 54, 56
Somatic Experiencing
   psychotherapy, 53–55
sound therapy, 49, 321. *See
   also* breathing practices
Spanish flu of 1918, 168
sphenoid bone, 225, 227,
   234–39, 255–57, 278
sphenosquamous suture,
   227, 234–36
spinal cord, 120, 121, 138,
   172, 186, 277. *See also*
   cerebral spinal fluid;
   cranial rhythmic impulse
   pathways of pain in, 294,
      296–97
   sexual arousal and, 149–
      51, 156
   trauma to, 181, 184, 297
spinal curves. *See* low back:
   excessive curve in
spinal nerves, 40, 120, 121,
   156, 178, 181
spinal stenosis, 133
spine, 117
   building blocks, 118–21
spiritual practice, 308. *See
   also specific practices*
sprains, 17, 180, 327, 335
Spurling, Morgan, 93
Still, Andrew Taylor, 11, 68
strabismus, 236
Stramonium, 337
stroke, 69, 81, 178
subarachnoid space (brain),
   272
Sullivan, Patricia, 41, 58–66,
   205, 208, 213, 216.

See also injury shock:
   a program for healing;
   motion: a program for
   restoring
surgery
   avoiding, 127, 132
   healing from, 12, 145–46,
      299
   hypermobility and, 199
   injury shock from, 33
Sutherland, William G., 55,
   222, 225–26, 288
sutures, 114, 115, 225–27,
   240–42
   allergies and, 347
   brain injury and, 281-82,
      288
   dura and, 47, 270
   occipitomastoid, 227–31,
      347
   sphenosquamous, 227,
      234–35
sweetened drinks, 101–2
swelling, 342. *See also*
   inflammation; pericarditis
   brain injury and, 246,
      260–61, 266–67, 276,
      283, 335
   homeopathy and, 332,
      335, 336
   inflammation and, 17, 69,
      71, 74, 79, 80, 91, 342
swimming, 12, 41, 49, 132,
   153, 173, 191, 193
sympathetic chain ganglia,
   40, 138, 142, 165–66, 236
sympathetic nervous system
   (SNS), 26, 29–31, 33, 34,
   39, 40, 83, 145. *See also*
   autonomic nervous system;
   fight-or-flight response
   breathing and, 35, 36
   case material, 42, 44, 45,
      71, 142, 165–67, 315
   interventions to calm, 49,
      208, 219, 278, 323, 324
   sacrum and, 138, 142
   sexual arousal and, 149–51
   sleep and, 90, 317, 318

   stress hormones and, 29, 36
   unable to calm down after
      accident, 334
Symphytum officinalis, 300

T
T cells, 77
tai chi, 49, 89, 132, 153,
   194, 289–91
tapping (EFT), 56–57
teeth, infected, 344
teeth grinding, 201
temperature imbalance, 341
temperature sensitivity, 340
temporal bone, 20, 189, 201,
   229, 233–34, 236, 241, 252
   case material, 20, 22,
      228–30, 234, 235,
      240–42
   and hearing, 233, 234
   osteopathic treatment, 22,
      55, 230, 232, 235,
      241–42
temporal lobe, 249, 252–54,
   299
temporomandibular joint
   (TMJ), 14, 201, 224
tentorium, 270, 271, 280
thirst, 248, 256, 329, 338
thoracic pain, 297. *See also*
   chest pain
thoracolumbar fascia,
   131–32
thumb sucking, 232
thyroid function, 339
   interventions, 341
   measuring, 341
   pituitary and, 152–53,
      255, 340
   trauma and, 340
thyroid gland, 340
   injury to, 339
thyroid hormones, 152–53,
   340–41. *See also* thyroid-
   stimulating hormone
thyroid-stimulating hormone
   (TSH), 340
tinnitus, 14, 201, 224, 226–
   28, 248, 253